MANAGING
OB/GYN
EMERGENCIES
SECOND EDITION

Edited by
John T. Queenan, M.D.
Professor and Chairman
Department of Obstetrics and Gynecology
Georgetown University School of Medicine
Washington, D.C.
Editor-in-Chief, CONTEMPORARY OB/GYN

Coordinating Editor
Evelyn C. Gross
Formerly: Editor, CONTEMPORARY OB/GYN
Currently: Editor, *Diagnosis* magazine

D1417893

MEDICAL ECONOMICS BOOKS
Oradell, New Jersey 07649

Library of Congress Cataloging in Publication Data

Main entry under title:

Managing ob/gyn emergencies.

"A Contemporary Ob/Gyn book."
Includes bibliographical references and index.
1. Pregnancy, Complications of.   2. Labor,
Complicated.   3. Gynecologic emergencies.   I. Queenan,
John T.   II. Title: Managing obstetrics/gynecology
emergencies.   [DNLM: 1. Emergencies.   2. Genital
diseases, Female—Therapy.   3. Pregnancy complications—
Therapy.   WQ   240   M267]
RG158.M35   1983   618.3'025   82-24936
ISBN 0-87489-344-5

ISBN 0-87489-344-5

Medical Economics Company Inc.
Oradell, New Jersey 07649

First Printing   April 1983
Second Printing   August 1985

Printed in the United States of America

CONTENTS

EDITORS		vii
CONTRIBUTORS		ix
PREFACE		xiii
John T. Queenan, MD		
TABLE: IMMEDIATE VERSUS IMMINENT EMERGENCIES		xv

Part I. OBSTETRICS

1.	ECTOPIC PREGNANCY	2
	Gregory C. Bolton, MD	
	Fredric L. Cohen, MD	
2.	ACUTE ABDOMEN	8
	Gail V. Anderson, MD	
	Alan Ball, PA-C	
3.	ACCIDENTAL INJURY	18
	Herbert J. Buchsbaum, MD	
4.	ACUTE RENAL FAILURE	24
	Kenneth A. Fisher, MD	
5.	SICKLE CELL CRISIS	31
	James N. Martin Jr., MD	
	John C. Morrison, MD	
6.	DIABETIC KETOACIDOSIS AND PREGNANCY	44
	John L. Kitzmiller, MD	
7.	PRETERM CERVICAL DILATION	56
	James H. Harger, MD	
	Steve N. Caritis, MD	
8.	SEVERE PREECLAMPSIA	65
	Robert C. Goodlin, MD	
9.	ECLAMPSIA	78
	Frederick P. Zuspan, MD	
	Kathryn J. Zuspan, MD	

10. THIRD-TRIMESTER BLEEDING 84
Robert W. Huff, MD

11. RUPTURED UTERUS 93
Mary Jo O'Sullivan, MD

12. HEMORRHAGIC SHOCK IN OBSTETRICS 100
Denis Cavanagh, MD
Robert A. Knuppel, MD
Donald E. Marsden, MD

13. COAGULOPATHY IN PREGNANCY 108
J. Patrick Lavery, MD

14. FETAL BRADYCARDIA 120
Edward J. Quilligan, MD

15. FETAL AND NEONATAL ANEMIAS 127
Martin L. Gimovsky, MD
Barry S. Schifrin, MD

16. SHOULDER DYSTOCIA 141
Lester T. Hibbard, MD

17. NEONATAL DISTRESS 148
John W. Scanlon, MD

18. POSTPARTUM HEMORRHAGE 156
Robert H. Hayashi, MD

19. GENITAL TRACT BIRTH TRAUMA 163
Bruce A. Work Jr., MD

20. POSTPARTUM ENDOMETRITIS 170
Philip B. Mead, MD

21. SEPTIC SHOCK 177
Patrick Duff, MD

22. SUDDEN SENSORIUM DERANGEMENTS 190
Charles E. Gibbs, MD

Part II. GYNECOLOGY

23. VASOVAGAL SYNCOPE 198
J. Stephen Naulty, MD
Gerard W. Ostheimer, MD

24. RESPONDING TO CARDIORESPIRATORY
COMPLICATIONS 205
Robert H. Hayashi, MD

25. ANOVULATORY BLEEDING 214
Leon Speroff, MD

26. VAGINAL HEMORRHAGE 219
Walter B. Jones, MD

27. RUPTURED PELVIC ABSCESS 224
David L. Hemsell, MD
F. Gary Cunningham, MD

28. LAPAROSCOPY 231
Richard M. Soderstrom, MD
Stephen L. Corson, MD

29. EVISCERATION AND DEHISCENCE 242
John T. Queenan, MD

30. ACUTE ADRENAL INSUFFICIENCY 248
William R. Gold Jr., MD

Part III. ANESTHESIA

31. ANESTHETIC EMERGENCIES 256
Raymond R. Schultetus, MD

32. COMPLICATIONS OF PARACERVICAL BLOCK 266
Thomas M. Warren, MD
Gerard W. Ostheimer, MD

INDEX 275

EDITORS

John T. Queenan, MD, is Professor and Chairman of the Department of Obstetrics and Gynecology, Georgetown University School of Medicine, and Obstetrician-Gynecologist-in-Chief and a member of the Division of Maternal-Fetal Medicine, Georgetown University Hospital, Washington, DC. Dr. Queenan also serves as Editor-in-Chief of CONTEMPORARY OB/GYN. In addition to his many publications in professional journals, he is author of *Modern Management of the Rh Problem* (Harper & Row, 1977); editor of *A New Life: Pregnancy, Birth, and Your Child's First Year* (Van Nostrand Reinhold, 1979) and *Management of High-Risk Pregnancy* (Medical Economics Books, 1980); and coeditor of *Protocols for High-Risk Pregnancies* (Medical Economics Books, 1982). Dr. Queenan is a Fellow of the American College of Obstetricians and Gynecologists and the American College of Surgeons.

Evelyn C. Gross is the former Editor of CONTEMPORARY OB/GYN and now serves as Editor of *Diagnosis*, a clinical magazine for primary-care physicians. She has also been a writer and editor of clinical information in such publications as *Medical World News* and *Contemporary Surgery*. With Mona Shangold, MD, Ms. Gross is the coauthor of a book for the public, *Women's Medical Problems*.

CONTRIBUTORS

Gail V. Anderson, MD, Professor and Chairman, Department of Emergency Medicine, and Professor of Obstetrics and Gynecology, University of Southern California School of Medicine; and Director of Emergency Medicine, LAC-USC Medical Center, Los Angeles

Alan Ball, PA-C, Emergency Medicine Physician's Assistant Resident, LAC-USC Medical Center, Los Angeles

Gregory C. Bolton, MD, Assistant Professor of Obstetrics and Gynecology, University of Pennsylvania School of Medicine, and Director of Family Planning, Pennsylvania Hospital, Philadelphia

Herbert J. Buchsbaum, MD, Professor of Obstetrics and Gynecology, Southwestern Medical School of the University of Texas, Dallas

Steve N. Caritis, MD, Associate Professor of Obstetrics, Gynecology, and Pediatrics, University of Pittsburgh School of Medicine and Magee-Women's Hospital

Denis Cavanagh, MD, Professor of Obstetrics and Gynecology, University of South Florida College of Medicine, Tampa

Fredric L. Cohen, MD, Clinical Instructor of Obstetrics and Gynecology, University of Pennsylvania School of Medicine and Pennsylvania Hospital, Philadelphia

Stephen L. Corson, MD, Director, Philadelphia Fertility Institute, and Assistant Clinical Professor of Obstetrics and Gynecology, University of Pennsylvania School of Medicine, Philadelphia

F. Gary Cunningham, MD, Professor and Interim Chairman, Department of Obstetrics and Gynecology, University of Texas Health Science Center, Dallas

Patrick Duff, MD, Clinical Assistant Professor of Obstetrics and Gynecology and Fellow, Maternal-Fetal Medicine, University of Texas Health Science Center, San Antonio

Kenneth A. Fisher, MD, Academic Director of Internal Medicine, University of Illinois at MacNeal Memorial Hospital, Berwyn

Charles E. Gibbs, MD, Professor of Obstetrics and Gynecology, University of Texas Health Science Center, San Antonio

Martin L. Gimovsky, MD, Assistant Professor of Obstetrics and Gynecology, University of Southern California School of Medicine, and Chief of Obstetrics, White Memorial Hospital, Los Angeles

William R. Gold Jr., MD, Assistant Professor of Obstetrics and Gynecology, Georgetown University School of Medicine, Washington, DC

Robert C. Goodlin, MD, Professor of Obstetrics and Gynecology and Director of Maternal-Fetal Medicine, University of Nebraska Medical School, Omaha

James Harger, MD, Assistant Professor of Obstetrics, Gynecology, and Pediatrics, University of Pittsburgh School of Medicine and Magee-Women's Hospital

Robert H. Hayashi, MD, Associate Professor of Obstetrics and Gynecology, University of Texas Health Science Center, San Antonio

David L. Hemsell, MD, Assistant Professor of Obstetrics and Gynecology and Director, Division of Gynecology, University of Texas Health Science Center, Dallas

Lester T. Hibbard, MD, Professor of Obstetrics and Gynecology, University of Southern California School of Medicine, Los Angeles

Robert W. Huff, MD, Professor of Obstetrics and Gynecology and Chief, Division of Obstetrics, University of Texas Health Science Center, San Antonio

Walter B. Jones, MD, Associate Professor of Obstetrics and Gynecology, Cornell University Medical College, and Associate Attending Surgeon, Memorial Sloan-Kettering Cancer Center, New York

John L. Kitzmiller, MD, Associate Professor of Obstetrics, Gynecology, and Reproductive Sciences, University of California—San Francisco School of Medicine, and Chief, Perinatal Service, Children's Hospital of San Francisco

Robert A. Knuppel, MD, MPH, Associate Professor of Obstetrics, Gynecology, and Comprehensive Medicine, University of South Florida College of Medicine, Tampa; and Director of Maternal-Fetal Medicine, Tampa General Hospital and Bayfront Medical Center, St. Petersburg

J. Patrick Lavery, MD, Associate Professor of Obstetrics and Gynecology and Director, Division of Maternal-Fetal Medicine, University of Louisville School of Medicine, Louisville, Kentucky

Donald E. Marsden, MD, Assistant Professor of Obstetrics and Gynecology, University of South Florida College of Medicine, and Fellow in Gynecologic Oncology, Tampa General Hospital

James N. Martin Jr., MD, Assistant Professor of Obstetrics and Gynecology, Division of Maternal-Fetal Medicine, University of Mississippi Medical Center, Jackson

Philip B. Mead, MD, Professor of Obstetrics and Gynecology, University of Vermont College of Medicine, Burlington

John C. Morrison, MD, Professor of Obstetrics and Gynecology and Director, Division of Maternal-Fetal Medicine, University of Mississippi Medical Center, Jackson

J. Stephen Naulty, MD, Assistant Professor of Anesthesia, Harvard Medical School and Brigham and Women's Hospital, Boston

Gerard W. Ostheimer, MD, Associate Professor of Anaesthesia, Harvard Medical School, and Director of Obstetric Anesthesia, Brigham and Women's Hospital, Boston

Mary Jo O'Sullivan, MD, Professor and Director of Obstetrics, University of Miami School of Medicine, Miami, Florida

John T. Queenan, MD, Professor and Chairman, Department of Obstetrics and Gynecology, Georgetown University School of Medicine, Washington, DC

Edward J. Quilligan, MD, Professor of Obstetrics and Gynecology and Director, Division of Maternal-Fetal Medicine, University of California—Irvine School of Medicine, Orange

John W. Scanlon, MD, Associate Professor of Pediatrics, Georgetown University School of Medicine, and Director of Neonatology, Columbia Hospital for Women, Washington, DC

Barry S. Schifrin, MD, Professor of Obstetrics and Gynecology, University of Southern California School of Medicine, Los Angeles

Raymond R. Schultetus, MD, PhD, Assistant Professor of Anesthesiology, University of Florida College of Medicine, Gainesville

Richard M. Soderstrom, MD, Clinical Professor of Obstetrics and Gynecology, University of Washington Medical School, and Chief of Obstetrics and Gynecology, The Mason Clinic, Seattle

Leon Speroff, MD, Professor and Chairman, Department of Obstetrics and Gynecology, University of Oregon Health Sciences Center School of Medicine, Portland

Thomas M. Warren, MD, Assistant Professor of Anesthesia, Indiana University School of Medicine, Indianapolis

Bruce A. Work Jr., MD, Professor of Obstetrics and Gynecology, University of Illinois College of Medicine at Chicago

Frederick P. Zuspan, MD, Professor and Chairman, Department of Obstetrics and Gynecology, The Ohio State University College of Medicine, Columbus

Kathryn J. Zuspan, MD, Resident, The Ohio State University College of Medicine, Columbus

PREFACE

In the United States and other developed countries, the ob/gyn patient has high expectations, and with good reason. When she has a well-trained physician and a good hospital behind her, all systems are poised for an excellent outcome. In fact, the only thing standing between her expectations and such an outcome is the unforeseen emergency. For the clinician, the emergency is the opportunity for failure. In highly developed countries, the standard of living and the medicolegal climate make a bad outcome particularly difficult to accept. We doctors must be dedicated to providing the best possible management of the unexpected.

Because ob/gyn emergencies have such an impact on outcome, CONTEMPORARY OB/GYN has devoted two entire issues to this subject. The first, in 1981, was so well received that the contents were published as a soft-cover book, which promptly sold out. In July 1982, the magazine's second "emergencies" issue was developed under the aegis of guest editor, Robert H. Hayashi, MD, associate professor of ob/gyn, University of Texas Health Science Center, San Antonio. With this second issue to complement the first, I thought the time had come to publish a more definitive book.

Perhaps some information about CONTEMPORARY OB/GYN would help the reader understand the scope of this book. We have a working editorial board that carefully considers which subjects will be of greatest practical interest to our readers. Then we select the outstanding authorities in these subject areas and invite them to write for us. We require our authors to focus on the problems of clinical practice. This gives us an extraordinary advantage in developing an authoritative book.

Most of the chapters in this second edition were prepared from the 1981 and 1982 "emergencies" issues of CONTEMPORARY OB/GYN. In addition, to broaden the scope of topics covered, a few pertinent articles were selected from subsequent issues of the magazine.

All the chapters in this edition of *Managing Ob/Gyn Emergencies* have been updated by the respective authors and further refined by the editors. As you read, I hope you will be critical. If you have suggestions for future directions our emergencies issues should take, I would welcome hearing from you. With your help, I plan to update this book regularly, so that it can be the standard reference work for emergencies in obstetrics and gynecology.

John T. Queenan, MD
Editor in Chief,
CONTEMPORARY OB/GYN

Immediate versus imminent emergencies

Immediate emergencies allow no time for review. You must react fast; seconds count. The imminent emergencies may be equally life-threatening, but you have a little time to organize a plan. Here, minutes count. The following table is a guide to the contents of this book, with page numbers in bold type for ready reference.

Immediate

Accidental injury   **18**

Eclampsia   **78**

Third-trimester bleeding   **84**

Ruptured uterus   **93**

Hemorrhagic shock in obstetrics **100**

Shoulder dystocia   **141**

Neonatal distress   **148**

Postpartum hemorrhage   **156**

Genital tract birth trauma   **163**

Sudden sensorium derangements   **190**

Vasovagal syncope   **198**

Responding to cardiorespiratory complications   **205**

Laparoscopy   **231**

Anesthetic emergencies   **256**

Complications of paracervical block   **266**

Imminent

Ectopic pregnancy   **2**

Acute abdomen   **8**

Acute renal failure   **24**

Sickle cell crisis   **31**

Diabetic ketoacidosis and pregnancy   **44**

Preterm cervical dilation   **56**

Severe preeclampsia   **65**

Coagulopathy in pregnancy   **108**

Fetal bradycardia   **120**

Fetal and neonatal anemias   **127**

Postpartum endometritis   **170**

Septic shock   **177**

Anovulatory bleeding   **214**

Vaginal hemorrhage   **219**

Ruptured pelvic abscess   **224**

Evisceration and dehiscence   **242**

Acute adrenal insufficiency   **248**

PART I
Obstetrics

1

Ectopic Pregnancy

GREGORY C. BOLTON, MD, and
FREDRIC L. COHEN, MD

CLINICAL SIGNIFICANCE: With an incidence of about 1:200 pregnancies, ectopic pregnancy remains the number one cause of death in the first trimester. Prompt recognition and treatment will avoid catastrophe. Once symptoms appear, rupture and massive hemorrhage may quickly follow.

The leading cause of maternal mortality during the first trimester of pregnancy, ectopic pregnancy remains very difficult to diagnose. This is primarily because it is relatively asymptomatic in the early weeks of pregnancy. The onset of symptoms often heralds acute rupture and sudden massive hemorrhage. Early diagnosis, aggressive surgical management, and adequate blood and fluid replacement could save 75% of these patients, most of whom have visited a physician days before the actual rupture. Ectopic pregnancy therefore remains not only a diagnostic challenge but also a therapeutic emergency.

The overall incidence of extrauterine implantation of the fertilized ovum (blastocyst) in the US is from 1:84 to 1:230. In the past decade alone, while the annual number of maternal deaths decreased, the number of ectopic pregnancies increased from 15,000 to 40,000 a year. The increase is attributable to the rising incidence of sexually transmitted disease that corresponds with more sex partners, and the double-edged sword of modern antibiotic therapy. The proportion of all maternal deaths secondary to ectopic pregnancies is now 10%. (In nonwhite patients, ectopic pregnancy has become the single largest cause of maternal death.)

Major sites of extrauterine implantation include all segments of the fallopian tube (90%), the ovary (0.1%), uterine cornua (0.6%), cervix (0.1%), and peritoneal cavity (1.3%) (Figure 1-1). Most tubal gestations occur in the ampullary and isthmic portions of the tube.

WHAT CAUSES EXTRAUTERINE PREGNANCY?

Although no single factor accounts for all cases, the increased incidence of salpingitis correlates well with the rising incidence of ectopic pregnancy. Partial occlusion of the fallopian tube allows conception to occur but often prevents passage of the fertilized egg into the uterine cavity. The success of current antibiotics in treating pelvic inflammatory disease often prevents total tubal occlusion. Occlusion tends to be more common in nongonococcal than in gonococcal salpingitis, probably because of the gonococcus's greater sensitivity to a wide variety of antibiotics. Following an infectious insult, the tubal lumen forms synechial bands that, along with agglutination of the tubal cilia, result in varying degrees of occlusion. One prospective study showed histologic evidence of chronic salpingitis in 50% to 55% of patients who have had infections. The likelihood that tubal occlusion will occur is known to increase with each subsequent infection: 12% of patients are at risk with the first infection, 30% with the second infection, and 75% with the third episode.

FIGURE 1-1

---

*Sites and frequency of ectopic pregnancies**

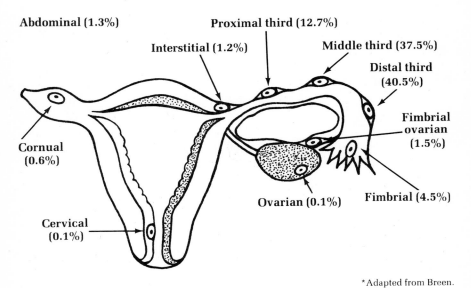

Abdominal (1.3%)

Proximal third (12.7%)

Interstitial (1.2%)

Middle third (37.5%)

Distal third (40.5%)

Fimbrial ovarian (1.5%)

Cornual (0.6%)

Cervical (0.1%)

Ovarian (0.1%)

Fimbrial (4.5%)

*Adapted from Breen.

The widespread use of IUDs also seems to have influenced the rate of extrauterine pregnancy. This association was first recognized by Grafenberg in 1929. A summary of the published literature on ectopic pregnancy, by Tatum and Schmidt, revealed that 1:23, or 4.3%, of pregnancies occurring with an IUD in place were ectopic. The IUD seems to reduce uterine implantation of the ovum far more effectively than it reduces either tubal or ovarian implantation. In short, it does not protect against ectopic implantation in predisposed patients. IUD users also seem to be at greater risk immediately after the IUD is removed, and so should avoid pregnancy for 2 to 3 months after removal. The 1980 Women's Health Study Collaborative drew the following conclusions on the relationship between IUDs and ectopic pregnancy:

● In the aggregate, women who have used an IUD in the past but are not using it now have the same risk of ectopic pregnancy as women who have never used one.

● Current use of any form of contraception, including the IUD, decreases one's risk of ectopic pregnancy.

● IUD users have three times the risk of ectopic pregnancy oral contraceptive users have, and a risk equal to barrier contraceptive users.

Progesterone-only OCs increase the risk of ectopic pregnancy. This is thought to be secondary to these agents' minimal propulsive effects on the oviduct at the ampullary-isthmic junction and to an increased incidence of ovum trapping.

Finally, our increased ability to restore tubal patency surgically increases the incidence. Women who have had such repair are at high risk of ectopic pregnancy. The common denominator in extrauterine pregnancy is delay of fertilized ovum transport from the site of ovulation to the uterine cavity.

MAKING THE DIAGNOSIS

Accurate diagnosis and prompt management depend on clinical suspicion and careful assessment of symptoms and physical findings. Essentially, any woman—regardless of childbearing age or method of birth control, including tubal ligation—who complains of an irregular bleeding pattern and pain needs evaluation for ectopic pregnancy. The classic triad of pain, bleeding, and adnexal mass is present in 75% of cases, but this figure varies according to how willing the patient in pain may be to let you examine her, the diagnostic skill of the examiner, and the duration of the pregnancy. Pain is almost always the most important feature and the symptom that first causes the patient to seek medical attention. Bleeding patterns and menstrual history vary from normal to highly irregular. Some form of bleeding takes place around the time of the expected menses in 50% of patients, and about 50% of women have a 5- to 10-week period of amenorrhea before other clinical signs appear.

Over 50% of patients have "normal menses" 4 to 8 weeks before admission, and up to 20% have no history of a missed period. Pain is present for less than 24 hours in 45% of cases, from 1 to 7 days in 30%, and more than 1 week in 25%. The location of the pain varies; there is adnexal tenderness in 95% of patients, bilateral tenderness in 43%, and pain on the side opposite the ectopic in 24% (Figure 1-2).

Pregnancy testing is of variable diagnostic value. Radioimmunoassay and radioreceptor assay have increased our accuracy in detecting an early pregnancy, but they can't identify its location.

Ultrasonic examination is helpful if the technique is performed correctly. An intrauterine gestational sac can be located consistently after 5 weeks' gestation. The presence of an intact sac should preclude suspi-

FIGURE 1-2

*Location and frequency of pain reported by patients with ectopic pregnancies**

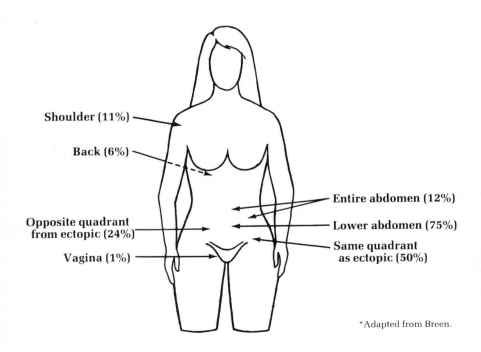

Shoulder (11%)
Back (6%)
Opposite quadrant from ectopic (24%)
Vagina (1%)
Entire abdomen (12%)
Lower abdomen (75%)
Same quadrant as ectopic (50%)

*Adapted from Breen.

cion of ectopic pregnancy, although dual pregnancy—intrauterine and ectopic—has been reported.

Culdocentesis is helpful if ultrasound is not available, and it is a quick, easy way to identify intraperitoneal bleeding before hospital admission. The simple procedure of inserting a spinal needle attached to an aspirating syringe into the cul-de-sac between the uterosacral ligaments can be carried out in almost any situation when the diagnosis is in doubt.

If the patient does not desire to keep an intrauterine pregnancy, D&C can be useful for evaluating endometrial tissue. The presence of decidua and the absence of chorionic villi, along with pain and an adnexal mass, mandate visual inspection of the adnexa before an ectopic pregnancy can be ruled out.

Diagnostic laparoscopy is probably the major improvement in our ability to diagnose pelvic disease within the past decade. Its use is essential, except when precluded by hemodynamic instability; emergency laparotomy is indicated in such cases. Laparoscopy has replaced the more difficult and cumbersome technique of culdoscopy and often saves patients an unnecessary exploratory laparotomy. A laparotomy is still mandatory in the presence of hemoperitoneum when culdocentesis is positive and diagnostic laparoscopy inadequate, so that the source and extent of the bleeding cannot be accurately defined.

SURGICAL APPROACHES

The primary treatment for ectopic pregnancy remains surgical. The clinician must consider the location of the ectopic pregnancy, the patient's hemodynamic stability, and her desire for more children. Salpingectomy, the classic treatment for removal of ectopic pregnancy, is still the procedure of choice in most cases. Salpingectomy obviates any chance of recurrence, especially in conjunction with ipsilateral cornual resection. However, when fimbrial ectopic pregnancy or distal tubal abortion is found, a tubal extraction or "milking" procedure may evacuate the ectopic products without disrupting the integrity of the tube. If you can accomplish this easily without damaging tubal structure, while achieving adequate hemostasis, you may be able to preserve tubal function. When the pregnancy occurs in the patient's remaining tube, or when the contralateral tube is obviously seriously compromised from preexisting disease, you may wish to consider a conservative approach to removing the fetus.

In experienced hands, salpingostomy—linear exposure of the unruptured ectopic sac—with removal and subsequent restoration of tubal integrity can preserve reproductive capability. Another conservative procedure involves partial salpingectomy with later anastomosis of proximal and distal segments of tube. Such attempts at conservation should be considered only in cases of unruptured ectopic pregnancy and only in consultation with surgeons experienced in and adept at such fertility procedures. The risk of recurrent ectopic pregnancy is definitely increased after any tubal surgery, and such patients need special follow-up in subsequent pregnancies.

SUGGESTED READING

- Breen JL: A 21 year survey of 654 ectopic pregnancies. Am J Obstet Gynecol 106:1004, 1970
- Brenner PF: Ectopic pregnancy. JAMA 243:7, 673, 1980
- Kitchin JD: Ectopic pregnancy: Current clinical trends. Am J Obstet Gynecol 134:870, 1979
- Stromme WB: Conservative surgery for ectopic pregnancy, a 20 year review. Obstet Gynecol 41:215, 1973

2

Acute Abdomen

GAIL V. ANDERSON, MD, and
ALAN BALL, PA-C

CLINICAL SIGNIFICANCE: Normal anatomic and physiologic changes during pregnancy complicate the diagnosis of various abdominal problems. When these changes are considered, findings are usually sufficient to make the correct diagnosis. Assuming that abdominal symptoms are due to pregnancy may delay diagnosis and treatment of an acute abdominal crisis, with catastrophic consequences.

The approach to any surgical problem of a pregnant or puerperal patient should be the same as for a nonpregnant patient, with prompt surgical intervention when indicated. The risk of precipitating labor with diagnostic laparotomy is negligible, provided unnecessary surgical maneuvers are avoided.[1] Spontaneous abortion is most likely to occur if surgery is performed before 16 weeks' gestation or when there is peritonitis and fluid in the peritoneal cavity.

DIAGNOSING APPENDICITIS

Appendicitis is the most common acute abdominal problem during pregnancy.[2, 3] It occurs slightly more often in the second trimester than in the first and third. Signs during pregnancy are fewer and milder.

The acute focal stage begins with an obstructive insult of the appendiceal lumen that is traceable to hypertrophied submucosal follicles following a viral infection (60%), fecalith (35%), foreign body (4%), or stricture (0.5%). The patient feels visceral pain in the periumbilical or epigastric areas.[4] As mucus accumulates and is turned to pus by bacterial and leukocytic action, distention, edema, and ulceration proceed to acute suppurative appendicitis. Pain is confined to the right lower quadrant in nonpregnant patients and those in early pregnancy. Venous distention and obstruction, ischemia, and bacterial invasion of the wall of the appendix cause irritation of the overlying parietal peritoneum and produce point tenderness.

Whether the pain is in the right iliac fossa depends on gestation. The enlarging uterus displaces the cecum and appendix upward, laterally, and often posteriorly. At term, the appendix is well above the iliac crest. The long axis changes counterclockwise from a downward to an upward direction.[5]

Once peritonitis sets in, in the wake of perforation, the pregnant patient may be moribund within 24 hours. During late second and third trimesters, the bulk of the uterus displaces the omentum upward, preventing "walling off" of the infection and allowing it to disseminate faster. The presence of pus after perforation causes irritability in the uterus, which forms the medial border of any appendiceal abscess or local peritonitis. This process induces preterm labor. With infarction, gangrene, or peritonitis, fetal mortality increases markedly.

You can elicit Alder's sign (fixed tenderness) by finding the point of maximal tenderness on the abdominal wall and turning the patient on her left side without changing the position or pressure of your fingers. The pain produced by the pressure will be reduced if the lesion is intrauterine and has fallen away from your fingers. If the pain is unaltered, the lesion is extrauterine. A few patients will not perceive the pain if the appendix is not in contact with the parietal peritoneum.

Leukocytosis is not helpful. During pregnancy, there is a physiologic increase in white blood cells to 11,000 to 16,000/mL. On x-ray, the most frequent sign is air-fluid levels or gaseous distention of the cecum or the adjacent small bowel, interpreted as a local adynamic ileus. (While x-rays of pregnant patients should be avoided, particularly during the first trimester, they sometimes must be done to establish the diagnosis.) Convex lumbar scoliosis, psoas obliteration, and appendicolith are also seen.[6] None of these is pathognomonic for appendicitis.

It is helpful to differentiate acute appendicitis from acute salpingitis (rare in pregnancy). Nausea and vomiting accompany both but are more frequent in appendicitis. The tenderness in salpingitis is usually bilateral and is accompanied by a higher temperature elevation (103°F) than is acute unruptured appendicitis (100°F). Guarding or rebound tenderness is less likely in salpingitis, and bowel sounds are usually normal.

URINARY TRACT INFECTIONS

Acute pyelonephritis, the most serious medical complication of pregnancy, is frequently confused with appendicitis when it involves the right side. Chills and fever (103° to 104°F) accompanied by costovertebral angle pain are the most common initial symptoms. Chills seldom herald the onset of appendicitis, and the temperature is rarely as high as 103°F. Urinary frequency, dysuria, nausea, and vomiting are common in pyelonephritis. As a rule, there is no abdominal muscle rigidity, while in acute appendicitis, local rigidity is often present. An uncentrifuged urine sample that shows the presence of pyuria and bacteriuria is usually sufficient to incriminate the urinary tract as the source of the problem.[7, 8]

Significant transient reversible renal dysfunction, possibly caused by endotoxemia, has been reported in a fifth of pyelonephritis cases. Exercise care when using nephrotoxic drugs and any drug excreted by the kidneys, if transient dysfunction becomes evident.

Urolithiasis is less common than pyelonephritis as a cause of abdominal pain in pregnancy. Pain is usually on the right side. Urolithiasis is differentiated from pyelonephritis by urinary findings. Pain associated with renal stones radiates to the groin or genitalia. However, if symptoms of pain referable to the kidney persist (especially on the left side), renal stones should be considered.

OVARIAN CYSTS

Complications of ovarian cysts during pregnancy and the puerperium are second to appendicitis in frequency. Torsion occurs in one pregnancy in a thousand and spontaneous rupture in approximately 2% of all ovarian cysts.[9, 10]

Ovarian cysts—and sometimes normal ovaries and tubes—may become ischemic because of torsion resulting from pressure and displacement during pregnancy and labor. Typically, there is acute lower abdominal pain on the affected side. Crampy, intermittent discomfort may occur initially if torsion is partial or self-limited, and patients may have recurrent episodes. The pain may radiate to the flank or thigh. Vomiting is frequently an early manifestation of torsion; in appendicitis it occurs later. A tender mass may be palpable in the left or right lower quadrant, adjacent to the uterus.

Acute rupture of an ovarian cyst is more common in the pregnant than the nonpregnant woman. The initial symptom is usually acute severe pain; there may be some evidence of peritonitis. Acute peritonitis results from rupture of a dermoid cyst, and subacute granulomatous peritonitis and dense adhesions result from continued leakage.

Elective operations on the ovary should be deferred until the 16th week or after, because of the increased incidence of spontaneous abortion before that time. However, ovarian cysts large enough to be discovered during pregnancy should be removed soon after discovery because the risk of complications outweighs the risk of laparotomy.[11]

TUBO-OVARIAN ABSCESS AND SALPINGITIS

Pregnancy and salpingitis or tubo-ovarian abscess rarely coexist. It is generally safer to seek another diagnosis.

Distinguishing between salpingitis and tubo-ovarian abscess with impending rupture is the principal problem in managing pelvic inflammatory disease. Salpingitis usually is accompanied by a vaginal discharge. There may be a history of infection by intercourse; a recent gynecologic or contraceptive procedure; a latent focal flare-up or nearby focus (such as appendicitis); or spread of bacteria from another focus of infection via the blood or lymphatic system.

The gonococcus is the usual cause of acute salpingitis; staphylococcal, streptococcal, or *Escherichia coli* infections occur less often. Patients with acute salpingitis usually consult a physician later than those with acute appendicitis. Symptom onset is closely related to the menstrual cycle.

The initial complaint is usually pelvic pain, often progressing from chronic to severe. In most instances, unruptured abscesses "point" to the pelvis and are managed quite successfully by colpotomy or proctotomy and insertion of a larger "dog-ear" drain into the abscess cavity. However, an unruptured abscess, felt as a unilateral or bilateral tender pelvic mass, not responding to conservative management, may rupture into the peritoneal cavity. Rupture is heralded by a sudden increase in pain, rapidly followed by generalized peritonitis, manifested by spiking temperature, tachycardia, and marked abdominal tenderness with muscle spasm. Shock will follow if ileus treatment is not instituted promptly. Culdocentesis frequently yields purulent material. *E. coli* is recovered most frequently and may be associated with β-hemolytic streptococci, *Staphylococcus aureus*, *Klebsiella*, *Proteus*, or *Bacteroides fragilis*. There is no place for "conservative" (nonsurgical) management of a ruptured tubo-ovarian abscess.[12]

Major complications stem directly from a delay in treatment and incomplete operation.[12, 13] Patients with tubo-ovarian abscess seldom become pregnant, and the abscess continues to be a source of ill health. Therefore, complete removal of uterus, tubes, and ovaries is advisable.[12, 14] Insertion of rubber drains through an open vaginal cuff to allow thorough drainage further decreases the chance of complications.

Before and during surgery, give colloids and crystalloids IV, along with blood and plasma, to maintain adequate volume, as indicated by estimated blood loss, hematocrit, urine output, urine specific gravity, clinical state of hydration, and central venous pressure (CVP). Monitoring the CVP is the best way to maintain hydration and oxygen-carrying capabilities and prevent fluid overload.

Give large doses of hydrocortisone preoperatively and 24 hours postoperatively to severely ill patients or those debilitated by prolonged illness or who have vascular collapse secondary to sepsis. It is not necessary to taper the dose of hydrocortisone or to give ACTH when steroids are administered for such a short period.

ACUTE INTESTINAL OBSTRUCTION

Adhesions are the most common cause of intestinal obstruction in both the general and pregnant populations. Incarcerated hernias and bowel neoplasms are the next most common causes in the general population, and volvulus and intussusception in pregnancy. Because the most frequent causes of adhesions are appendectomies and gynecologic procedures, consider obstruction in symptomatic patients who have had abdominal surgery.[15] Bowel obstruction is an unusual complication during pregnancy, but delay in diagnosis can lead to episodes of maternal hypoxia and hypotension that can be fatal for the fetus.

Adhesions are most likely to precipitate obstruction during three time periods: in the fourth to fifth month, when the uterus changes from a pelvic to an abdominal position, causing traction on previous adhesions; in the eighth to ninth month, when the fetal head descends into the pelvis; and in the period immediately after delivery, when a sudden change in uterine size drastically alters the relation of adhesions to the surrounding bowel. According to Goldthrop, most cases of intestinal obstruction secondary to adhesions occur during the first pregnancy after an operation.[15] The average time between onset of symptoms and hospital admission is 3.5 days, and between admission and operation, 2.8 days.[16]

Diagnosis is based on a classic triad of colicky abdominal pain, vomiting increasing in frequency and amount, and absolute constipation. Remember, constipation is common in pregnancy—obstipation is not.[17]

The degree and suddenness of obstruction govern onset and severity of symptoms. An obstruction high up in the small bowel will produce early symptoms of frequent, violent vomiting associated with pain and shock. Distention is not an early feature and the vomitus will be green and bilious unless obstruction is proximal to the ampulla of Vater. Symptoms of lower small bowel obstruction are less severe, with less pain and shock, and include delayed and feculent vomiting. Obstruction in the upper jejunum diminishes urine output.

Pain in large bowel obstruction is much less acute than in small bowel blockage, and shock is less frequent and severe, except with volvulus or intussusception. Distention is an early manifestation of large bowel obstruction; vomiting occurs later. The length of time between bouts of pain can help locate the obstruction. A 4- to 5-minute period between attacks indicates small bowel obstruction; a 10- to 15-minute period between attacks indicates large bowel obstruction. During the third trimester, you can rule out early labor by auscultating and palpating the uterus during the bout of pain, as you may hear "rushes" of high-pitched bowel sounds.

Radiographically, air-fluid levels and distended loops of small bowel indicate small bowel obstruction. "Hoop loops," transverse loops, "string-of-beads sign," and "coffee bean sign" may also be seen. In large bowel obstruction, the bowel is distended, with or without cecal distention, and air-fluid levels may be demonstrated. There may be secondary obstruction of the small bowel due to an incompetent ileocecal valve.

Intussusception during pregnancy is one of the most serious complications of bowel obstruction. Passage of a stool consisting of blood-streaked mucus—the "currant jelly" stool—is diagnostic. Uterine size may allow palpation of the sausage-shaped tumor.[18]

Midgut volvulus is secondary to a congenital defect either in the rotation of the midgut or in the attachment of the bowel to the posterior abdomen, or both. Torsion at the point of fixation, by the enlarging uterus, can cause partial obstruction and proximal distention. The decreased abdominal space prevents spontaneous detorsion. Sudden reduction in uterine size and a changed position of abdominal organs can also cause this problem. Barium enema seems to be the best way to identify it. Immediate surgery is mandatory, as bowel infarction is rapidly fatal.

To gain the best possible exposure and access to the bowel at operation, cesarean section may be necessary. However, it need not be done routinely.

ACUTE CHOLECYSTITIS

Acute or chronic gallbladder disease is associated with gallstones in 85% to 95% of cases. Bile stasis, bacterial infection, or other factors account for the rest. The increased incidence of cholecystitis in pregnancy may be secondary to accelerated stone growth. There are three possible causes:

● Increased progesterone slows gallbladder emptying.
● A 50% increase in esterified and free blood cholesterol during pregnancy increases the amount of cholesterol in the bile.
● The bile salt pool decreases.

Women taking exogenous estrogens in oral contraceptives or for postmenopausal replacement therapy are at a higher risk for gallstones, as are pregnant patients. The hormones affect cholesterol metabolism and smooth muscle tone of the gallbladder.

Acute and chronic symptoms seem to be the same for pregnant and nonpregnant patients. Right upper quadrant tenderness, the most frequent sign, is usually produced by cystic duct obstruction. Jaundice may accompany common duct obstruction. The WBC is not of diagnostic value. The pain, described by the patient as lancing, colicky, or just a "deep ache," may be excruciating. It usually begins in the midepigastrium and radiates to the right upper quadrant around the sides to the back or directly to the scapula. Most patients describe a steady pain lasting 15 to 60 minutes. In nonpregnant patients, the gallbladder may be palpable, with a positive Murphy sign. The gallbladder can rarely be palpated in pregnancy. Nausea and vomiting or anorexia may accompany the onset of symptoms.

Oral cholecystograms and IV cholangiography, while helpful in nonpregnant patients, are contraindicated in pregnancy. Radiopaque calculi are most often seen, as is a soft tissue mass. Sometimes there is a local ileus or basal chest change.

The postpartum period seems to be a time of greater susceptibility to gallstone attack than is gestation itself. Attacks during the puerperium are generally more severe than during pregnancy.

Management is initially conservative, with intermittent nasogastric suctioning, administration of crystalloids IV, narcotics, and antibiotics if sepsis is evident or if conservative therapy has produced no improvement after four days. Surgery is indicated for uncontrollable chronic disease or for an acute episode with peritonitis. The second trimester is best for surgery because the risk to the fetus is less and the uterus is not enlarged enough to encroach on the operative field. Surgery is more often necessary after delivery.

PEPTIC ULCER DISEASE

We define peptic ulcer disease as the formation of ulcerations 1.0 mm to 1.0 cm or greater in diameter in the duodenal bulb, postbulbar area, distal antrum, or the pyloric channel of the upper GI tract. Pregnancy ameliorates peptic ulcer disease in two ways. Progesterone appears to lower gastric acid secretion and increase the production of gastric mucus. And histamine is inactivated or blocked by plasma histaminase, which is synthesized by the placenta and rises dramatically during pregnancy.

Attacks are characterized by moderate to severe burning, cramping, boring, or pressing pain. Discomfort lasts from 15 to 60 minutes, is relieved by food or antacid, and is exacerbated by ingestion of aspirin, coffee, or alcoholic beverages. Vomiting is rare unless an ulcer is present in the pyloric channel. Melena or hematemesis may be present secondary to erosion.

Complications arise from bleeding at the base of an ulcer, luminal obstruction secondary to edema or fibrosis in the region of the ulcer, or perforation into the peritoneal cavity or the pancreatic bed. Manage bleeding by endoscopy, nasogastric suction, cold isotonic saline lavage, and blood replacement.

Perforation has a 100% mortality if treated by medical means alone. Symptoms of perforation can be divided into three stages:

1. Prostration, or primary shock. There is great generalized abdominal pain, anxious and ashen appearance, subnormal temperature, small and weak pulse, shallow respirations, nausea and vomiting, and pain in one or both shoulders.

2. Reaction, or masked peritonitis. The abdominal pain decreases, vomiting ceases, appearance improves, temperature is normal, pulse normal, respirations still shallow, abdominal wall very rigid and tender and/or flat. Movement induces pain.

3. Frank peritonitis with toxic shock. Vomiting becomes more frequent. The abdomen is distended and tender. The pulse is rapid and small, respirations labored and rapid, and the facial expression reflects pain and anxiety.

The diagnosis often can be made before frank peritonitis sets in and surgery becomes necessary. If complications develop late in the third trimester, cesarean section may be necessary to obtain better exposure and to protect the fetus from potential distress secondary to peritonitis and maternal hypotension.[19]

Radiographically, perforated peptic ulcer is best diagnosed by a finding of pneumoperitoneum. There may also be air-fluid levels, free fluid, and elevated diaphragm.

There is an increased frequency of peptic ulcer disease and exacerbation of symptoms and complications around the menopause. A differential diagnosis includes cholecystitis, acute pancreatitis, acute appendicitis, ischemic coronary artery disease, ischemic bowel disease, and stomach cancer.

ACUTE PANCREATITIS

In the nonpregnant patient, acute pancreatitis is usually associated with chronic alcoholism, gallstones, surgery, trauma, metabolic disorders, infections, drugs, connective tissue disease, penetrating duodenal ulcer, or obstruction of the ampulla of Vater. During pregnancy, the cause is usually gallstones (36%), infection (25%), preeclampsia (9%), chlorothiazides (8%), or alcohol consumption (1%). Stasis, increased concentration of cholesterol in bile, and changes in the physicochemical nature of bile salts—all factors believed important in the formation of biliary calculi—occur in normal pregnancy. Pancreatitis commonly occurs in conjunction with or secondary to gallbladder disease. Lymphatic transmission of inflammatory disease within the pancreaticobiliary system may be involved.

Initially, inflammation of the pancreas liberates proteolytic enzymes that begin to digest pancreatic and peripancreatic tissues. This process liberates other active enzymes, continuing the process of autodigestion. Necrotizing pancreatitis develops. It may resolve with medical management or may continue, with associated symptoms of systemic deterioration, including circulatory collapse, renal and respiratory failure, and hypocalcemia. While calcium levels normally are somewhat depressed during pregnancy, hypocalcemia accompanying severe pancreatitis is a poor prognostic sign. Death has occurred in most patients whose serum calcium levels fell below 7.0 mg/dL.[20]

Fever without other complications is unusual and the WBC is generally not helpful. The incidence of proteinuria is very high. Blood electrolyte derangements reflect the severity of vomiting. Liver function tests will be abnormal when there is concomitant biliary tract disease.

Epigastric pain and guarding may be significant, but the diagnosis is made by confirming an elevation of the serum amylase and diastase (urinary amylase). Serum amylase levels peak 6 to 12 hours after the onset of symptoms and return to normal within 24 to 72 hours. However, the diastase levels remain elevated for 7 to 10 days.

Radiographically, the most reliable x-ray finding is the "sentinel loop sign," in which one or more loops of jejunum are seen in the left upper quadrant of the abdomen. There may also be a localized ileus of the stomach or duodenum. Another occasional finding is the "colon cut-off sign," where the large bowel is dilated in either the hepatic or splenic flexure. Pleural effusion, left greater than right, has also been reported.

Management centers on putting the pancreas to rest: nothing taken orally, intermittent nasogastric suction, analgesics (meperidine is the drug of choice), IV fluids, and antiemetics. Anticholinergics, glucagon, and antibiotics do not appear to be of therapeutic benefit.

Most complications are associated with the severe necrotizing or hemorrhagic type of pancreatitis, and are secondary to local inflammation and the necrotic effects of pancreatic enzymes on peripancreatic tissues, or a remote effect of circulating enzymes. Laparotomy is indicated only when the diagnosis is not definite or toxic pancreatic exudate must be removed with a wide sump drain. There is no reason to terminate pregnancy, as there is no proof that pregnancy adversely affects the prognosis.

The differential diagnosis in women of childbearing age includes perforated viscus, especially from peptic ulcer, cholecystitis, acute intestinal obstruction, renal disease, dissecting aortic aneurysm, pneumonia, and diabetic ketoacidosis.

REFERENCES

1. Saunders P, Milton PJD: Laparotomy during pregnancy: An assessment of diagnostic accuracy and fetal wastage. Br Med J 13:165, 1973
2. King RM, Anderson GV: Appendicitis in pregnancy. Calif Med 97:158, 1962
3. Lowthian J: Appendicitis during pregnancy. Ann Emerg Med 9:431, 1980
4. DeVore GR: Acute abdominal pain in the pregnant patient due to pancreatitis, acute appendicitis, cholecystitis, or peptic ulcer disease. Clin Perinatol 7:349, 1980

5. Farquharson RG: Acute appendicitis in pregnancy. Scott Med J 25:36, 1980

6. Lee PWR: The plain x-ray in the acute abdomen: A surgeon's evaluation. Br J Surg 63:763, 1976

7. Gilstrap LC, Cunningham FG, Whalley PG: Acute pyelonephritis in pregnancy: An anterospective study. Obstet Gynecol 57:409, 1981

8. Cope A: *The Early Diagnosis of the Acute Abdomen.* New York: Oxford University Press, 1972

9. Munro A, Jones PF: Abdominal emergencies in the puerperium. Br Med J. 691: 1975

10. Stern JL, Buscema J, Rosensheim NB, et al: Spontaneous rupture of benign cystic teratomas. Obstet Gynecol 57:363, 1981

11. Hamlin E Jr, Bartlett MD, Smith JA: Acute surgical emergencies of the abdomen in pregnancy. N Engl J Med 244:128, 1951

12. Anderson GV, Bucklew WB: Abdominal surgery and tubo-ovarian abscesses. West J Surg Obstet Gynecol 70:67, 1962

13. Nebel WA, Lucas WE: Management of tubo-ovarian abscess in pregnancy. Obstet Gynecol 32:382, 1968

14. Hunt SM, Kimchloe BW, Schriver PC: Tubo-ovarian abscess in pregnancy. Obstet Gynecol 43:57, 1974

15. Hill LM, Symmonds RE: Small bowel obstruction in pregnancy. Obstet Gynecol 49:170, 1977

16. Milne B, Johnstone MS: Intestinal obstruction in pregnancy. Scott Med J 24:80, 1979

17. Crouch M: The acute abdomen in women. Practitioner 222:457, 1979

18. Svesko VS, Pisani BJ: Intestinal obstruction in pregnancy. Am J Obstet Gynecol 71:157, 1960

19. Becker-Anderson H, Husfeldt V: Peptic ulcer in pregnancy. Acta Obstet Gynecol Scand 50:371, 1971

20. Corlett RC, Mishell DR: Pancreatitis in pregnancy. Am J Obstet Gynecol 113:281, 1972

3

Accidental Injury

HERBERT J. BUCHSBAUM, MD

CLINICAL SIGNIFICANCE: About 7% of gravidas sustain trauma of some kind. The response of mother and fetus is variable, depending on the type of injury sustained and the effects of the anatomic and physiologic alterations of pregnancy.

Because more pregnant women are participating in physical activities, they are increasingly exposed to vehicular, work-related, and even sports-induced injuries. As a result, accidental injury is becoming a more frequent—and important—complication of pregnancy.

One study, by a prepaid medical group in California, found that 7% of women sustain some form of injury, from minor to catastrophic, during pregnancy. If this percentage were to hold nationwide, applied to the more than 3 million live births annually in the US, the result would be nearly 250,000 injured gravidas per year. In Minnesota, trauma is now the most common cause of nonobstetric maternal deaths, accounting for 20% of the mortality in this category. Similar figures have been published for California.

In dealing with the injured gravida, remember that the two lives involved respond differently to trauma. The management of specific injuries is often left to the trauma specialist, who will generally take the same approach used for the nongravid patient. This chapter emphasizes the anatomic and physiologic alterations of pregnancy that might modify the type of injury the mother sustains and alter her response to the trauma. Physiologic alterations may also modify diagnosis and management, as well as interpretation of clinical laboratory studies.

PHYSIOLOGIC CHANGES OF PREGNANCY

Pulse. The heart rate increases throughout pregnancy, reaching a level as much as 15 bpm above the nonpregnant rate. Tachycardia is pathognomonic of hypovolemic shock (rate greater than 100 bpm).

Blood pressure. There is no physiologic elevation of blood pressure during pregnancy. However, pregnancy-induced hypertension affects many primigravidas.

Venous pressure. Peripheral venous pressure increases in the legs but remains unchanged in the arms during pregnancy. This differential increase has been ascribed to the gravid uterus's obstructing venous return, but the effect of pregnancy on central venous pressure remains unclear. One recent report suggests a progressive rise, while another suggests a progressive drop, throughout pregnancy.

Blood volume. There is a physiologic increase in total volume that begins in the first trimester and continues up to 34 to 36 weeks. Plasma volume increases proportionately more than red cell mass, with a fall in hematocrit the result.

Leukocyte count. Leukocytosis following trauma suggests acute hemorrhage; a marked elevation is found when the liver or spleen is ruptured. In caring for an injured gravida, however, remember that a certain degree of leukocytosis is physiologic in pregnancy. It is progressive, and may reach levels of 18,000 to 20,000 WBC/cu mm during labor.

GI tract. Delayed emptying of the stomach and prolonged intestinal transit time are normal in pregnancy. In the nonpregnant woman, transit time from the stomach to the ileocecal valve is significantly increased during the luteal phase, suggesting that higher progesterone levels may play a role in altering transit time during pregnancy.

Liver and spleen. There is no evidence that the spleen or liver enlarges during pregnancy. However, altered tissue mechanisms may cause the spleen to descend from its protected site behind the rib cage, loosening supportive ligaments and increasing its susceptibility to trauma with subsequent rupture.

Hydronephrosis. Pregnancy-related hydroureter and hydronephrosis are almost always evident on an IV pyelogram at the end of the first trimester. These changes are more prominent on the right than on the left, suggesting a mechanical etiology, as the left ureter is cushioned by the sigmoid colon.

IMMEDIATE MANAGEMENT

Table 3-1 summarizes the key points of emergency treatment. During evaluation and early management, the injured gravida—particularly the unconscious patient near term—should be put on her left side to displace the uterus from the inferior vena cava. There is both clinical and experimental evidence that the pressure of the uterus may compromise venous return and even cause premature separation of a normally implanted placenta. The uterus can also be displaced laterally by a uterine displacer or by a pillow under the patient's right hip.

After determining ventilatory and cardiovascular status and evaluating consciousness, institute emergency resuscitative measures, if necessary. Insert a large-bore IV catheter into a peripheral vein and a subclavian or Swan-Ganz catheter for central venous pressure monitoring. After acute blood loss, start fluid replacement with crystalloid solution to maintain maternal blood volume until blood is available for transfusion. Physiologic hypervolemia of pregnancy spares the mother the immediate adverse effects of hypovolemic shock by compromising uterine blood flow, which may be reduced by as much as 10% to 20%, while maternal blood pressure remains unchanged. The mother's vital signs may not change until she has sustained a 30% reduction in circulating blood volume. Maternal blood pressure is therefore not a satisfactory measure of fetal well-being, since the mother maintains her own homeostasis at the fetus's expense.

Draw blood for typing and cross-matching. Order CBC, SMA-6 and SMA-12, and specialized studies, such as serum amylase measurements, as clinically indicated.

With gastric emptying delayed and intestinal transit time prolonged, any gravida who has sustained major abdominal trauma or who is unconscious should have a nasogastric tube placed. Equally important is

---

TABLE 3-1

Early management of the injured gravida

Position patient on her left side

Determine ventilatory and cardiovascular status. Institute cardiopulmonary resuscitation as needed. Monitor vital signs

Start IV infusions. Insert central and peripheral venous catheters

Draw blood for typing, cross-matching, and laboratory determinations

Insert nasogastric tube. Place Foley catheter in bladder

Obtain complete history and perform physical examination

Obtain diagnostic studies—x-rays, clinical procedures

Institute tetanus prophylaxis

the placement of an indwelling catheter in the urinary bladder. Difficulty in passing a catheter may suggest disruption of the urethra, while blood in the urine suggests rupture of the bladder. Both injuries are common accompaniments of pelvic fracture. The indwelling catheter will allow adequate monitoring of urinary output and will also permit a retrograde cystogram to be performed.

X-RAY STUDIES

X-rays are important in diagnosing and managing fractures, but their value is less defined when soft tissue injuries of the abdomen are involved. The interpretation of maternal x-rays during pregnancy must take into consideration physiologic connective tissue alterations. Separation of the symphysis and ureteral dilation are two examples. While no x-ray study that might help manage a maternal injury should be withheld, the significance of whole-body irradiation of the fetus must be carefully evaluated. No threshold dose for radiation injury to the fetus has been established; the deleterious effect is related to dose and period of gestation. Only those films that would alter management should be ordered, with great care to avoid duplication. When x-ray studies are necessary, their use should be coordinated. (A scout film of the abdomen should not be repeated when an IVP is ordered.) When x-rays are taken of the extremities, the abdomen should be shielded.

DIAGNOSING INTRAPERITONEAL HEMORRHAGE

Needle paracentesis and culdocentesis are techniques widely used to detect intraperitoneal hemorrhage resulting from blunt abdominal trauma. Peritoneal catheter lavage, a more accurate technique for the pregnant patient, has recently found widespread acceptance. Increased anteroposterior diameter of the abdominal cavity in late pregnancy, compartmentalization of the peritoneum by the uterine ligaments, and small bowel displacement into the upper abdomen reduce the effectiveness and increase the risks of paracentesis and culdocentesis.

The open lavage technique described by Rothenberger and colleagues appears to be uniquely suited to the diagnosis of intraperitoneal hemorrhage in the gravid patient. Under local anesthesia, a small incision is made into the peritoneum and a renal dialysis catheter is advanced toward the pelvis. If you aspirate over 10 mL of nonclotting blood, consider the test positive. If no blood is returned, 1 liter of lactated Ringer's solution is infused through the catheter and later removed by gravity drainage. The criteria for interpreting the test are shown in Table 3-2.

POSTMORTEM CESAREAN SECTION

Although rare, postmortem cesarean section is sometimes indicated. Over 150 such operations have resulted in the birth of live infants. The possibility of success correlates directly with the time interval between maternal death and delivery as well as with the cause of maternal death. Fetal outcome is likely to be good if the interval is less than 10 but no more than 20 minutes. When the cause of maternal death has not compromised the fetus, a successful outcome is also more likely.

A postmortem delivery may be performed with only a scalpel. Make a vertical incision in the abdominal wall and a classic vertical incision in the uterus. Equipment and personnel should be available to resuscitate the baby.

The question of consent is often raised in this era of medicolegal concerns. No US physician has ever been successfully prosecuted for performing a postmortem cesarean, even against the expressed wishes of the next of kin. In this situation, the rights of the child demand that no time be wasted in obtaining consent.

Maternal injury has become a significant factor in perinatal mortality. The sensitivity and response to trauma vary in the mother and fetus. Recognition of the physiologic alterations in the pregnant patient is essential to proper diagnosis and management of the injured gravida.

TABLE 3-2

*Criteria for interpreting diagnostic peritoneal lavage**

Positive
Aspiration of more than 10 ml of blood
Grossly bloody lavage fluid
Lavage fluid or urine returned through Foley catheter or chest tube
Red blood cell count >100,000/cu mm
White blood cell count >500/cu mm
Amylase >175/dL (Somogyi units)

Indeterminate (test should be repeated)
Red blood cell count >50,000 and <100,000/cu mm
White blood cell count >100 and <500/cu mm
Amylase >75 and <175/dL (Somogyi units)
Dialysis catheter fills with blood

Negative
Red blood cell count <50,000/cu mm
White blood cell count <100/cu mm
Amylase <75/dL (Somogyi units)

*Reprinted, with permission, from Rothenberger DA, Quattlebaum FW, Zabel J, et al: Diagnostic peritoneal lavage for blunt trauma in pregnant women. Am J Obstet Gynecol 129:479, 1977

SUGGESTED READING

- Brinkman CR III, Mofid M, Assali NS: Circulatory shock in pregnant sheep. Am J Obstet Gynecol 118:77, 1974
- Buchsbaum HJ: *Trauma in Pregnancy*. Philadelphia, WB Saunders, 1979
- Buchsbaum HJ, White AJ: The use of subclavian central venous catheters in gynecology and obstetrics. Surg Gynecol Obstet 136:561, 1973
- Greiss FC: Uterine vascular response to hemorrhage during pregnancy. Obstet Gynecol 27:549, 1966
- Pachter HL, Hofstetter SR: Open and percutaneous paracentesis and lavage for abdominal trauma. Arch Surg 116:318, 1981
- Rothenberger DA, Quattlebaum FW, Zabel J, et al: Diagnostic peritoneal lavage for blunt trauma in pregnant women. Am J Obstet Gynecol 129:479, 1977
- Weber CE: Postmortem cesarean section: Review of the literature and case reports. Am J Obstet Gynecol 110:158, 1971

Acute Renal Failure

KENNETH A. FISHER, MD

CLINICAL SIGNIFICANCE: With one in every 2,000 to 5,000 pregnancies affected, gravidas make up a significant 10% to 25% of all patients with acute renal failure. The condition is the major cause of acute cortical necrosis.

Any deterioration of renal function, with or without oliguria, poses a serious obstetric problem. Obstetrician and nephrologist must work closely together. The nephrologist is best equipped to deal with the metabolic aberrations caused by renal failure, while the obstetrician has the skills to treat the underlying systemic pathology. In most cases, the patient's survival depends on managing these problems successfully.

Contrary to what clinicians used to believe, pregnancy without further complications does not exacerbate pre-existing renal disease—even in systemic lupus erythematosus.[1] Increasing proteinuria, which is secondary to the physiologic increase in glomerular filtration rate, was in good part responsible for this misconception.[2] However, severe hypertension, especially if uncontrolled, can cause a permanent decrease in renal function. Also, the pregnant woman is susceptible to any of the renal diseases seen in the general population.[3] Still, most problems that are known to be associated with renal function in pregnant women are related to one of the various complications of pregnancy.

DIAGNOSING THE SPECIFIC SYNDROME

Two diseases associated with pregnancy—preeclampsia-eclampsia and postpartum renal failure—can lead to renal failure without additional obstetric complications. Preeclampsia-eclampsia, a systemic hypertensive disease of unknown etiology, is associated with a relatively specific renal lesion.[4] This disease can be complicated by acute renal failure, which is frequently the result of tubular necrosis (usually reversible). Occasionally, renal failure is caused by bilateral cortical necrosis. This often progresses to chronic renal failure. Preeclampsia is difficult to diagnose clinically, especially in the multipara. Differentiating pre-eclampsia clinically from nephrosclerosis (hypertensive kidney) or other renal disease is also difficult.[5] These entities, when superimposed on preeclampsia, may increase the incidence of acute renal failure.[6]

Postpartum renal failure, another pregnancy-specific syndrome, frequently results in kidney failure. This relatively rare syndrome may be associated with microangiopathic hemolytic anemia.[7] It usually does not resolve, thereby requiring dialysis or transplantation to maintain life. Two pathologic patterns have emerged. One resembles thrombotic microangiopathy;[7] the other is a nephrosclerotic picture much like scleroderma.[8] Whether these two lesions represent a different time course in the same disease or separate diseases is not yet known. Some authors, who do not consider postpartum renal failure a specific disease, have classified various lesions under this heading.[9] Experience with heparin therapy in these patients has been inconsistent, and if a subset of patients exists who would benefit from such therapy, they are yet to be defined.

Other pregnancy-associated entities can lead to acute renal failure as the result of the additional complications of coagulation defects, ischemia, or infection (Table 4-1). Abruptio placentae, prolonged intrauterine death, and amniotic fluid embolism probably cause renal failure through alterations in coagulation. Infection, as a result of puerperal sepsis, pyelonephritis, chorioamnionitis, or septic abortion (early in pregnancy), may cause renal failure, with or without associated disseminated intravascular coagulation. Ischemic renal damage may accompany postpartum hemorrhage, placenta previa, and hyperemesis gravidarum. Renal failure associated with fatty liver and jaundice of pregnancy probably results from the same mechanism as any severe hepatic failure.

In the obstetric patient, acute renal failure is usually due to bilateral cortical necrosis or acute tubular necrosis. Most cases of bilateral cortical necrosis progress to chronic renal failure.[10] The condition often seems to be associated with abruptio placentae, prolonged intrauterine fetal death, or uterine hemorrhage.[6] Some authors suggest a hypercoagulable state causes this association. The extent of necrosis varies; it is most severe in the superficial cortex and frequently spares the juxtamedullary area. Extensive renovascular fibrin thrombi are seen throughout the infarcted area.[11]

Vascular hyperreactivity (with preferential cortical ischemia), glomerular changes, intraluminal obstruction, back-leak of luminal contents, and abnormalities in prostaglandin metabolism have all been demonstrated in acute tubular necrosis. Which of these mechanisms is paramount in a particular type of patient is unknown. Damage is limited to the tubular cells. The extent of cell necrosis is quite variable and there may be great disparity between the severity of the lesion—frequently quite mild—and the clinical course.[12]

Most of the mortality from acute renal failure in pregnant patients is due to the severity of the underlying process rather than to the renal failure itself. Many studies have described lab tests designed to help differentiate between prerenal and parenchymal renal disease.[13] Recent research into the nature of acute renal failure has demonstrated its multifactorial nature and the possibility of lessening its severity with therapeutic maneuvers such as saline loading, mannitol, or loop diuretics. However, these laboratory models do not exactly duplicate human disease and the therapeutic interventions must be initiated within a narrow time period. Hence, we usually don't give large doses of a loop di-

---

TABLE 4-1

Conditions associated with acute renal failure in pregnancy

Placenta previa

Abruptio placentae

Postpartum hemorrhage

Hyperemesis gravidarum

Preeclampsia-eclampsia

Abortion
   Septic
   Hemorrhage
   Toxins

Puerperal sepsis

Chorioamnionitis

Pyelonephritis

Disseminated intravascular coagulation
   Sepsis-endotoxemia
   Preeclampsia-eclampsia
   Massive hemolysis

Association with fatty liver of pregnancy

Amniotic fluid embolism

Other causes seen in nonpregnant state
   Acute glomerulonephritis
   Subacute bacterial endocarditis
   Other infections

Acute postpartum renal failure

---

uretic. Instead, we concentrate on the underlying disease process, using a composite of the total clinical picture.

If the disease is prerenal, try to correct the situation with appropriate fluids. Once this is done, acute renal failure should not ensue. If acute renal failure has already taken place, no known therapeutic intervention has yet been proven to reverse this process immediately. (It is also important to rule out postrenal obstruction, even though it's seen only rarely in pregnant women.)

WHAT THERAPY TO CHOOSE

The first and most important step in therapy is to diagnose and correct the underlying disease process. This is probably the most important factor in patient survival and it is here that the obstetrician must assume a leading role. Consider the various disease processes listed in Table 4-1 and make the appropriate diagnosis. If the patient is hypertensive, consider the diagnosis of preeclampsia. Once you have made this diagnosis, delivery is mandatory if renal function deteriorates.

If hypovolemia is present, it must be aggressively monitored and treated (Table 4-2), and the cause diagnosed and corrected. Treat serious infections with appropriate antibiotics. Usually, a broad-spectrum antibiotic should be used first, with careful adjustment of dosage if renal function is impaired. Locate and drain any abscess.

Use prothrombin time, partial thromboplastin time, platelet count, and factor VIII assay to diagnose disseminated intravascular coagulation, and correct the underlying causes. Heparin therapy is controversial; many authorities prefer to concentrate on the underlying cause.

If you find none of the above entities, consider the other possibilities listed in Table 4-1. If the patient is to survive, you must diagnose and control the underlying disease process.

Adjust drug dosage and fluid administration to compensate for loss of renal function. Evaluate fluid status, electrolyte and acid-base balance, and the presence of uremia. The decision to dialyze usually rests on these criteria. The recent trend, especially in pregnancy, is to dialyze early. This keeps the internal milieu as normal as possible. The clinical parameters used to determine fluid overload are listed in Table 4-2.

Electrolyte and acid-base status require careful monitoring. Be especially on guard for rapid development of hyperkalemia and acidosis, as a good deal of tissue breakdown or sequestered blood may occur as part of the underlying pathology. Although acute hyperkalemia may be treated with sodium bicarbonate, insulin and glucose, ion exchange resins, or calcium gluconate, dialysis is frequently the treatment of choice.

Once you are sure the patient requires artificial renal support, you must decide whether to choose hemo- or peritoneal dialysis. Usually, multiple factors enter into the decision (Table 4-3).

You should choose hemodialysis if the patient has had recent abdominal surgery, because peritoneal dialysis fluid tends to leak. Hemodialysis is also preferable for obese patients, because the peritoneal dialysis catheter may cause infection. Peritoneal dialysis is undesirable for patients with an active pulmonary process, because it tends to decrease diaphragmatic movement, and for patients who are massively catabolic, because it may not be able to maintain a normal internal environment. Peritoneal dialysis is also indicated if blood access sites are not easily available, but not if the patient's nutritional status is poor, because of the loss of protein.

Peritoneal dialysis is a better choice if the patient's cardiac output is inadequate, since hemodialysis needs a 200- to 300-mL/minute blood flow. Because hemodialysis requires a more highly trained support group, peritoneal dialysis is indicated if technical support is inadequate. If there is a bleeding diathesis, choose peritoneal dialysis,

---

TABLE 4-2

Clinical parameters for judging fluid status

Blood pressure

Pulse

Skin turgor

Mucous membrane appearance

Neck vein distention

Lung rales

Heart sounds
   Second sound in pulmonic area
   Protodiastolic gallop—S_3

Central venous pressure
   Swan-Ganz catheter if necessary (unusual)

Ascites

Peripheral edema

Chest x-ray for:
   Heart size
   Pulmonary venous pattern
   Azygous vein dilation
   Alveolar filling pattern
   Effusions

Hematocrit changes

TABLE 4-3

Criteria for choosing hemo- or peritoneal dialysis

Choose hemodialysis
If the patient has had recent abdominal surgery
If the patient is obese
If there is an active pulmonary process
If the patient is massively catabolic
If the patient's nutritional status is poor

Choose peritoneal dialysis
If the patient's cardiac output is inadequate
If technical support is inadequate
If there is a bleeding diathesis
If access sites are not easily available
If the patient is HAA positive

which requires less alteration of the clotting system than hemodialysis. Finally, peritoneal dialysis is preferable if the patient is HAA positive, because there is less chance of spread to staff.

Rapidly accumulating evidence indicates that nutritional status is important not only to combat infection, repair wounds, and replace lost protein, but also to accelerate the repair process of acute tubular necrosis.[14] Early nutrition is becoming more accepted as part of the therapeutic regimen, given orally if possible, parenterally when necessary. Early dialysis, which permits control of fluids and chemistries, enables the patient to receive adequate nutrition. The patient being dialyzed has little need for the special amino acid mixes recommended by some pharmaceutical manufacturers. Dialysis offers the alternative of less specific nutrition, even relatively normal meals if the patient can manage them.

REFERENCES

1. Hayslett JP, Lynn RP: Effect of pregnancy in patients with lupus nephropathy. Kidney Int 18:207, 1980

2. Katz AI, Davison JM, Hayslett JP, et al: Pregnancy in women with kidney disease. Kidney Int 18:192, 1980

3. Singson E, Fisher K, Lindheimer MD: Acute poststreptococcal glomerulonephritis in pregnancy: Case report with an 18 year follow-up. Am J Obstet Gynecol 137:857, 1980

4. Spargo B, McCartney CP, Winemiller R: Glomerular capillary endotheliosis in toxemia of pregnancy. Arch Pathol 68:593, 1959

5. Fisher KA, Luger A, Spargo BH, et al: Hypertension in pregnancy: Clinical-pathological correlations and remote prognosis. Medicine 60:267, 1981

6. Grunfeld J, Ganeval D, Bournerias F: Acute renal failure in pregnancy. Kidney Int 18:179, 1980

7. Robson JS, Martin AM, Ruckley VA, et al: Irreversible postpartum renal failure: A new syndrome. Q J Med 37:423, 1968

8. Schoolwerth AC, Sandler RS, Klahr S, et al: Nephrosclerosis postpartum and in women taking oral contraceptives. Arch Intern Med 136:178, 1976

9. Ferris TF: Postpartum renal insufficiency. Kidney Int 14:383, 1978

10. Kleinknecht D, Grunfeld JP, Cia-Gomez P, et al: Diagnostic procedures and long-term prognosis in bilateral renal cortical necrosis. Kidney Int 4:390, 1973

11. Spargo BH, Seymour AE, Ordonez NG: *Renal Biopsy Pathology*. New York, John Wiley & Sons, 1980, p 286

12. Lindheimer MD, Katz AI: *Kidney Function and Disease in Pregnancy*. Philadelphia, Lea & Febiger, 1977

13. Miller TR, Anderson RJ, Linas SL, et al: Urinary diagnostic indices in acute renal failure. Ann Intern Med 89:47, 1978

14. Toback FG: Amino acid enhancement of renal regeneration after acute tubular necrosis. Kidney Int 12:193, 1977

5

Sickle Cell Crisis

JAMES N. MARTIN JR., MD, and
JOHN C. MORRISON, MD

CLINICAL SIGNIFICANCE: One black American in 600 has sickle cell disease. During pregnancy, this hemoglobinopathy is associated with significant morbidity and mortality in mothers and babies. Vaso-occlusive crises can occur at any time during pregnancy, including labor and delivery, and in the postpartum period. Improved outcomes depend on prevention or rapid treatment.

During pregnancy, women with sickle hemoglobinopathies have a high risk of morbidity and mortality. Perinatal morbidity and mortality also are high. The clinical hallmark of these inherited hematologic disorders is the usually acute, painful, recurring vaso-occlusive attack known as a sickle cell crisis. Many obstetrics services have significantly reduced or eliminated such episodes by giving prophylactic exchange transfusions throughout pregnancy. Even so, those who care for these patients must be prepared to respond quickly with a well-founded management plan, for a sickle crisis may occur at any time during pregnancy, labor and delivery, or postpartum.

Homozygous sickle cell anemia (HbS-S), the most common of the severe hemoglobinopathies, is an inherited hematologic disorder affecting approximately one in every 600 black Americans. When deoxygenation occurs in patients with this disease, their normally rounded, slightly elliptical red blood cells assume half-moon or sickle shapes (Figure 5-1). The disease is incurable and along with other severe variants— hemoglobin S-C disease (HbS-C) and sickle cell thalassemia (HbS-thal)—is found almost exclusively among persons of African or Mediterranean descent. It causes widespread organ damage, a shortened life span, and a multitude of medical and perinatal complications.

Some events that initiate sickle cell crisis are viral and bacterial infection, fever, acid-base imbalance, dehydration, trauma, blood loss, anesthesia, emotional disturbance with severe stress, strenuous physical activity, exposure to cold, antivenin injections, alcohol intoxication, extreme fatigue, high-altitude nonpressurized flights, and drug overdose.

TYPES OF CRISES

In a broad sense, the term "sickle cell crisis" includes all the acute events seen in sickle cell disease. Crises can be divided into two major groups, the vaso-occlusive and the hematologic (Table 5-1). During

---

FIGURE 5-1

Red blood cells from a sickle cell patient

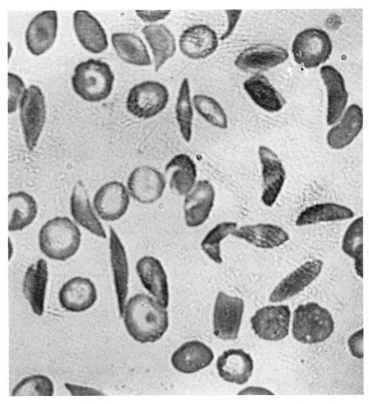

When deoxygenation occurs, normally shaped, rounded, slightly elliptical red blood cells are converted to half-moon or sickle-shaped cells.

pregnancy, most crises are vaso-occlusive, occur most often in the latter half of pregnancy, and produce the well-known scenario of recurring sudden attacks of pain involving the abdomen, chest, vertebrae, and extremities. The clinical manifestations for each patient usually follow a repetitive pattern from one crisis to the next. Some pregnant patients will have generalized pain; others exhibit more localized syndromes, as microcirculations involving bone or joints, the chest and lungs, intra-abdominal organs such as the liver and kidneys, or the central nervous system become obstructed.

Hematologic crises, infrequent in pregnancy, are characterized by reticulocytopenia and a rapid decline in the packed red cell volume. Their outstanding clinical feature is a marked pallor not associated with any significant degree of icterus. Affected patients generally have pale conjunctivas, are weak, and may show evidence of cardiac failure. Aplastic crisis, the most common hematologic type, is self-limited and is usually associated with infection. Other hematologic crises are hemolytic and are associated with hereditary spherocytosis or glucose 6-phosphate dehydrogenase deficiency; splenic sequestration crises, confined most often to childhood; and megaloblastic crises, secondary to folate depletion. Today's emphasis on folate supplementation for all known sickle cell patients, especially during pregnancy, has helped minimize the occurrence of megaloblastic crises.

DIFFERENTIAL DIAGNOSIS

Diagnosing sickle cell vaso-occlusive crisis in pregnancy requires clinical acumen. Most women with hemoglobinopathies are known to have the condition by the time they become pregnant. For undetected disease, the most accurate diagnostic test is hemoglobin electrophoresis. When confronted with a possible sickle crisis, you must determine whether this is an uncomplicated vaso-occlusive episode, a crisis associated with an infection, malingering, or a surgical or obstetric condition. Pain does not always mean a vaso-occlusive crisis; a patient may have any one of a wide variety of other medical or surgical conditions

---

TABLE 5-1

Sickle cell crisis classification

Vaso-occlusive crises	Hematologic crises
Abdominal	Aplastic
Central nervous system	Hemolytic
Pulmonary	Megaloblastic
Skeletal	Splenic sequestration

(Table 5-2) or one of several pregnancy-associated conditions. The diagnosis therefore is one of exclusion and may become clear only after a failed trial of conservative management.

Approximately 20% to 33% of adult sickle crises are associated with apparent or occult infection. Pneumococcal infection, especially in the lungs and meninges, is particularly common in young patients. During the reproductive years, gram-negative bacteria such as *Escherichia coli* and *Salmonella* replace the pneumococcus as the major offending organisms. *Mycoplasma* may also cause pneumonia in these patients. Pneumonia, urinary tract infection, puerperal endomyometritis, and osteomyelitis are the infections that are most frequently encountered.

There are several possible explanations for the sickle patient's increased susceptibility to infection. Studies have suggested decreased serum IgM, impaired serum opsonizing capacity, or a defective alternative pathway for complement activation may be the cause. There may be a deficiency of the phagocytosis-promoting tetrapeptide tuftsin.[1, 2] Recent investigations have shown inhibited neutrophil migration in the sera of children with sickle cell crisis and impaired leukocyte postphagocytic oxidative metabolism.[3, 4] Recurrent episodes of perivascular hemorrhage and infarction during the first decade of life usually destroy the spleen's filtering capacity and immunologic function. The

---

TABLE 5-2

Some differential diagnostic considerations in vaso-occlusive crises

Abdominal
Appendicitis
Cholecystitis
Cholelithiasis
Duodenal ulcer disease
Intestinal obstruction
Intussusception
Pancreatitis
Perforated viscus

Gynecologic/obstetric
Abruptio placentae
Degenerating leiomyomas
Ectopic pregnancy
Threatened abortion
Ruptured uterus
Torsion of ovary or cyst
Toxemia

Pulmonary
Embolus and infarction
Pneumonia

Renal
Colic
Cystitis
Pyelonephritis

General
Drug addiction
Gouty arthritis
Thrombophlebitis

presence of Howell-Jolly bodies on a peripheral blood smear attests to the presence of functional asplenia.

USEFUL LAB TESTS

Laboratory aids to differential diagnosis can help identify patients who are experiencing a vaso-occlusive crisis when there is no potentially serious infection. Although the total WBC count and the number of segmented leukocytes usually increase during infection and vaso-occlusive crisis, only a significant bacterial infection consistently increases band (nonsegmented) leukocytes to levels above 1,000/cu mm.[5] Leukocyte alkaline phosphatase activity has been reported greatly increased secondary to bacterial infection, compared with a normal range for vaso-occlusive crisis alone.[6] Serum lactate dehydrogenases are elevated, especially isoenzymes 1 and 2 (α-hydroxybutyrate dehydrogenase), in the steady state of sickle cell disease. The levels rise significantly during vaso-occlusive episodes, in proportion to the severity of the crisis. It may be possible to differentiate between true infarctive crisis and some other condition by determining these levels, if the patient's own baseline value is available for comparison.[7, 8] Platelet counts and coagulation factors are not helpful in differential diagnosis but may be useful for overall clinical management. Augmented platelet activation and turnover, hypercoagulability, and hyperviscosity characterize crises and are secondary to an acute phase protein reaction common to both vascular stasis and infection.[9]

MANAGING A CRISIS

Patients should be cared for in centers where expertise and equipment are optimal. Because none of the specific antisickling agents under investigation has been approved for routine use, management is mainly supportive and symptomatic, with meticulous medical and obstetric care. Basic goals of therapy at any time during pregnancy and the puerperium include managing pain, alleviating dehydration, and treating intercurrent infections and other complications. The most important therapy is some form of partial exchange transfusion to decrease the amount of HbS in the circulation. Our comprehensive plan includes both general and specific recommendations for antepartum, intrapartum, and postpartum crises.

The essentials of optimal sickle cell crisis management in the nonlaboring pregnant patient include the following factors:

Environment. The patient should be hospitalized in a quiet, comfortable area of the obstetric unit where family support and medical care are both available. Encourage relaxation at bed rest and give mild sedation. In other words, make the patient as comfortable as possible.

Fluid and electrolyte replacement. Vigorous hydration is a cornerstone of therapy, especially if the patient is febrile. Since these patients may have hyposthenuria and increased insensible fluid losses, dehydration and hyperosmolarity are common problems. If there are no signs of congestive heart failure, we infuse 1 liter of Ringer's lactate or isotonic saline over a 2-hour period and continue fluid replacement at 125 mL/hour. We avoid urinary catheterization, to minimize risk of infection. Also, we avoid central venous pressure lines unless we suspect impending cardiovascular failure or unless the patient also has severe pregnancy-induced hypertension.

Alkali therapy is rarely used in fluid and electrolyte management. While there appears to be local acidosis in the capillary beds where sickling occurs, systemic acidosis rarely develops.[10] It is not surprising that administering alkali is no more effective than hydration alone.[11] Also, it is arguable whether the recently reported practice of treating patients in sickle cell crisis with a potent antidiuretic and hypotonic IV solutions is appropriate, efficacious, or safe for the parturient and her fetus.[12] Finally, fresh frozen plasma may be a useful adjuvant to fluid therapy for vaso-occlusive crisis.[13] In addition to expanding blood volume and enhancing flow, fresh frozen plasma may stimulate plasma prostacyclin regeneration with subsequent vasodilatory and antiplatelet effects.[14]

Analgesia. A wide range of analgesics appropriate to the subjective needs of the parturient in crisis can achieve pain relief without respiratory depression. Because the liberal use of salicylates imposes an acid load, we prefer acetaminophen as the antipyretic and mild analgesic of choice. Meperidine and a sedative or ataractic agent such as a phenothiazine derivative usually are adequate for alleviating severe pain. Morphine is used infrequently in view of its tendency to cause smooth-muscle constriction. As soon as the painful symptoms have begun to abate, we substitute non-narcotic agents up to and after discharge. To avoid drug abuse or addiction, we proscribe outpatient use of any narcotic or mood-altering chemical.

Antibiotics. During initial assessment, we search for possible occult infection, a complication that occurs in approximately 25% of parturients with vaso-occlusive crisis. We recommend early treatment, when indicated, because infection accounts for about a third of all deaths in pregnant patients with sickle cell disease. We discourage prophylactic use of antibiotics as part of general crisis management. However, when physical findings and laboratory test results are highly suggestive of a crisis-associated infection, we obtain appropriate cultures and begin antibiotics immediately.

Oxygen administration. Because its efficacy is doubtful, we do not advocate conventional oxygen therapy unless the parturient in crisis has evidence of a respiratory infection, a low PaO_2 level (less than 70 mm), or is in labor. If this therapy is needed, 3 liters of oxygen per minute by nasal prongs is usually sufficient. In general, the best way to remedy hypoxemia is to eliminate the underlying factors.

FHR monitoring. Fetal loss is a substantial risk for mothers with sickle cell disease. It may occur during or immediately after a vaso-occlusive crisis. Electronic fetal monitoring throughout crisis treatment will alert the obstetric health-care team to potential fetal distress or death. Be cautious about responding too quickly to ominous late decelerations or other worrisome FHR patterns; they may be seen transiently during crisis but resolve soon after the mother's condition begins to improve.[15]

Blood. The most important therapeutic maneuver for interrupting sickle cell crisis in pregnancy is partial exchange transfusion. This temporarily diminishes erythropoiesis, improves the oxygen-carrying capacity of circulating blood, and reduces the concentration of HbS by substituting HbA-containing red cells for the HbS-containing cells. The older, manual, or "push-pull" techniques of phlebotomy infusion recently have been replaced by automated erythrocytapheresis, using an IBM 2997 cell separator (Figure 5-2).[16] This technique removes both HbS-containing red cells and irreversibly sickled cells by extracorporeal differential centrifugation. The patient's own plasma—including leukocytes, platelets, and clotting factors—can simultaneously be returned to her circulation along with buffy-coat-poor washed donor erythrocytes (BCPWDE). The goal of either partial exchange method is to increase the HbA concentration by at least 40%. A great advantage of the newer method is the controlled, close monitoring of withdrawal and return rates to protect the patient from overload or hypovolemia. This is particularly important for the patient in crisis who also has congestive heart failure or acute renal failure. A simple manual transfusion is helpful when the patient's initial packed red cell volume is dangerously low (PCV < 15%, hemoglobin < 6 gm/dL).

Another advantage of the automated method is the greatly reduced transfusion time it requires. In slightly over 2 hours, the newer method exchanges the same blood volume that took 12 to 24 hours to replace with manual methods. We have observed that crisis pain usually begins to abate within 60 minutes of the time a partial exchange transfusion is begun. The treatment decreases HbS concentration, erythropoiesis, blood viscosity, and chance of sickling. It increases HbA concentration and the patient's sense of well-being, and is useful in associated anemia and congestive heart failure.

FIGURE 5-2

Automated erythrocytapheresis

This method of performing a partial exchange transfusion uses an IBM 2997 cell separator.

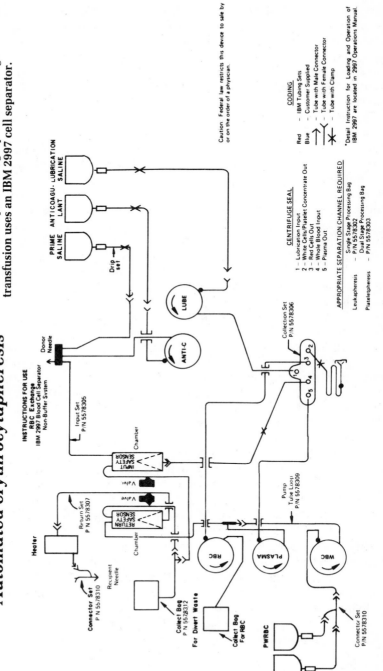

Blood smears performed during the transfusion to detect the presence of sickling usually become negative by the end of the second hour. Soon after the partial exchange (blood volume average of 1,400 to 1,800 mL) by this method, the transfused patient will have blood values of more than 50% HbA, a PCV greater than 25%, and a hemoglobin level above 9 gm/dL. Each patient's specific hematologic needs should be evaluated before transfusion, and the procedure calibrated to achieve the desired results.

Other automated modalities have been used to transfuse red blood cells. The Haemonetics model 30 is a discontinuous automated device that is cumbersome to use and time-consuming. Also, it is difficult to measure exactly the amounts of blood infused and removed. The other currently available machine for cell separation is the Fenwall CS-3000. It is efficiently employed for cell separation and removal of white blood cells (leukapheresis) and platelets (plateletpheresis), but there is some doubt as to its usefulness for red cell or plasma exchange.

If automated erythrocytapheresis is not available in a referral center for high-risk pregnancy management, or if a pregnant patient with sickle cell crisis must be treated temporarily in a less than optimal setting, a partial exchange transfusion using a manual protocol such as that outlined in Table 5-3 is the next best alternative.[17] Performed in 4-hour increments until the desired HbA concentration is reached, this method involves an infusion of a balanced electrolyte solution such as Ringer's lactate, followed by a phlebotomy and exchange transfusion of BCPWDE.

TABLE 5-3

Protocol for manual partial exchange transfusion

Type and cross-match 6 units packed red cells; measure HbA and PCV

Start IV, right arm. Give 1,000 mL ¹⁄₆ M lactate or normal saline, infusing 200 to 400 mL in first hour

Then phlebotomize 500 mL blood into Vacutainer from opposite arm (30 minutes)

Give 2 units (150 to 300 mL/unit) buffy-coat-poor washed red cells (under pressure and warmed) over next 2 hours

Repeat procedure in afternoon and allow overnight equilibration

If next morning PCV $\geq$ 35% and HbA $\geq$ 40%, discharge; if not, repeat procedure until desired levels obtained

---

It is critically important that blood banking techniques be monitored carefully to minimize the potential for blood transfusion complications (Table 5-4). Use all volunteer donor blood and wash the red cells to reduce the risk of hepatitis. BCPWDE reduces the risk of transfusion reactions. Blood for transfusion should be screened thoroughly for contamination with hepatitis and syphilis pathogens, or other hemoglobinopathies. Blood for transfusion should be fresh or stored less than 5 days in citrate-phosphate-dextrose solution. This will assure normal oxygen delivery and normal 2,3-diphosphoglycerate levels.

Minimizing any possible minor blood group incompatibility to prevent formation of cold agglutinins or minor antibodies is critical to the survival of these patients, who are likely to require transfusion at a later time for another crisis, after trauma or pregnancy. Preventing this isosensitization is of utmost importance and demands a very high standard of blood banking. Use blood negative for as many paternal antigens (Kell, Duffy) as possible, to minimize the risk of erythroblastosis fetalis.

Rarely, a pregnant patient with sickle cell crisis will fail to respond to medical management and transfusion. Other likely causes should then be considered (Table 5-2). If surgical exploration is required, the patient will be in optimal condition after medical management and exchange transfusion.

INTRAPARTUM CRISIS TREATMENT

The juxtaposition of sickle crisis and onset of labor presents the obstetrician with many challenging problems. It may be difficult to determine whether the parturient is in true labor or is having abdominal symptoms of crisis or a placental abruption, and whether simple or exchange transfusion is indicated before delivery. The following impor-

---

TABLE 5-4

Possible complications of blood transfusion

Circulatory overload	Iron overload
Erythroblastosis fetalis	Post-transfusion isoimmunization
Febrile reaction	
Immune intravascular hemolysis	Post-transfusion hepatitis
	Premature labor
Incompatibility	Urticaria

tant management concepts should be added to those listed in the previous section:

Oxytocics. There is no contraindication to the use of ecbolic agents during labor or postpartum.

Transfusion. A simple or a partial exchange transfusion can be administered during labor. Give a simple transfusion of 2 to 4 units of HbA BCPWDE to help abort the crisis and lessen the insult of blood loss at delivery.

Oxygen. Place the patient in the left lateral position, giving oxygen by mask or nasal prongs. Oxygen administration for patients in labor and in sickle crisis seems reasonable but has not been critically evaluated.

Maternal monitoring. Do frequent vital sign assessments; order coagulation studies, primarily to monitor platelet counts and fibrinogen levels; check blood films for evidence of sickling; determine serial maternal blood gases. Avoid central venous lines and Foley catheters, to reduce infectious morbidity.

Fetal monitoring. Electronic monitoring of the FHR and maternal contractions is very important to help assess the labor pattern and fetal tolerance to labor. We discourage indiscriminate use of the intrauterine pressure catheter, to minimize the possibility of endomyometritis. Fetal scalp blood sampling may be helpful.

Analgesia and anesthesia. Intermittent IV analgesia with pudendal block and nitrous oxide for vaginal delivery seems most prudent. For vaginal delivery during sickle crisis, conduction anesthesia is usually to be avoided, although it may be safe and satisfactory for the same patient when she is not in crisis. For cesarean births, conduction anesthesia may be preferable to general anesthesia, particularly if no crisis is present.

Delivery. Midline episiotomy and low forceps to shorten the second stage of labor, along with efforts to minimize blood loss, usually yield excellent results. A perinatal team approach to delivery is especially important. Communication and cooperation are critical. In addition to the obstetrician, well-trained anesthesia personnel should monitor the patient's vital signs and attend to any of her anesthetic-related needs during delivery and immediately postpartum. If general anesthesia must be used, it should be skillfully delivered to effect proper oxygenation and maintenance of normal Pa_{O_2}, pH, and cardiac output. Maintain adequate circulatory volume with blood and fluid replacement and avoid hypothermia in air-conditioned delivery and recovery rooms. Pediatric personnel skilled in infant resuscitation should be present to rapidly assess the neonate, who may have suffered during the delivery from its compromised mother or have life-threatening complications of its own.

POSTPARTUM CRISIS TREATMENT

Sickle cell crisis may develop during the puerperium, especially as a consequence of massive hemodynamic changes after delivery. The principles outlined for antepartum crisis treatment continue to apply. Watch vigilantly for possible infection, particularly endomyometritis and urinary tract infection. Encourage early ambulation and use of properly applied antithrombotic stockings. Optimal hydration, avoidance of hyperviscosity, and maintenance of HbA at high levels by transfusion may be most critical in the immediate postpartum and postoperative period, especially since there is a great risk of congestive heart failure and pulmonary emboli.

Investigators are striving to develop a safe pharmacologic treatment for sickle cell disease. Earlier enthusiasm for urea and cyanate has waned as the result of findings of ineffectiveness and toxicity.[18-21] The quest is being conducted primarily on three research fronts, with pharmacologic agents designed to effect disruption of intermolecular bonding (urea, dichloromethane), decreased deoxygenation of HbS (cyanate, dimethyl adipimidate), and prevention of sickling by interaction with the red cell membrane (zinc, phenothiazines).

Sickle cell crisis is a serious obstetric emergency. However, the combined life spans of mother and fetus have improved considerably over the past few years, primarily because of better management of complications and improvements in pregnancy care. There is reason to believe that adherence to the management principles we have described offers increasing hope that vaso-occlusive episodes can be effectively managed for better pregnancy outcomes.

REFERENCES

1. Bjornson AB, Lobel JS, Lampkin BC: Humoral components of host defense in sickle cell disease during painful crisis and asymptomatic periods. J Pediatr 96:259, 1980
2. Johnston RB, Newman SL, Struth AG: An abnormality of the alternate pathway of complement activation in sickle-cell disease. N Engl J Med 288:803, 1973
3. Boggs DR, Hyde F, Srodes C: An unusual pattern of neutrophil kinetics in sickle-cell anemia. Blood 41:59, 1973
4. Kaplan SS, Nardi M: Impairment of leukocyte function during sickle cell crisis. J Reticuloendothel Soc 22:499, 1977
5. Buchanan GR, Glader BE: Leukocyte counts in children with sickle cell disease. Am J Dis Child 132:396, 1978

6. Wajima T, Draus AP: Leukocyte alkaline phosphatase in sickle cell anemia. N Engl J Med 293:918, 1975

7. White JM, Muller MA, Billimoria F, et al: Serum α-hydroxybutyrate levels in sickle-cell disease and sickle-cell crisis. Lancet 1:532, 1978

8. Roth EF Jr, Bardfeld PA, Goldsmith SJ, et al: Sickle cell crisis as evaluated from measurements of hydroxybutyrate-dehydrogenase and myoglobin in plasma. Clin Chem 27:314, 1981

9. Richardson SGN, Matthews KB, Stuart J, et al: Serial changes in coagulation and viscosity during sickle-cell crisis. Br J Haematol 41:95, 1979

10. Ringelhann B, Konotey-Ahulu FID: Sickle cell crisis and acid-base balance. Clin C Acta 34:64, 1971

11. Schwartz E, McElfresh AE: Treatment of painful crises of sickle cell disease: A double-blind study. J Pediatr 64:132, 1964

12. Rosa RM, Bierer BE, Thomas R, et al: Study of induced hyponatremia in the prevention and treatment of sickle-cell crisis. N Engl J Med 303:1138, 1980

13. Huehns ER, Davies SC, Brozovic M: Fresh frozen plasma for vaso-occlusive crises in sickle cell disease. Lancet 1:1310, 1981

14. Stuart MJ, Blinder E, Sills R: Abnormal vascular prostaglandin I_2 (PGI_2) synthesis in sickle cell anemia. 18th Meeting of the International Society of Haematology (Montreal), August 1980, abstract 1612

15. Cruz AC, Spellacy WN, Jarrell M: Fetal heart rate tracing during sickle cell crisis—A cause for transient late decelerations. Obstet Gynecol 54:647, 1979

16. Morrison JC, Douvas SG, Martin JN Jr: Methods of exchange transfusion in pregnant patients with sickle hemoglobinopathies. Unpublished data

17. Morrison JC, Schneider JM, Whybrew WD, et al: Prophylactic transfusions in pregnant patients with sickle hemoglobinopathies: Benefit versus risk. Obstet Gynecol 56:274, 1980

18. Cooperative Urea Trials Group: Clinical trials of therapy for sickle cell vaso-occlusive crisis. JAMA 228:1120, 1974

19. Harkness DR, Roth S: Clinical evaluation of cyanate in sickle cell anemia. Prog Hematol 9:157, 1975

20. Charache S, Duffy TR, Jander N, et al: Toxic-therapeutic ratio of sodium cyanate. Arch Intern Med 135:1043, 1975

21. Peterson CM, Tsairis P, Ohnishi A, et al: Sodium cyanate induced polyneuropathy in patients with sickle cell disease. Ann Intern Med 81:152, 1974

Diabetic Ketoacidosis and Pregnancy

JOHN L. KITZMILLER, MD

CLINICAL SIGNIFICANCE: A high fetal death rate makes diabetic ketoacidosis a dire complication. But with good care, the incidence should be minimal in insulin-dependent pregnant women. While hormonal and metabolic changes of pregnancy increase the diabetic's chances of developing ketoacidosis, understanding the pathogenesis can help prevent the condition. Knowledge of the complex pathophysiology is essential to treatment.

In pregnancy, ketoacidosis (KTA) is a true emergency. Fetal death rates as high as 90% have been reported. Maternal death in these relatively young patients should be rare, but the average mortality per episode of KTA among all US diabetics in 1975 was 10%.[1] The metabolic changes of pregnancy increase the potential for acidosis in insulin-dependent patients.[2]

The purpose of this review of KTA is to relate clinical signs and symptoms to important physiologic aspects, point out areas of ignorance concerning effects of pregnancy and effects on the fetus, indicate the association with betamimetics and corticosteroids, and emphasize measures to prevent this severe disorder.

PATHOGENESIS

Four factors may contribute to ketoacidosis in diabetics: a relative insulin deficiency, an excess of stress hormone, fasting, and dehydration.[3] We used to think ketoacidosis was caused by insulin withdrawal or an absolute deficiency of it; however, most diabetics with KTA don't have subnormal plasma insulin concentrations (lower than 6 μU/mL). On the other hand, since none of the patients with KTA studied have had insulin levels above 50 μU/mL, and since nondiabetics can achieve plasma concentrations higher than 50 μU/mL when blood glucose levels exceed 250 mg/dL, a relative deficiency has been suggested as a cause of KTA.[4] But when insulin infusions produce sufficient circulating plasma concentrations, KTA does not develop, despite the presence of other risk factors.[5]

Schade and Eaton reviewed the evidence that too much stress hormone contributes to the development of KTA.[4] In all the cases, at least one stress hormone (glucagon, catecholamines, or cortisol) was elevated early. It may be argued that the elevation is a result, not the cause, of the acidosis..However, in one study of stress-induced KTA, the elevation preceded metabolic decompensation.[6] In diabetics, stress hormones elevate plasma glucose and ketone anions. Pharmacologic blockade of these hormones retards KTA when diabetics are taken off insulin.[4] The degree of acidosis diabetics develop correlates with plasma norepinephrine concentrations and cortisol secretion, but not with plasma insulin levels.[3] The most common precipitating cause of KTA is a stress, such as infection or dehydration, rather than omission of insulin.[7] KTA can be produced in animals only if their pituitary or adrenal glands are intact.[4] When insulin is withdrawn from patients who don't secrete endogenous glucagon or ACTH-growth hormone, the acidosis is greatly delayed. These findings support the concept that excess stress hormone is important in pathogenesis.

Whether it results from the nausea and vomiting that accompany certain infections or from the ketoacidotic state itself, fasting increases the production of hepatic ketone bodies and decreases the disposal of ketone anions.[8] The exact cause in diabetics has not yet been determined. It may be related to the rise in the secretion of glucagon and catecholamines induced by fasting.

When there is too little insulin or too much glucagon, sodium is lost through the kidneys.[3] Water can be lost through osmotic diuresis, vomiting, and diaphoresis. Dehydration exacerbates the developing KTA by reducing the glomerular filtration rate and urine flow, which reduces excretion of glucose and ketone anions. Also, dehydration reduces the distribution of glucose and ketone anions, so that plasma concentrations rise. Rehydration tends to reduce plasma glucose and ketone anion concentrations.[9]

The increased tendency to ketoacidosis during pregnancy may be related to a state of relative insulin resistance, plus enhanced lipolysis and ketogenesis.[2] Production of ketone acids increases during pregnancy because more substrate free fatty acids (FFA) are available. Also, hormonal effects stimulate the uptake and β-oxidation of FFA in liver cells. Plasma glucagon levels are higher in the basal, postabsorptive state during pregnancy,[10] and catecholamine and cortisol secretion in response to stress is unchanged.

PATHOPHYSIOLOGY

Glucose accumulates in extracellular fluid (ECF) as a result of a relative deficiency of insulin and an excess of stress hormone. Initially *hyperglycemia* is related to hepatic overproduction (a rise in gluconeogenesis) coupled with underuse of glucose. Excessive FFA is released, because insulin is not exerting its normal effect on adipose cells and also because of elevated catecholamines and glucagon. This FFA excess provides increased substrate for hepatic *ketogenesis.* Another result of the glucagon excess and insulin deficiency is that they stimulate the carnitine acyltransferase-dependent uptake of FFA by the mitochondria and β-oxidation of FFA in liver cells. The resultant ketonemia is probably also related to reduced uptake of ketone acids by muscle in the insulin-deficient state, which also leads to less regeneration of bicarbonate and contributes to the acidosis.

The osmotic diuresis secondary to glucosuria causes an excessive water loss. Despite *dehydration* and *hyperosmolarity,* about two-thirds of patients with KTA are *hyponatremic.* Insulin deficiency and excess glucagon exacerbate urinary loss of sodium. A major factor in hyponatremia is the shift of intracellular water to the extracellular space, because without adequate insulin cells are impermeable to glucose. Elevated blood triglycerides, sometimes found in patients with KTA, can also cause factitious hyponatremia. This can be ruled out by study of the plasma.

Urinary and GI losses lead to a marked *deficit in total body potassium,* usually ranging from 3 to 10 mEq/kg. However, the pretreatment plasma concentration of potassium is generally normal or elevated, because of the contraction in blood volume that characterizes KTA. In addition, there is an acidosis-induced shift of potassium into the ECF, as hydrogen ions from organic acids are buffered intracellularly. The potential for hyponatremia and hypokalemia to develop in patients with KTA must be a major consideration when treatment plans are being formulated.

The catabolic state and the acidosis of KTA also increase urinary excretion of phosphorus. There is an intracellular *phosphorus deficit* as well, because cellular uptake of phosphorus is impaired in parallel with decreased glucose uptake.

Despite their phosphorus depletion (approximately 1 mmole/kg), only 10% to 12% of patients with KTA are initially hypophosphatemic. The combination of phosphorus depletion, hyperglycemia, and acidosis impairs the synthesis of 2,3-diphosphoglycerate (2,3-DPG) within red blood cells, and 2,3-DPG levels are subnormal in KTA. Theoretically, this could impair oxygen delivery to tissues by increasing the affinity of hemoglobin for oxygen. The exact clinical effect, however, remains controversial.

HOW TO RECOGNIZE KTA

The possibility of ketoacidosis is suggested by a number of signs and symptoms, which can be confirmed by laboratory diagnoses. Polydipsia and polyuria are early symptoms of severe hyperglycemia. The main consequence of severe hyperglycemia is volume and electrolyte depletion, secondary to glucose-induced osmotic diuresis.

Signs of volume depletion include poor tissue turgor, soft or sunken eyeballs, hypotension, tachycardia, and hypothermia. Malaise, fatigue, stupor, drowsiness, and hyperventilation (deep, sighing Kussmaul respiration) indicate acidosis. The face may appear flushed. Nausea and vomiting, which are almost always present, cause further volume and electrolyte depletion. The characteristic fruity odor on the patient's breath comes from the large amounts (up to 12 mmoles/liter) of acetone in the blood, formed by decarboxylation from acetoacetic acid.

A biochemical definition based on lab tests and the work of Kitabchi and co-workers is given in Table 6-1.[11] About 15% of patients with KTA initially have moderate glucose levels of 300 to 350 mg/dL;[12] the rest are higher. The elevated organic acids found in KTA (β-hydroxybutyrate, acetoacetate, and sometimes lactate) completely dissociate at body pH. The hydrogen ions are buffered by intracellular proteins or alkaline salts of bone, or enter the ECF and combine with and deplete HCO_3^-. They are eliminated indirectly in the lungs or excreted as ammonium or titratable acid in the urine.

Acidosis occurs when the body buffer base is reduced and respiratory compensation and renal excretion cannot maintain a normal pH. Acetone does not contribute to the acidosis. Some authors consider KTA present when plasma HCO_3^- is less than 10 mEq/liter and arterial blood pH is less than 7.25. I prefer Kitabchi's criteria (Table 6-1).

TABLE 6-1

*Biochemical definition of diabetic KTA**

Plasma glucose > 300 mg/dL

Plasma HCO_3 < 15 mEq/liter

Arterial pH < 7.30

Serum acetone positive at 1:2 dilution

*Adapted from Kitabchi et al.[11]

Usually, the ketone anion concentration of plasma exceeds 7 mmoles/liter, often with a ratio of β-hydroxybutyrate to acetoacetate of 3:1. You can do a semiquantitative determination for ketones immediately using nitroprusside tablets (Acetest) or strips (Ketostix) on diluted (1:1) plasma or serum. The nitroprusside reaction estimates the concentration of acetoacetic acid and acetone in the blood, but cannot detect β-hydroxybutyrate. When KTA is accompanied by lactic acidosis and deficient oxygenation, the altered intracellular redox state favors conversion of acetoacetate to β-hydroxybutyrate (Figure 6-1). Therefore, it is possible that reagent testing may underestimate the degree of KTA.

Determining the so-called anion gap (unmeasured anions in plasma) is important when assessing acid-base disorders.[13, 14] The gap is calculated by subtracting the sum of plasma Cl^- and HCO_3^- (the major anions) from Na^+ (the major cation). The normal value for nonpregnant adults is 12 ± 2 mEq/liter. Determinations during pregnancy vary. Newman found 139.2 mEq/liter − (103.7 + 21.2 mEq/liter) = 14.3 mEq/liter,[15] but Kirschbaum reported 139.1 mEq/liter − (109.2 + 23.9 mEq/liter) = 6.1 mEq/liter for the midtrimester.[16]

In diabetic KTA, the anion gap is usually increased because of the increase of organic acid anions in the plasma. The degree to which the anion gap is widened reflects the magnitude of the acid load, and approximates the decrease in serum HCO_3^-.[17] In severe cases, before treatment, apparently more hydrogen ions than ketone anions accumulate in intracellular fluid. So, by the law of mass action, the rise in plasma unmeasured anions should be greater than the fall in plasma

---

FIGURE 6-1

Biochemical transformations important in acidosis

$$H^+ + HCO_3^- \rightleftharpoons H_2CO_3 \rightleftharpoons CO_2 + H_2O$$

$$pH = 6.1 + \log \frac{[HCO_3^-]}{[CO_2] + [H_2CO_3]}$$

$$\text{Acetoacetate} + NADH + H^+ \rightleftharpoons \beta\text{-hydroxybutyrate} + NAD^+$$

$$\text{Pyruvate} + NADH + H^+ \rightleftharpoons \text{lactate} + NAD^+$$

HCO_3^- This concept has been confirmed by measurements in patients, and was reviewed recently by Halperin and associates. These authors discuss the mechanism by which so-called hyperchloremic metabolic acidosis, present in nearly all KTA patients on admission, is related to indirect loss of sodium bicarbonate.[17]

During mid- and late pregnancy, the diabetic's tendency to slip into KTA is enhanced, and the acidosis may be more severe than symptoms such as moderate vomiting would suggest. White[18] and Pedersen[19] found acidosis could develop during pregnancy at relatively low levels of hyperglycemia (180 to 300 mg/dL). Pedersen pointed out that acidosis can develop rapidly during pregnancy, against the physiologic background of compensated respiratory alkalosis.[19] He found KTA most common at 20 to 36 weeks' gestation, when insulin resistance increases.

MANAGEMENT

The keystones of treatment are providing enough insulin to correct the acidosis and carefully balancing fluids and electrolytes. When you suspect KTA, take the following steps:
- Do a urinalysis and obtain venous blood for a CBC and glucose, BUN, and electrolyte determinations and to estimate serum ketones.
- Measure pH and blood gases in arterial blood.
- Begin to treat immediately when a comatose patient has arterial pH below 7.25, heavy glucosuria, and a strongly positive reaction for ketones in serum diluted 1:1. Don't wait for lab measurements of glucose and electrolytes.
- If possible, measure plasma osmolality, because values above 340 to 350 mOsM correlate with the degree of stupor and coma.
- Beyond 25 weeks' gestation, institute continuous FHR monitoring.

If enough obstetricians were to collect and report the effects of KTA on FHR, an adequate data base might be developed. Then FHR patterns might be useful in guiding fetal resuscitation.

Look for predisposing factors such as infection or psychogenic stress, to prevent recurrence of KTA. Chart changes in vital signs, laboratory data, quantities of insulin, fluid, and electrolyte treatment.[20]

CHOICE OF INSULIN TREATMENT

Large intermittent doses of regular insulin (50 to 100 units every 2 to 4 hours) were formerly thought necessary for treating KTA, apparently because of a postulated state of insulin resistance. In the mid 1970s, however, evidence suggested that relatively low-dose intermittent IM or continuous IV insulin regimens were equally successful.

Studies of plasma insulin levels indicated that a maximal biologic effect was obtained with levels of 20 to 200 $\mu U/mL$. Low-dose immunoreactive insulin levels (60 to 200 $\mu U/mL$), produced by doses of 2 to

10 units/hour IV, achieved the same effect as higher doses of insulin with blood levels of 400 to 1,200 μU/mL. Several studies showed there is less danger of producing hypoglycemia and hypokalemia with low-dose infusions.[11, 12] With less risk of treatment-induced hypoglycemia, there should be less danger of cerebral edema due to osmotic shifts.[12]

With a low-dose regimen, blood glucose should decline at rates of 75 to 100 mg/dL/hour and should reach 200 to 300 mg/dL in 4 to 6 hours of treatment.[12] The decrease will vary from patient to patient and will be retarded about 50% when infection is present. Correcting acidosis will take about twice as long, 8 to 10 hours. Acetone can persist in the blood for many hours after acidosis is corrected, and the serum ketone test will remain positive.

Although most patients respond to a low-dose regimen, correction of hyperglycemia and acidosis could be delayed if the dosage of insulin is too low. It is often difficult to predict who might not respond, so observe all patients closely. If there is no response, begin more aggressive insulin treatment.

Immediate insulin treatment. A protocol for regular insulin administration to treat KTA during pregnancy modified from Kitabchi and coworkers, is listed in Table 6-2. The IV loading dose is important in achieving a decline in ketones in the first 2 hours of therapy. The loading dose should be repeated in 1 hour if the plasma glucose has not declined by 10%. *The end point of treatment is correction of the acidosis.* If pH doesn't rise in 3 or 4 hours, then give much larger doses IV. With this regimen, it took mean intervals of 4.3 $\pm$ 1.1 hours to achieve a glucose level of 250 mg/dL; 6.7 $\pm$ 1.5 hours to achieve pH greater than 7.3; and 17.9 $\pm$ 2.8 hours to achieve HCO_3^- greater than 15 mEq/liter.[11]

Diluting IV insulin infusions with protein-containing solutions—to minimize the loss of insulin by adsorption to glassware and plastic tubing—is unnecessary. Instead, to saturate the binding sites, run 50 to 100 mL of a solution containing 5.0 units/dL of insulin through the tubing before connecting it to the patient.[21]

In the days of high-dose intermittent insulin therapy, White reported that pregnant patients required about twice as much insulin as nonpregnant patients to correct KTA and that recovery was delayed. Because hormonal changes of pregnancy produce a state of relative insulin resistance, you would expect higher IV doses might be required. However, no studies of KTA have compared pregnant women with the rest of the diabetic population, probably because careful preventive management in most perinatal centers today has decreased the incidence of KTA. The importance of prevention cannot be overemphasized.

IV fluids. Correcting dehydration and hypovolemia is primary. Infuse 2 liters of electrolyte solution during the first 2 to 3 hours. The average fluid deficit is 3 to 5 liters (Table 6-2). Formerly, hypotonic solutions were recommended, but administering sodium ions may offset a decline in ECF osmolality, as blood glucose is shifted intracellularly secondary to the insulin effect. Patients with elevated serum osmolality (greater than 320 mOsM) should be given 0.5 N saline for initial infusions. To prevent hypoglycemia, infuse 5% dextrose in water at 3 mL/kg/hour when the plasma glucose reaches 250 to 300 mg/dL.

Proper fluid management is necessary to prevent shock or cerebral edema. The combination of severe hypovolemia and reduced myocardial contractility, secondary to acidosis, may produce shock. Hypotensive patients need rapid infusions of large volumes of isotonic electrolyte solution, or even plasma volume expanders.[9] Central hemodynamic monitoring should guide fluid administration.

Initial hyponatremia may identify patients at risk for cerebral edema. Despite hyperglycemia, these patients' plasma osmolality will increase only mildly. When hyperglycemia is corrected with insulin, plasma os-

---

TABLE 6-2

*Treatment dosages for diabetic KTA**

A. Regular insulin

1. 0.4 unit/kg IV loading dose (30 to 40 units)

2. 5 to 10 units/hour IV

3. Repeat loading dose in 1 hour if plasma glucose does not decrease by 10%

4. End point is correction of acidosis. If there is no decrease in ketones or rise of pH in 3 to 4 hours, give 50 units/hour

B. Fluids

1. Ringer's lactate or normal saline, 2 liters over 2 to 3 hours; average deficit, 3 to 5 liters. Or give 10 mL/kg/hour

2. If serum > 320 mOsM, use 0.5 N saline

3. When plasma glucose is 250 to 300 mg/dL, add D_5W at 3 mL/kg/hour

C. Potassium

1. If serum K is normal or low, start 10 to 40 mEq/hour IV as KPO_4

2. If serum K is high, wait 1 to 4 hours for serum level to start to fall

D. Bicarbonate

1. If pH < 7.10, add 89.2 mEq $NaHCO_3$ to each liter of 0.5 N saline

2. Stop infusion when pH reaches 7.20

*Adapted from Kitabchi et al.[11]

molality falls more than intracellular osmolality, the osmotic gradient may reverse, and intracellular water can increase and produce cerebral edema. The identity of the intracellular osmoles remains unknown, but is probably unrelated to osmotically active sugars such as sorbitol. Insulin treatment does increase water, sodium, and potassium in the brain. Kreisberg reviewed and refuted other theories proposed to explain this cerebral edema.[12] Animal data support the hypothesis of the unfavorable osmotic gradients. Large pharmacologic doses of corticosteroids or mannitol have been recommended if signs of cerebral edema develop despite appropriate fluids and electrolytes, although data proving benefits are scarce.

CONTINUING TREATMENT

Patients with KTA have a marked deficit of body potassium, even though plasma potassium concentrations generally are normal or elevated when first measured. Levels can drop rapidly within the first 4 hours of insulin treatment. Kreisberg attributes this to four factors: dilution from rehydration; continued urinary loss (20% to 50% of potassium administered is excreted in urine); correction of acidosis and re-entry of potassium into the intracellular compartment; and insulin-mediated cellular uptake of glucose and potassium.[12]

Begin infusing neutral potassium phosphate once the serum plasma level of potassium has reached the upper normal range (4.5 to 5.5 mEq/liter). However, if the initial concentration is normal or reduced, then immediately start giving 10 to 40 mEq/hour. When large amounts of bicarbonate are administered as therapy for severe acidosis, more potassium phosphate will be needed.[20]

Plasma phosphate concentration declines from the initial normal or high levels during the first 4 to 5 hours of KTA treatment, probably from insulin's effect on phosphorus uptake and its use in intracellular phosphorylation reactions. Phosphate levels may go below 2 mg/dL in about 40% of KTA patients. Patients with levels below 1 mg/dL could exhibit serious metabolic disturbances. Until theoretical arguments about phosphate repletion and its effects on red cell glycolytic intermediates (2,3-DPG) and oxygen transport are resolved, administer phosphate with the potassium.

Giving alkali for diabetic KTA is controversial. Prompt correction of the acidosis could reduce morbidity and mortality and avoid potentially harmful effects on myocardial function. However, there are two problems with bicarbonate therapy. When HCO_3^- is administered, plasma CO_2 increases and enters the CSF more readily than HCO_3^- does, because of differential permeability of CO_2 and HCO_3^- across the blood-brain barrier. In theory, this therapy could produce a transient but paradoxical intracerebral acidosis. However, measurements of pH in the

CSF of patients treated with bicarbonate do not differ from those in the untreated.[12] Another potential problem is that bicarbonate therapy could further change oxygen dissociation toward increased affinity and reduce oxygen unloading to tissues. Most investigators reserve bicarbonate therapy for patients with very severe acidosis (blood pH less than 7.10). A suggested regimen is to add 89.2 mEq $NaHCO_3$ to each liter of 0.5 N or normal saline. Bicarbonate infusion should be stopped when pH reaches 7.20.

FETAL RESPONSE TO KTA

The possible mechanisms of the often disastrous fetal response to ketoacidosis have not been studied in detail. Since ketone acids cross the placenta readily in either direction and without limit, it is assumed that the fetus also develops profound acidosis. Presumably, fetal cardiac arrest could also result from a state of potassium depletion, although in normal pregnancy the transplacental potassium gradient is from fetus to mother. White found fetal susceptibility to ketoacidosis greatest in the second trimester.[18] There is an anecdotal report of "fetal resuscitation" with maternal bicarbonate therapy.[22] However, whether administered bicarbonate crosses the placenta in the form of HCO_3^- or as CO_2 is still controversial.[23]

SIDE EFFECTS OF CORTICOSTEROIDS AND BETAMIMETICS

If diabetics are given synthetic corticosteroids to induce surfactant production in the fetal lung, or β-adrenergic agents to suppress uterine contractions, the side effects of the drugs may place them at risk for ketoacidosis. In nondiabetic pregnant women, IV β-adrenergics promptly raise plasma FFA, ketone acids, and insulin, and somewhat increase blood glucose and lactate. The metabolic changes are secondary to the adrenergic effects of catecholamines, which stimulate hepatic glycogenolysis, adipose lipolysis, and insulin secretion. Corticosteroids produce insulin resistance. Severe hyperglycemia, KTA, and fetal death have been reported in chemical- and insulin-dependent diabetic women treated with either or both classes of drugs. In most of the cases, a high IV insulin infusion rate (often >10 units/hour) was needed to reverse metabolic decompensation. Anticipate this need when diabetic women are treated for premature labor. The closed-loop, glucose-controlled insulin infusion system (Biostator) is quite useful in these patients.

MEASURES TO PREVENT KTA

Patients must be taught to detect the early onset of psychogenic stresses or such infections as influenza, gastroenteritis, and pyelonephritis. Polyuria and polydipsia are warning signs, as is the appearance of heavy glycosuria and ketonuria. Self-monitoring of blood glucose should prevent loss of control to the stage of ketoacidosis. When warning signs are suspected, patients must contact their physicians immediately. Pedersen stressed that the glycosuria of pregnancy can lead to a carbohydrate deficiency that would exacerbate ketoacidosis. This could be prevented by proper intake of carbohydrates.[19]

Schade and Eaton reviewed several preventive measures for diabetics at risk of ketoacidosis.[3] In patients with incipient KTA, switching to regular insulin every 4 hours may prevent insulin deficiency. They advise giving a maximum dosage of 20 units of regular insulin subcutaneously for a 4+ double-voided urine test. An excess of stress hormone can be minimized by giving appropriate antibiotics for infections and aspirin and fluids for chills, fever, and dehydration. As Pedersen has emphasized, the fasting state should be avoided when incipient KTA is suspected. Antiemetics may prevent vomiting. Patients should be encouraged to take clear liquids with easily absorbed sucrose added. Suppressing diaphoretic losses of fever and administering insulin prudently are other measures that reduce or prevent dehydration. Again, patients at risk should be treated with intermittent or continuous doses of regular, rather than intermediate, insulin. Schade and Eaton recommend hospitalizing diabetics who lose more than 5% of their usual body weight (indicating severe dehydration), have a respiration rate above 36/minute, or are disoriented.[3] Pregnant patients with persistent severe hyperglycemia should also be admitted.

REFERENCES

1. Report of the National Commission on Diabetes to the Congress of the United States. US Dept of Health, Education, and Welfare publication NIH 76-1022, vol 3, pt 2, 1975, pp 88-97

2. Kitzmiller JL: The endocrine pancreas and maternal metabolism. In Tulchinsky D, Ryan KJ (eds): Maternal-Fetal Endocrinology. Philadelphia, WB Saunders, 1980, pp 58-83

3. Schade DS, Eaton RP: Prevention of diabetic ketoacidosis. JAMA 242:2455, 1979

4. Schade DS, Eaton RP: The pathogenesis of diabetic ketoacidosis—A reappraisal. Diabetes Care 2:296, 1979

5. Felig P, Wahren J, Sherwin R, et al: Insulin, glucagon, and somatostatin in normal physiology and diabetes mellitus. Diabetes 25:1091, 1976

6. Schade DS, Eaton RP: Human model for stress-induced ketoacidosis. Clin Res 27:50, 1979

7. Hockaday TDR, Alberti KGMM: Diabetic coma. Br J Hosp Med 7:183, 1972

8. Owen OE, Reichard GA Jr: Ketone body metabolism in normal, obese and diabetic subjects. Isr J Med Sci 11:560, 1975

9. Page MM, Alberti KGMM, Greenwood R, et al: Treatment of diabetic coma with continuous low-dose infusion of insulin. Br Med J 2:687, 1974

10. Kitzmiller JL, Tanenberg RJ, Aoki TJ, et al: Pancreatic alpha cell response to alanine during and after normal and diabetic pregnancies. Obstet Gynecol 56:45, 1980

11. Kitabchi AE, Young R, Sacks H, et al: Diabetic ketoacidosis: Reappraisal of therapeutic approach. Annu Rev Med 30:339, 1979

12. Kreisberg RA: Diabetic ketoacidosis: New concepts and trends in pathogenesis and treatment. Ann Intern Med 88:681, 1978

13. Narins RG, Emmett M: Simple and mixed acid-base disorders: A practical approach. Medicine 59:161, 1980

14. Rose DR: *Clinical Physiology of Acid-Base and Electrolyte Disorders.* New York, McGraw-Hill, 1977, pp 435-447

15. Newman RL: Serum electrolytes in pregnancy, parturition, and puerperium. Obstet Gynecol 10:51, 1957

16. Kirschbaum T, in Assali N (ed): *Biology of Gestation.* New York, Academic Press, vol 2, 1966, pp 143-178

17. Halperin ML, Bear RA, Hannaford MC: Selected aspects of the pathophysiology of metabolic acidosis in diabetes mellitus. Diabetes 30:781, 1981

18. White P: Pregnancy and diabetes. In Marble A, White P, Bradley RF, et al (eds): *Joslin's Diabetes Mellitus.* Philadelphia, Lea & Febiger, 1971, pp 581-598

19. Pedersen J: *The Pregnant Diabetic and Her Newborn.* Baltimore, Williams & Wilkins, 1977, pp 88-97

20. Felig P: Diabetic ketoacidosis. N Engl J Med 290:1360, 1974

21. Peterson L, Caldwell J, Hoffman J: Insulin adsorbance to polyvinylchloride surfaces with implications for constant-infusion therapy. Diabetes 25:72, 1976

22. LoBue C, Goodlin RC: Treatment of fetal distress during diabetic ketoacidosis. J Reprod Med 20:101, 1978

23. Chang A, Wood C: Fetal acid-base balance. I. Interdependence of maternal and fetal pCO_2 and bicarbonate concentration. Am J Obstet Gynecol 125:61, 1976

7

Preterm Cervical Dilation

JAMES H. HARGER, MD, and
STEVE N. CARITIS, MD

CLINICAL SIGNIFICANCE: In 5% to 10% of pregnancies, the cervix dilates before term—because of either progressive uterine contractions or structural problems (incompetence) that allow dilation without contractions. Distinguishing between causes is essential to preventing preterm delivery—still the major cause of perinatal morbidity and mortality in the US.

Prematurity has long been the leading cause of perinatal morbidity and mortality. Despite extensive study, it remains a problem that often defies prediction and treatment. The difficulty in handling it lies in the very nature of the problem. When a woman shows signs of cervical dilation or effacement between 20 and 37 weeks' gestation, the clinician must make rapid decisions about diagnosis and management. If you act too slowly, labor may progress too far to be stopped by any method. Hasty intervention, however, may expose mother and fetus to greater hazard, and may even accelerate delivery.

DIAGNOSIS

When making the differential diagnosis of preterm cervical dilation, effacement, or both between 20 and 37 weeks' gestation, consider the following: normal cervical changes associated with advancing pregnancy, error in estimating gestational age, true preterm labor, or cervical incompetence (Table 7-1). Some multiparas may have appreciable cervical dilation after 20 weeks' gestation. A smaller number of nulliparas also show dilation before term. In Floyd's study of patients who delivered after 36 weeks' gestation, the cervix in 15% of primigravidas and 36% of multigravidas was dilated at least 1 cm at 6 months.[1] Further, 32% of the multigravidas showed dilation of 2 cm. Floyd concluded that a dilated cervix doesn't necessarily indicate impending delivery.

BUSINESS REPLY MAIL

FIRST CLASS   PERMIT NO. 7330   DES MOINES, IA

POSTAGE WILL BE PAID BY ADDRESSEE

Bon Appétit
P.O. Box 10707
Des Moines, Iowa 50347-0707

FOR
TRANK

F16 1-1
1-2   PP5
21-1   17B

~~$30.00~~
only $14.95

Bon Appétit

12 issues (1 year)

Save $15.05 (over ½ off the newsstand price)

Name _____

(please print)

Address _____ Apt._____

City _____ State _____ Zip _____

□ 12 issues for $14.95
□ Payment enclosed
□ Bill me later

The regular one year subscriber rate is $15.00.

Please allow 6-8 weeks for mailing of first issue. For all foreign orders, including Canadian, add $10.00. No credit orders outside the U.S. Payment must accompany order in U.S. currency.

OFFER EXPIRES MARCH 31, 1987. NEW SUBSCRIBERS ONLY, PLEASE.

Save $15.05

JPWB4

This conclusion is supported by Parikh and Mehta, who performed digital exams of the cervix in 655 pregnant women at 21 to 36 weeks' gestation.[2] They classified the cervix as "open" if it was dilated at least one fingertip—about 1.5 to 2.0 cm. The investigators observed that 16% of primigravidas and 17% of multigravidas had an "open cervix" at 21 to 28 weeks' gestation. An "open cervix" in the second trimester is often interpreted as indicating early labor if Braxton-Hicks contractions are noticed, and otherwise as cervical incompetence. Without therapeutic intervention, the women with an open cervix had a premature delivery rate of 13.9%, not significantly different from the 11.1% rate of those with a closed cervix.

Schaffner and Schanzer[3] at William Beaumont General Hospital, El Paso, Texas, performed digital cervical exams on 299 women at 28 to 32 weeks' gestation and found that 27.4% had dilation of at least 2 to 3 cm. This degree of dilation was twice as common in multigravidas as in primigravidas, but birth weights and gestational ages at delivery were similar whether or not the mother had had early cervical dilation. Women who had dilation of at least 2 to 3 cm at 28 to 32 weeks delivered infants under 2,500 gm at a rate of 6.1%, compared with 6.9% when dilation was 1 cm or less at 28 to 32 weeks. The risk of premature rupture of membranes was unaffected by parity or cervical dilation.

When a woman is admitted with suspected preterm cervical dilation, the first priority is to identify premature labor. To do this, the clinician should answer the following questions: Are the contractions characteristic of labor or are they Braxton-Hicks? Is the cervical dilation constant in that patient, or does it represent a progressive change due to preterm labor or cervical incompetence? If a labor-inhibiting drug such as rito-

---

TABLE 7-1

Factors to consider in diagnosing preterm dilation

Normal or physiologic cervical dilation

Error in gestational age
Term infant
Small-for-gestational-age infant

Premature labor
Idiopathic
With chorioamnionitis
With concealed abruption

Cervical incompetence

---

drine or terbutaline is given to a patient with cervical incompetence, the therapy will benefit neither the patient nor her fetus, and will expose her unnecessarily to complications from these potent drugs (Table 7-2).[4, 5] If a cerclage is performed when cervical dilation is due to premature labor, the labor may be accelerated and a cervical laceration or uterine rupture sustained. And if the cervical changes are physiologic, neither therapy will help, but both will subject the woman to the risks of labor-inhibiting drugs or to the 2% risk of pregnancy loss that follows cervical cerclage.[6]

When making a diagnosis of preterm cervical dilation, the physician is often caught in a dilemma: Hasty diagnosis may result in treatment of women who don't need it, but indecision may delay therapy too long for it to succeed. Several controlled studies of labor-inhibiting drugs bear out this point. The diagnosis of preterm labor was incorrect in about 40% to 60% of patients; about 40% of the untreated controls did not deliver in the period specified in the experimental protocol.[5] What criteria can the physician use, then, to decide quickly when therapy should be instituted?

The information needed for this decision should be drawn from three types of evaluation: careful history taking, physical examination upon admission, and brief longitudinal monitoring after admission.

History taking. A careful history of the present pregnancy is essential to determine gestational age and cause of the cervical dilation. Obviously, if the fetus is older than first suspected, no delay in delivery may be necessary. To obtain a complete history, you will need to answer the following questions: When did the last menstrual period begin? Was it a normal period, at the expected time, and was it typical in amount of menstrual flow and dysmenorrhea? Were oral contraceptives used just

---

TABLE 7-2

Effects and complications of β-adrenergic agonists

Fetal	Maternal
Hyperglycemia	Chest pain
Tachycardia	Hyperglycemia
	Hypokalemia
	Hypotension
	Pulmonary edema
	Tachycardia
	Increased myocardial O_2 consumption

---

before or even after this last period? How long is the patient's normal cycle? If it's more than 30 to 33 days, gestational age should be adjusted to account for delayed ovulation. What was the date of the first positive urine pregnancy test? When was quickening first noticed? Quickening is subjective, but should be recorded on every obstetric patient's chart to help assessment during emergencies.

Of course, if routine ultrasound scanning has been done, the results will be very helpful in determining gestational age. Symptoms reported by the patient may help to direct the diagnosis. Some studies show that about a third of women with cervical incompetence report increases in pelvic pressure and urinary frequency, as well as a watery vaginal discharge for 1 to 3 days prior to diagnosis.[7] Because these symptoms often involve only slight variations from normal, clinicians should be aware that frequent questioning may make the patient anxious and yield misleading answers.

Prior obstetric and gynecologic history may also provide some important clues to the diagnosis. It's important to know if there is a family history of premature deliveries. Further, since infants with some types of congenital anomalies may be more likely to be born prematurely, a family history of congenital anomalies not only is pertinent but also provides direction for sonographic evaluation of the fetus.

If the patient's mother had vaginal bleeding when pregnant with her, or if she had one or more pregnancy losses prior to that pregnancy, there is a greater chance that your patient is a DES daughter. If that is the case, many studies indicate there is an increased risk of spontaneous abortion and preterm labor, in addition to a greater chance of morphologic uterine abnormalities.[8, 9]

Some studies imply—but do not prove—that a prior history of D&C, suction curettage for therapeutic abortion, or a cone biopsy of the cervix means a greater chance of cervical incompetence. A history of deep cervical lacerations at delivery, Dührssen's incisions, or progressively earlier and earlier second-trimester deliveries without labor also are consistent with, but do not necessarily prove, cervical incompetence.

On the other hand, a history of preterm labor or a history of second-trimester deliveries with uterine contractions and vaginal bleeding would be more suggestive of preterm labor as the cause of the current cervical dilation. Hypertension, chronic glomerulonephritis or pyelonephritis, other chronic medical disorders, and heavy smoking also increase the risk of preterm labor.

Physical examination. Inspect the patient thoroughly but quickly at the time of admission. How large is the uterus? Has it enlarged normally since the original bimanual exam? Determining cervical dilation is easy, but recognizing effacement is quite subjective. Some examiners use the term to indicate softness of the cervix while others use it only to signify cervical shortening and thinning.

When examining a patient with preterm cervical dilation, carefully determine the status of the membranes, using an alkaline reaction to Nitrazine paper or other pH indicator, ferning in dried fluid, and Nile blue staining of fetal fat cells. If you don't see fluid in the posterior vaginal fornix or flowing from the external os during the speculum exam, apply fundal pressure to extrude amniotic fluid from the cervix. Measure fundal height and estimate fetal weight to confirm gestational age. Palpate to determine whether there are uterine contractions and tenderness, indicating chorioamnionitis or abruptio placentae. Listen for fetal heart sounds, and note the presence and degree of vaginal bleeding.

Longitudinal monitoring. Finally, do a brief longitudinal evaluation of the fetal condition and uterine status while awaiting laboratory data. Objective information about gestational age can be obtained by ultrasound measurements of fetal biparietal diameter and long-bone lengths.[10] Such measurements are most accurate when made at 20 to 28 weeks' gestation, but ultrasound information before 20 weeks may also be useful.

An electronic fetal monitor will inform you of the health of the fetus. The tocodynamometer will furnish information about the frequency and duration of uterine contractions, though bedside clinical assessment by hand often provides important information about uterine tenderness and intensity of contractions. Progressive cervical dilation means you must take action, though the nature of that action depends on etiology and contraindications to various treatments.

Initial laboratory work should include a urinalysis and a complete blood count with differential. If urinary tract infection is present, hydration and appropriate antibiotic therapy may forestall preterm labor. If you find fever and leukocytosis and no evidence of infection elsewhere, give strong consideration to chorioamnionitis, even if the membranes are intact. This diagnosis may be hard to make, since uterine tenderness is not always present or may be difficult to ascertain in the presence of contractions.

Transabdominal amniocentesis guided by real-time ultrasound may provide additional useful information, some of which may be pertinent to fetal lung maturity. Fetal and maternal tachycardia and the presence of many leukocytes or bacteria in amniotic fluid increase the suspicion of chorioamnionitis. It is very important to make this diagnosis because it is a contraindication to labor-inhibiting drugs and also to cervical cerclage (Table 7-3).

In cases of vaginal bleeding or uterine tenderness with or without vaginal bleeding, consider the possibility of a concealed abruptio placentae. To help rule this out, periodically obtain platelet counts and serum fibrinogen levels. These will help detect evidence of disseminated intravascular coagulation (DIC).

If physical examination shows signs of peritonitis, acute appendicitis, acute pancreatitis, intraperitoneal abscess, or acute cholecystitis, order the appropriate confirmatory tests and ultrasound scans.

MANAGEMENT

Therapy for preterm cervical dilation depends on the cause of the condition. In a sense, however, treatment begins when you place the woman at bed rest for observation and electronic fetal monitoring. Bed rest often decreases the frequency of both Braxton-Hicks contractions and true labor.

If the preterm cervical dilation is ascribed to premature labor, rule out chorioamnionitis and abruptio placentae before beginning therapy with labor-inhibiting drugs. To inhibit labor, we now prefer IV ritodrine at an initial dose of 100 μg/minute. Advance the dosage by 50 μg/minute every 20 minutes up to the maximum required to decrease the frequency of contractions, but never use more than 350 μg/minute.

β-Adrenergic agonists such as ritodrine or terbutaline may cause fetal and maternal tachycardia and hyperglycemia, maternal hypokalemia, hypotension, increased myocardial oxygen consumption, chest pain, and even pulmonary edema (Table 7-2).[4, 5] β-Agonist infusions require close monitoring of maternal vital signs and serum glucose and potassium concentrations.

Since pulmonary edema has been associated most often with increased maternal intravascular volume, limit IV infusion of crystalloids and use β-agonists with great care and attention in twin pregnancies. If the patient reports dyspnea or chest pain, discontinue the infusion until you can evaluate these complaints. Whether or not you encounter side

TABLE 7-3

When therapy is contraindicated

CONDITION	β-ADRENERGIC AGONISTS	CERVICAL CERCLAGE
Abruptio placentae	X	X
Cervical insufficiency	X	
Chorioamnionitis	X	X
Fetal distress	X	X
Maternal heart disease	X	
Preterm labor		X
Ruptured membranes		X

effects and complications, reduce the infusion rate of the β-adrenergic agent as soon as possible to the lowest rate that inhibits labor (contractions more than 10 minutes apart).

If the β-adrenergic agent produces unacceptable side effects, or if the patient has contraindications to these agents (Table 7-3), consider the use of IV magnesium sulfate. Steer and Petrie's study showed the efficacy of this drug, which has few side effects.[11]

Depending on the patient's weight, we administer a loading dose of magnesium sulfate 4 to 6 gm IV over 2 to 5 minutes. Patients may feel uncomfortably warm and flushed during administration of the initial dose and may vomit, especially if you give the initial bolus too rapidly. These effects are almost always transitory, however, and do not persist with the maintenance infusion of 2 to 3 gm/hour. Since magnesium ion is excreted in the urine, measure urine output and check deep tendon reflexes frequently. In view of the lesser efficacy and greater risks of IV ethanol for labor inhibition, we see no indications for its use today.

If IV drugs succeed in inhibiting labor when the patient has advanced cervical dilation, advise her to maintain reduced activity until 36 to 38 weeks' gestation. The value of chronic administration of oral tocolytic agents is unproven, but recent studies show treated women have a reduced risk of recurrent preterm labor, compared with those receiving placebo.

If cervical incompetence is the cause of advanced dilation, you may arrest further dilation with bed rest. Once you diagnose cervical incompetence, take the patient to the operating room as soon as possible for a cerclage. No published series has shown the McDonald or Shirodkar technique to be superior; we use the McDonald purse-string suture with swaged-on No. 5 silk sutures because this approach requires the least operating time and causes the least cervical trauma.[6]

To facilitate cerclage, place the patient in lithotomy position with the operating table in 30° Trendelenburg position and secure her with shoulder braces. In this position, aspiration of gastric contents is a significant risk, so rapidly induce general endotracheal anesthesia, which has the added benefit of relaxing the myometrium. This effect allows the membranes to recede or be pushed back into the lower uterine segment if the amniotic sac is protruding. Sher recommends using the bulb of a Foley catheter with the tip cut off as the safest way to replace prolapsed membranes without rupturing them.[12]

Place the McDonald suture as high on the cervix as possible. Insert your index finger into the cervix to guide the depth of the needle and to protect the amniotic sac from being pierced by the needle. Finally, tie the suture snugly, but not so tightly that the cervix is completely closed. There is no reason to believe that a second parallel purse-string suture adds anything but operating time or surgical trauma.

Postoperatively, keep the patient at bed rest for 24 to 72 hours. We do not advise therapy with progestins or labor-inhibiting drugs since there is no evidence that these agents significantly reduce the risk of labor or of ruptured membranes.[6, 13] The use of oral or parenteral antibiotics at this time to prevent infection has also never proved helpful.

Recent studies by the authors and by Olatunbosun and Dyck have yielded fetal survival rates of 59% and 83%, respectively, when selected patients had cerclage procedures under emergency conditions.[6, 14] In 3 of 10 patients in our series, the bulging or prolapsed membranes ruptured during surgery. This did not occur in Olatunbosun and Dyck's series of 12 women.

Long-term therapy for patients with preterm cervical dilation who do not deliver is not well established. We recommend encouraging women who have had emergency cervical cerclage to maintain reduced activity until the suture is removed electively at 36 to 38 weeks' gestation.

If the patient develops manifestations of labor, vaginal bleeding, chorioamnionitis, or ruptured membranes, remove the cerclage suture immediately. If the emergency cerclage fails to delay delivery long enough to prevent a poor outcome, study the patient postpartum. Use hysterosalpingography, peripheral leukocyte karyotyping, and other tests to determine what caused the loss. Study the fetus as well, using photographs, x-rays, and postmortem examination to detect any significant abnormalities and to permit effective counseling about future pregnancies. Neonates who die after failure to inhibit labor should be similarly studied.

In cases of abruptio placentae and chorioamnionitis, do not prevent cervical dilation, but rather hasten delivery. If fetal distress is apparent after viability is attained, usually at 26 to 28 weeks' gestation, deliver the patient as soon as possible.

SUMMARY

The most effective therapy in a particular case of preterm cervical dilation is at best difficult to determine. It is rendered even more so by the urgency with which optimum therapy is required. Pay attention to the details of diagnosis and therapy and you may be able to improve outcome considerably.

REFERENCES

1. Floyd WE: Cervical dilation in the mid-trimester of pregnancy. Obstet Gynecol 18:380, 1961
2. Parikh MN, Mehta AC: Internal cervical os during the second half of pregnancy. J Obstet Gynaecol Br Commonw 68:818, 1961
3. Schaffner F, Schanzer SN: Cervical dilation in the early third trimester. Obstet Gynecol 27:130, 1966

4. Katz M, Robertson PA, Creasy RK: Cardiovascular complications associated with terbutaline treatment for preterm labor. Am J Obstet Gynecol 139:605, 1981

5. Caritis SN, Edelstone DI, Mueller-Heubach E: Pharmacologic inhibition of preterm labor. Am J Obstet Gynecol 133:557, 1979

6. Harger JH: Comparison of success and morbidity in cervical cerclage procedures. Obstet Gynecol 56:543, 1980

7. Toaff R, Toaff ME: Diagnosis of impending late abortion. Obstet Gynecol 43:756, 1974

8. Barnes AB, Colton T, Gundersen J, et al: Fertility and outcome of pregnancy in women exposed in utero to diethylstilbestrol. N Engl J Med 302:609, 1980

9. Kaufmann RH, Binder GL, Gray PM, et al: Upper genital tract changes associated with exposure in utero to diethylstilbestrol. Am J Obstet Gynecol 128:51, 1977

10. O'Brien GD, Queenan JT: Growth of the ultrasound fetal femur length during normal pregnancy. Am J Obstet Gynecol 141:833, 1981

11. Steer CM, Petrie RH: A comparison of magnesium sulfate and alcohol for the prevention of premature labor. Am J Obstet Gynecol 129:1, 1977

12. Sher G: Congenital incompetence of the cervical os. Reduction of bulging membranes with a modified Foley catheter. J Reprod Med 22:165, 1979

13. Block MF, Rahhal DK: Cervical incompetence: A diagnostic and prognostic scoring system. Obstet Gynecol 47:279, 1976

14. Olatunbosun OA, Dyck F: Cervical cerclage operation for a dilated cervix. Obstet Gynecol 57:166, 1981

Severe Preeclampsia

ROBERT C. GOODLIN, MD

CLINICAL SIGNIFICANCE: Severe preeclampsia with multiple organ
  dysfunction is rare in blacks; native Americans have an
  increased incidence. Multiple organ involvement may occur without hypertension. When severe preeclampsia is
  associated with multiple organ dysfunction, suspect maternal liver hematoma or fetal involvement.

A patient was transferred to the University of Nebraska Medical Center
after spontaneous abortion at 22 weeks' gestation. Her earlier pregnancy
had been normal, as was her present one until the onset of seizures 2
days before admission. In the referring hospital, after delivering a 428-
gm stillborn fetus, she developed severe hypertension with thrombocytopenia, oliguria, and jaundice. She was semicomatose on admission to
our institution. Because her respiratory problems were associated with
fluid overload, she was managed in the medical ICU.

Consultants all felt confident of their diagnoses. The obstetric team's
was eclampsia (type B EPH gestosis—edema, proteinuria, and hypertension). The hematologists' was thrombotic thrombocytopenic purpura (TTP); the gastroenterologists', fulminating hepatitis; and the ne-
phrologists', hemolytic uremic syndrome (HUS). After dialysis and
plasma volume expansion, the patient recovered and appeared well 2
months after discharge.

This case illustrates how the severely preeclamptic patient can have
symptoms that mimic those of many different diseases. Conversely,
symptoms of many other serious diseases can mimic those of severe
preeclampsia.

A 1972 review of the records of all women referred to Stanford University Hospital for hemodialysis for renal failure revealed a surprising
fact: Most had been diagnosed as preeclamptic during their pregnancies, even when it was known they had renal disease. Few had had anything but the most superficial medical work-up for their preeclampsia.[1]

This suggests that obstetricians not only should be aware of the wide diversity of symptoms that severe preeclampsia produces but also should know that other diseases can cause the same symptoms. It isn't always in the patient's best interests to presume that delivery will resolve her medical problems.

Women with severe preeclampsia may have several different symptom complexes. The term EPH gestosis is widely used in Europe; it implies that abnormalities other than simple hypertension are present. We have suggested using *type A EPH gestosis* for the more widely recognized form of severe preeclampsia, and *type B* for the form with multiple organ defects.[2] Figure 8-1 shows the differences in frequency of symptoms in types A and B. The high incidence of thrombocytopenia and liver disease with type B is expected, since one or the other is required for its diagnosis; the high perinatal mortality reflects both the

FIGURE 8-1

Findings in EPH gestosis (severe preeclampsia)

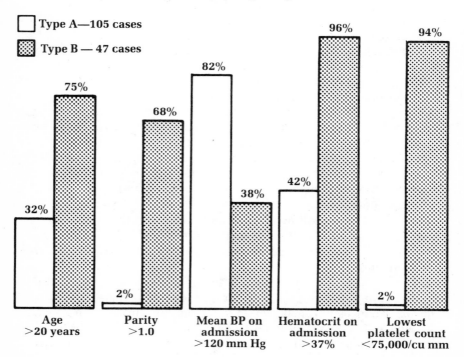

Type A—105 cases

Type B — 47 cases

| | Age >20 years | Parity >1.0 | Mean BP on admission >120 mm Hg | Hematocrit on admission >37% | Lowest platelet count <75,000/cu mm |

incidence of delivery before 32 weeks and the fetal involvement in the maternal disease process.[2]

Obstetricians are well aware of the differential diagnosis when hypertension predominates; but when the primary symptoms include liver dysfunction or thrombocytopenia, or when seizures are the major symptom, the picture becomes confused. Tables of differential diagnosis with suggested discriminating tests are provided for each of the major entities discussed here.

HYPERTENSION

The differential diagnosis for a young woman with acute severe hypertension in the third trimester includes essential hypertension and renal disease, but it's also wise to rule out systemic lupus erythematosus (SLE) and, as almost every medical student knows, pheochromocytoma

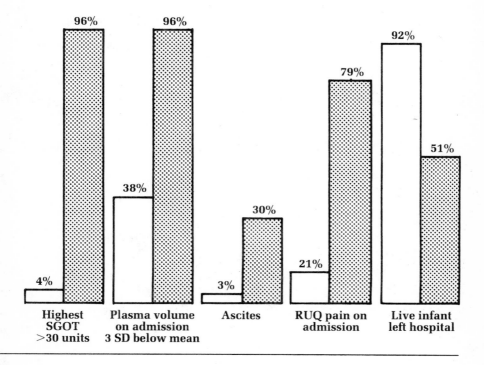

(Table 8-1). Routinely testing all pregnant women with hypertension for serum antinuclear antibodies (ANA) may prove valuable in diagnosing unsuspected SLE.

PROTEINURIA

For pregnant women spilling albumin into their urine in quantities greater than 1 gm/24 hours but less than 5 gm/24 hours, the differential diagnosis is somewhat limited (Table 8-2). Chesley has suggested that women with preeclampsia usually have significant proteinuria and that

---

TABLE 8-1

Differential diagnosis for hypertension (normal platelets and liver enzymes)

CONDITION	TEST
Severe preeclampsia (type A EPH gestosis)	Resolves with pregnancy Increased uric acid (serum)
Coarctation of aorta	X-ray of chest Increased arm-leg systolic pressure differences
Essential hypertension	Large-cuff sphygmomanometer
Obesity	History
Pheochromocytoma	Regitine response Increased urinary catecholamines
Polycystic disease	Positive ultrasound of kidney
Renal disease Acute glomerulonephritis	RBC in urine Decreased creatinine clearance
Chronic glomerulonephritis	Ultrasound; decreased renal size Decreased creatinine clearance
Nephrotic syndrome	Elevated triglycerides Low serum albumin
Chronic undifferentiated renal disease	Decreased renal function
Diabetic nephropathy	Diabetic history
Systemic lupus erythematosus	Positive serum ANA and positive Coombs

when they do not, the diagnosis is doubtful.[3] When proteinuria is severe enough to be confused with the nephrotic syndrome (greater than 5 gm/24 hours), the differential diagnosis becomes even more difficult. The nephrotic complication of preeclampsia is common, but there are also women with nephrotic syndrome apparent only in pregnancy.[4]

Regardless of the underlying disease, the obstetrician should focus on the amount of protein lost in the urine, which correlates with fetal death. Lost protein should be replaced. In many cases, nephrotic syndrome in pregnancy is never clearly diagnosed because these women apparently recover postpartum. The underlying pathology can be determined only by renal biopsy. Most often the nephrotic syndrome is due to preeclampsia.

THROMBOCYTOPENIA

For pregnant women with acute thrombocytopenia, the list for differential diagnosis is long (Table 8-3). Platelets are nearly always decreased in preeclampsia; documenting such decreases usually requires getting platelet counts in each trimester—counts in normal pregnant women may vary from 75,000 to 350,000/cu mm.[2] In severe preeclampsia (type B EPH gestosis) and thrombocytopenia, the more severe the disease process, the greater the degree of thrombocytopenia.

The literature suggests that type B EPH gestosis occurs mostly in white Americans, having been described only rarely among blacks.[5] In type B EPH gestosis, it is sometimes impossible to distinguish clearly among TTP, HUS, idiopathic thrombocytopenic purpura (ITP), and fulminating hepatitis of pregnancy. The presence of antibodies to platelets points to a diagnosis of ITP, but with all these conditions the pregnant woman may have severe hypertension, seizures, fetal growth retardation, or renal involvement; delivery more or less resolves the acute medical problem. HUS is usually manifested only after delivery. It may be that HUS, TTP, and type B EPH gestosis represent the same disease process and that differential diagnosis depends upon whether the patient is pregnant and whether her primary physician is an obstetrician, a hematologist, a nephrologist, or a gastroenterologist.

Obstetricians often diagnose disseminated intravascular coagulation (DIC) when thrombocytopenia and hypertension coexist, despite normal serum fibrinogen levels. Abnormalities of the microcirculation, such as severe vasoconstriction or platelet adhesions, may produce schistocytes and cause microangiopathic hemolytic anemia (MAHA). Brain first described MAHA and demonstrated the origin of the schistocytes. He used an artificial circulation system in which blood was pumped through fibers small enough in diameter so that red cells were looped over the fibers like clothes hung on a clothesline. When the red cells were severed, schistocytes were produced.[6]

Despite distinguished basic research demonstrating the presence of DIC in animals under conditions resembling preeclampsia, most pregnant women with thrombocytopenia do not have DIC and should not be treated with heparin. Obstetric patients with MAHA are markedly hypovolemic, and their thrombocytopenia responds to plasma volume expansion.[2] Improvement after plasma infusion suggests prostacyclin (PGI_2) defects in women with EPH gestosis.

TABLE 8-2

Differential diagnosis of proteinuria

CONDITION	TEST
Minor quantity	
Exercise	History
Postural	History
Febrile	History
Vaginal contamination	History
Major quantity	
Primary renal disease	
When protein is 0.1 to 2.0 gm/24 hours:	
Chronic interstitial nephritis	Renal biopsy, urinalysis
Nephrocalcinosis	Differential urinary protein clearance
When protein > 2.0 gm/24 hours:	
Acute or chronic glomerulonephritis	Serum complement, antistreptolysin O titer (ASOT) urinalysis, renal biopsy
Intercapillary glomerulosclerosis	Serum complement, ASOT urinalysis, renal biopsy
Membranous glomerulonephritis	Serum complement, ASOT urinalysis, renal biopsy
Lipid nephrosis	Serum complement, ASOT urinalysis, renal biopsy
Acute tubular necrosis	History
Renal vein thrombosis	Scintigrams
Nephrotoxic and allergic disorders	
Reaction to heavy metals (Hg, Ag)	History
Poison ivy	Differential urine protein analysis
Reaction to trimethadione	History

While the list of disorders thought to cause DIC in pregnancy is long, evidence for intravascular coagulation in the pathogenesis of these disease states varies, as Ratnoff notes, according to the "degree of conviction" of the investigators.[7] The thrombocytopenia that develops in association with preeclampsia probably represents either aggregation of platelets at the placental site or their destruction within the constricted microcirculation.

CONDITION	TEST
Reaction to paramethadione	History
Snake bite	History
Reaction to tetracyclines (degraded)	History
Systemic illness	
Diabetes mellitus	History
SLE	ANA
Multiple myeloma	Bence Jones proteins
Syphilis	Serology
Malaria	Peripheral smear
Sickle cell anemia	History—hemoglobin electrophoresis
Hemolytic uremic syndrome	History
EPH gestosis (severe preeclampsia)	Resolves with delivery
Nephrotic syndrome	Blood lipids 75 gm protein/ 24 hours
Sarcoidosis	Chest x-ray with skin test
Hypercalcemic nephropathy	Electrolytes
Hypokalemic nephropathy	Electrolytes
Aminoacidopathies	Specific urinalysis
Fanconi syndrome	History
Urinary tract infections	
Lower tract (cystitis)	Urine culture
Upper tract (pyelonephritis)	Blood and urine cultures
Urinary bleeding	Cystoscopy

Routine tests should include (when appropriate) CBC, BUN, serum protein electrophoresis, serum triglyceride levels, serum albumin, serum complement, serum ANA, 24-hour urine for total protein and creatinine clearance, urine culture.

A relatively frequent cause of thrombocytopenia in pregnant women is trauma, particularly when large hematomas develop in the pelvis or legs. Although the differential diagnosis must include possible abruptio placentae, hematomas can, by themselves, explain much of the apparent coagulation disorder. This is about the only time when a live fetus is associated with laboratory evidence of DIC.

LIVER DISEASE

When the primary manifestation of illness is liver dysfunction, differential diagnosis is especially complex (Table 8-4). Early in this century, acute yellow atrophy was considered a form of preeclampsia; as so of-

---

TABLE 8-3

Differential diagnosis for thrombocytopenia

CONDITION	TEST
Disorders of production	
Decrease due to marrow hypoplasia, idiopathic drug, chemical, ionizing radiation	
Marrow replacement	Bone marrow, history
Leukemia	Peripheral smear
Metastatic tumor	History, physical findings
Myeloma	Bence Jones protein
Lymphoma	History, physical findings
Ineffective production	
Vitamin B_{12}, folate deficiency ·	Serum levels
Alcohol	History
Uremia	BUN
Disorders of destruction	
Isoimmune thrombocytopenia	
Primary ITP	Antibody
Secondary ITP	Antibody, history of drugs, etc.
Vasculitis	
Polyarteritis nodosa	Angiographic studies
SLE	ANA
Dermatomyositis	Biopsy
Rheumatic fever	Rheumatoid factor

ten happens, the early investigators may have been correct. It is not unusual for a caucasian woman with type B EPH gestosis to have the markedly elevated serum transaminase levels typical of liver damage. Indeed, we recently described impending gestosis in five pregnant women who had thrombocytopenia, liver dysfunction, and right upper quadrant pain, but who had yet to develop such signs of preeclampsia as edema, proteinuria, and hypertension. The implication is that EPH may appear relatively late in the disease process of EPH gestosis.[8]

We believe that type B EPH gestosis has a wide spectrum of clinical findings—from only thrombocytopenia and elevated serum glutamic-oxaloacetic transaminase (SGOT) levels with right upper quadrant pain

CONDITION	TEST
Infectious hepatitis B	Serum HBV
Streptococcal infection	Cultures
Viral infections	Cultures
Drug allergy (antibiotics, phenothiazines, heparin)	History
Malignancy	History
Accelerated consumption	
Septicemia with shock	DIC screen, blood culture
Abruptio placentae	Dead fetus
Dead fetus syndrome	Dead fetus
Microangiopathic hemolytic anemia	Schistocytes in peripheral smear
Hemolytic uremic syndrome	Postpartum renal failure
Thrombotic thrombocytopenic purpura	Gingival biopsy
Post-transfusion thrombocytopenia	Transfusion 7 to 10 days previously
Type B EPH gestosis (severe preeclampsia)	Resolves with delivery
Sequestration	
Splenomegaly	Ultrasound
Hypersplenism	Ultrasound

Tests should (when appropriate) include CBC, urinalysis, ANA, rheumatoid factor, complement levels (C_3, C_4), hepatitis B antigen, serum protein electrophoresis, platelet aggregation, and antibody studies.

(and no other signs of preeclampsia), to severe hypertension, to liver hematomas and ruptures. On the other hand, Weinstein ascribes these type B EPH gestosis cases to a syndrome of hemolysis, elevated liver enzymes, and low platelet count (HELLP syndrome), all as a severe consequence of hypertension in pregnancy.[9] The important message is to search for liver hematomas, which apparently can be done accurately with ultrasound.

It is with type B disease that the differential diagnosis becomes confused, and specialists in internal medicine may sometimes assume control, ignoring the possibility of severe preeclampsia-eclampsia with marked hypovolemia. I have seen such patients explored for cholelithiasis or having intravenous dye studies to rule out gallbladder or renal disease, or both—with disastrous results.[10]

TABLE 8-4

Differential diagnosis of liver dysfunction (elevated serum transaminases, RUQ pain)

CONDITION	TEST
Type B EPH gestosis (severe preeclampsia)	Resolves with delivery
Acute viral hepatitis	Positive serum HAV antigens Positive serum HBV antigens
Choledocholithiasis with obstruction	Increased alkaline phosphatase, stones, fever
Cholestatic jaundice of pregnancy	Increased alkaline phosphatase, elevated serum bile salts
Fatty liver of pregnancy	Increased liver enzymes, renal failure, premature labor
Liver hematoma	Ultrasound
Infectious mononucleosis	Heterophil antibody
TORCH (toxoplasmosis, others, rubella, cytomegalovirus, herpes simplex virus) infections	TORCH titers
Toxic hepatitis (drug reactions caused by halothane, methyldopa, alcohol, etc.)	History

It is also difficult to make a diagnosis when a pregnant woman has an unexpected onset of seizures (Table 8-5). A young woman seen in the emergency room with convulsions may have associated proteinuria and hypertension, regardless of the underlying pathology. Depending on her physician's past experience, she may first be worked up for epilepsy, brain tumor, or eclampsia. Using a CT scanner should make the differential diagnosis much easier.

TABLE 8-5

Differential diagnosis for seizures or coma

CONDITION	TEST
Pre-existent epilepsy	History, EEG
Meningitis/encephalitis	EEG, CSF
Local anesthetics	History
Brain tumor	
Primary	CT scan
Metastatic	CT scan
Cerebrovascular	
Embolic stroke	CT scan, cardiac exam
Thrombotic stroke	CT scan, angiography
Cerebral venous thrombosis	CT scan
Subarachnoid hemorrhage	CSF, CT scan, angiography
Intracerebral hemorrhage	CT scan
Thrombotic thrombocytopenic purpura	Gingival biopsy
Hypertensive encephalopathy	BP, fundus
EPH gestosis	Resolves with delivery
Pituitary apoplexy	CT scan, endocrine studies
Metabolic	
Acidosis	Electrolytes
Hypoglycemia	Blood glucose
Liver disease	Serum NH_3 levels
Uremia	BUN
Water intoxication	Serum Na $<$ 115 mEq/liter
Pseudotumor cerebri (headache, papilledema, vision loss only)	CT scan, history

For example, two pregnant women were admitted to the hospital comatose and with obvious eclampsia, but postmortem examination showed only extensive intraventricular hemorrhage. In retrospect, the clue to the underlying disease process should have been that they were hyponatremic, apparently because of inappropriate antidiuretic hormone (ADH) excretion. Now that CT scanners are more readily available, this error is less likely to occur.

Some of these patients require a cerebrospinal fluid examination (those with suspected cerebral hemorrhage and hematoma or infection), but there is always a possibility of tentorial herniation following the tap. Such lumbar punctures should be done only after consultation with a neurologist and after a CT scan.

GENERAL COMMENTS

Diagnosis is sometimes confounded by a number of isolated symptoms about which women with severe preeclampsia may complain. Two such women were referred from our service to ophthalmologists, to rule out retinal detachment. Their relatively mild degrees of hypertension and proteinuria were ignored by the referring obstetricians, who focused on eye problems. We have also transferred to the medical service women at term who had heart failure. When this was corrected, the diagnosis of severe preeclampsia emerged. Patients have been admitted to the hospital on the GI service with GI hemorrhage, apparently another manifestation of preeclampsia.[11] The presence of ascites is difficult to evaluate since approximately 25% of our normal postpartum patients have significant amounts of peritoneal fluid at the time of postpartum tubal ligations. Nevertheless, patients with type B EPH gestosis, in contrast to others, often have significant ascites at cesarean section.

Some general laboratory signs are helpful when the diagnosis is uncertain. The normal pregnant woman's BUN should always be below 10 mg/dL and her hemoglobin should be relatively low before 36 weeks' gestation. We have found that 76% of women with severe preeclampsia are markedly hypovolemic, as suggested by increased hematocrit, decreased creatinine clearance, decreased amniotic fluid volume, elevated BUN, and evidence of fetal growth retardation.

Plasma uric acid levels rise in preeclampsia and not with other hypertensive disease, although the degree of rise does not necessarily reflect the severity of the disease process. Likewise, it's rare for a woman with severe preeclampsia to have normal platelet function. A markedly elevated SGOT level, severe thrombocytopenia, abnormal platelet function, or renal failure is consistent with the diagnosis of severe preeclampsia.

Neonatologists have made it much easier to manage cases of severe preeclampsia, since very early delivery often helps reduce maternal and neonatal morbidity and mortality. Nevertheless, the patient with type B EPH gestosis sometimes presents problems that are not necessarily solved by early delivery. The tables in this chapter, outlining differential diagnosis, have proved useful both for patient care and for discussions with medical consultants.

REFERENCES

1. Goodlin RC: Discussant of Rice GG: Hypermenorrhea in the young hemodialysis patient. Am J Obstet Gynecol 116:539, 1973

2. Goodlin RC, Cotton DB, Haesslein HC: Severe EPH gestosis. Am J Obstet Gynecol 132:595, 1978

3. Chesley LC: Hypertension during gestation: Concepts and perspectives. In Iffy L, Kaminetzky H (eds): *Principles and Practices of Obstetrics and Perinatology.* John Wiley, New York, 1981

4. Lindheimer MD, Katz AI: Pathophysiology of preeclampsia. Annu Rev Med 32:273, 1981

5. Goodlin RC, Quaife MA, Dirksen JW: The significance, diagnosis, and treatment of maternal hypovolemia as associated with fetal/maternal illness. Semin Perinatol 5:163, 1981

6. Brain JM: Microangiopathic hemolytic anemia. Annu Rev Med 21:133, 1970

7. Ratnoff OD: Hemorrhagic disorders: Coagulation defects. In Beeson PB, McDermott W, Wyngaarden JB (eds): *Cecil Textbook of Medicine,* 15th ed. Philadelphia, WB Saunders, 1979

8. Goodlin RC, Holdt D: Impending gestosis. Obstet Gynecol 58:743, 1981

9. Weinstein L: Syndrome of hemolysis, elevated liver enzymes and low platelet count. Am J Obstet Gynecol 142:159, 1982

10. Cotton DB, Haesslein HC, Goodlin RC: Effects of x-ray on a gravida with severe hemoconcentration: A case report. Int J Gynaecol Obstet 15:466, 1978

11. Goodlin RC: Severe pre-eclampsia—Another great imitator. Am J Obstet Gynecol 125:747, 1976

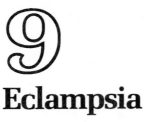

Eclampsia

FREDERICK P. ZUSPAN, MD, and
KATHRYN J. ZUSPAN, MD

CLINICAL SIGNIFICANCE: A true emergency with very real potential for death of mother or fetus, eclampsia has an incidence that probably ranges from 1.2:1,000 to 2.6:1,000 deliveries. Paramount in management is prevention of maternal/fetal morbidity and mortality by achieving adequate control of convulsions and hypertension.

The word means to strike forth or suddenly appear, but eclampsia rarely develops suddenly. Only our inability to perceive its subtle progression impedes early diagnosis. A catabolic disease that develops gradually, eclampsia is part of a continuum characterized by the increasing edema, acute hypertension, and proteinuria of preeclampsia, followed finally by the generalized eclamptic convulsion (Table 9-1). Eclampsia is a true emergency that can result in death of the mother or fetus.

Incidence figures are difficult to determine accurately. It probably ranges from 1.2:1,000 to 2.6:1,000 deliveries. Maternal mortality, worldwide, is between 0 and 17%; fetal mortality, between 10% and 37%. Management goals must be directed at controlling the convulsions and hypertension, since the underlying cause is unknown, and at effecting safe delivery.

Once eclampsia develops, it is a medical emergency that must be given the highest priority by a skilled health-care team. Before that, the aim of therapy is to prevent preeclampsia from progressing to the characteristic convulsions. The ultimate aim, of course, is prevention of maternal complications and delivery of a healthy baby.

PATHOPHYSIOLOGY OF ACUTE HYPERTENSION OF PREGNANCY

Vasospasms at the arteriole level produce hypertension and, ultimately, decrease uterine blood flow—especially in the uteroplacental bed, where the spiral arteries do not dilate as they normally would in response to pregnancy. Normally, the pregnant patient is resistant to pressor agents, but in preeclampsia, she develops increased vascular sensitivity and reactivity.

Patients with moderate to severe preeclampsia cannot handle ingested sodium appropriately, because of altered renal function. As preeclampsia develops, a renal vascular lesion, glomeruloendotheliosis, appears. Glomerular function diminishes and glomerular filtration rate declines from the normal 100 mL/minute or higher. This renal lesion disappears after delivery. It is usually associated with a significant proteinuria—more than 2 + on a dipstick urine test.

There is decreased volume in the vascular compartment because more solutes are present in the third space. Keep this decreased blood volume in mind as you follow the patient through serial hematocrit determinations. These will be higher than normal and should diminish with clinical improvement.

CNS alterations proceed from hyperactive reflexes, to clonus, to a generalized seizure. Fetal and maternal mortality correlate with the number of seizures.

DIAGNOSIS AND COMPLICATIONS

The only difference between eclampsia and severe preeclampsia is seizure and the fact that the eclamptic patient is usually sicker. The common clinical signs of both are weight gain of more than 5 to 6 pounds in a week, often accompanied by headaches, epigastric pain, and dis-

---

TABLE 9-1

Pathophysiology of eclampsia

NORMAL PREGNANCY	MILD PREECLAMPSIA
⬆ Aldosterone	⬆ Cardiovascular reactivity
⬆ Sodium retention	⬆ Vasospasm
⬆ Fluid retention	⬆ Blood pressure
⬆ Weight gain	Uteroplacental bed
	Vascular occlusion

SEVERE PREECLAMPSIA	ECLAMPSIA
Fibrin deposition	Convulsion
Renal lesion	
Proteinuria	
⬇ Vascular volume	
CNS irritability	
⬆ Amines	
⬇ PG dilators	

turbed vision, especially scotomas. Test results that are diagnostic may include the following:

- Systolic blood pressure of 160 or diastolic pressure of 110, recorded twice at 6-hour intervals with the patient at bed rest
- Proteinuria of 5 gm in 24 hours or 3 + to 4 + on dipstick
- Oliguria—urinary output of less than 400 mL in 24 hours
- Cerebral or eye disturbances, including eye ground changes
- Pulmonary edema or cyanosis.

A generalized seizure, associated with edema, hypertension, and (usually) proteinuria, confirms the diagnosis.

The three most serious complications are cerebrovascular accident or cerebral edema, placental abruption with or without hypofibrinogenemia or disseminated intravascular coagulation, and fetal death. Death is a risk for the mother when the brain, the liver and hemopoietic system, or the kidneys are compromised. Complications in the brain include cerebral hemorrhage; in the liver, disseminated intravascular coagulation and periportal necrosis; in the kidneys, glomeruloendotheliosis and severe oliguria.

CHOOSING THE TREATMENT

Therapy is much the same whether the patient is diagnosed as having eclampsia or severe preeclampsia. The extent of therapy is dictated by the degree of illness, and how worried the health-care team is about the patient's condition.

Regimens vary from country to country and from specialty to specialty. In the US, clinicians control blood pressure with IV hydralazine and treat convulsions with therapeutic doses of magnesium sulfate.[1-3] No one really knows whether the disease is the same in Europe and the US. We believe prominent academicians influence the mode of practice in their countries.

Here in the US, over the past 25 years, Pritchard and Zuspan have been major proponents of parenteral magnesium sulfate. Pritchard administers $MgSO_4$ IM while Zuspan prefers the IV route. Their methods and results are basically identical. Both have achieved at least 90% fetal salvage and reduced maternal mortality to near zero levels. These results, reported in 1965 (Zuspan and Ward) and 1967 (Pritchard and Stone), remain the best in the world literature.

THE CASE FOR MAGNESIUM THERAPY

Magnesium is the fourth most common cation in the body and the second most plentiful intracellular cation. Administered parenterally, it is excreted almost entirely in the urine; only 1% to 2% is recovered in the feces. Magnesium activates a host of enzyme systems critical to cellular metabolism and is a required cofactor for oxidative metabolism in vitro.

Magnesium and calcium have a complex interdependent influence on the excitability of the neuromuscular junction.

In pharmacologic doses, magnesium may have a curariform action on the neuromuscular junction, interfering with the release of acetylcholine from motor nerve terminals. Another hypothesis is that replacing calcium with magnesium changes membrane potential. This change would prevent convulsions by altering neuromuscular transmission and the excitability of the motor nerve terminal.

Magnesium excess at concentrations between 8 and 10 mEq/liter is expressed clinically by hypoactive deep tendon reflexes. Respiratory paralysis occurs at concentrations greater than 13 to 15 mEq/liter. Concentrations in excess of 25 mEq/liter produce cardiac arrest.

"Magnesium sulfate" refers to the hydrated form, $MgSO_4 \cdot 7H_2O$. The anhydrous salt contains twice as much magnesium as the hydrated. Magnesium sulfate has been used since 1906 for the treatment of both preeclampsia and eclampsia. Lazard first popularized IV magnesium sulfate in 1925. Eastman is credited with establishing the current IM regimen (Table 9-2). The eclampsia therapies listed in the table are only guidelines.

In planning therapy, take into consideration the patient's body weight and urinary output as well as the clinical severity of the disease. Use reflexes, respiration, and urinary output as bioassay parameters to monitor the patient. Reflexes should be hypoactive but present, respirations at least 14/minute, and urine output more than 100 mL/4 hours.

Sibai and colleagues found that convulsions recurred in 1% of eclamptic patients treated with Zuspan's regimen—a loading dose of 4 gm IV followed by a maintenance dose consisting of 1 gm/hour IV.[4]

Prevalent misconceptions are that $MgSO_4$ crosses the blood-brain barrier in large amounts and has hypotensive qualities. Magnesium sul-

---

TABLE 9-2

Specific eclampsia therapy

Magnesium sulfate
  Loading dose 4 to 6 gm over 10 minutes
  Then 1 to 2 gm/hour by infusion device

Antihypertensive drugs (if diastolic blood pressure is over 100)
  Hydralazine 5 mg bolus IV
  Then by regulated delivery system IV (100 mg in 250 mL saline)

Constant physician and nurse supervision

Early decision for delivery

fate does cross the placenta and is present in essentially the same concentrations in cord blood as in maternal blood. It is excreted by the fetus within 48 hours with no ill effect. It is not a hypotensive agent, though it does decrease intrinsic resistance in uterine vessels and may occasionally cause a transient decline in blood pressure, which soon returns to baseline levels. Whether magnesium also decreases uterine activity is being debated. It may do so in some individuals, causing a problem in induction of labor.

RECOMMENDED TREATMENT

Once eclampsia develops, both mother and fetus require intensive care. The following regimen should result in less than 1% maternal mortality and greater than 90% fetal salvage.

During convulsion
- Place padded tongue blade in mouth.
- Give magnesium sulfate 4 to 6 gm IV over 4 to 10 minutes to control the convulsions. Do not use diazepam or sodium amobarbital, because they depress mother and fetus.

After convulsion
- Insert a plastic airway and give the patient oxygen.
- Place patient in Trendelenburg position.
- Suction passages to remove secretions.
- If the stomach is full, empty stomach with nasogastric tube and instill antacid before removing the tube.
- Start IV with 5% dextrose in 0.25 N saline to replace urine output and insensible loss. Use 5% dextrose in 0.5 N saline if electrolyte levels are abnormal.
- Insert Foley catheter and record intake and output every hour.
- Order 24-hour urinalysis for protein, creatinine, and estriol.
- Check urine for specific gravity and for protein every 6 to 8 hours.
- Check serial hematocrits every 6 to 8 hours.
- Check baseline laboratory values—BUN, creatinine, electrolytes, and liver enzymes.
- Obtain a portable chest x-ray to rule out aspiration.
- Continue IV magnesium sulfate 1 gm every hour by infusion pump. (Increase magnesium sulfate if reflexes are hyperactive; decrease magnesium sulfate if reflexes are absent or if oliguria is evident.)
- Keep calcium gluconate or calcium chloride at bedside in case of magnesium overdose (dosage is 1 gm IV push).
- Check reflexes, urinary output, and respirations every hour. Expect a urine output of at least 30 mL/hour and respirations of 14/minute.
- Treat diastolic pressures of 100 or more with hydralazine in a 5-mg IV

bolus; then with a regulated IV dose—100 mg of hydralazine in 250 mL of normal saline in a plastic IV bag—to maintain a diastolic pressure of 80 to 90.

RULES FOR DELIVERING THE ECLAMPTIC PATIENT

1. Once magnesium sulfate and hydration are under way, evaluate maternal and fetal indications and make a decision concerning delivery within 4 hours. Do not wait for the patient's condition to stabilize.

2. Do amniocentesis to check for meconium and surfactant.

3. If the cervix is favorable, treat with amniotomy and begin IV oxytocin induction.

4. Do cesarean section when the fetus is severely premature (1,500 gm or less), when the cervix is unfavorable, or when there is a breech presentation. Do not use spinal anesthesia, because of the mother's decreased blood volume.

5. Spinal anesthesia is contraindicated in eclampsia and severe preeclampsia. Use local anesthetics or pudendal block for vaginal delivery.

6. For patients in labor, avoid barbiturates and narcotics that depress the fetus.

REFERENCES

1. Zuspan FP, Ward MC: Improved fetal salvage in eclampsia. Obstet Gynecol 26:893, 1965

2. Pritchard JA, Stone SR: Clinical and laboratory observations on eclampsia. Am J Obstet Gynecol 99:754, 1967

3. Zuspan FP: Problems encountered in the treatment of pregnancy induced hypertension. Am J Obstet Gynecol 131:591, 1978

4. Sibai BM, Lipshitz J, Anderson GD, et al: Reassessment of intravenous $MgSO_4$ therapy in preeclampsia-eclampsia. Obstet Gynecol 57:199, 1981

10

Third-Trimester Bleeding

ROBERT W. HUFF, MD

CLINICAL SIGNIFICANCE: Complicating 3% of pregnancies, this bleeding requires prompt, aggressive management. Whether it is due to placental abruption or placenta previa, maternal and perinatal mortality and morbidity are serious risks.

About 3% of pregnancies are complicated by bleeding in the third trimester. The causes may be such diverse entities as heavy bloody show, cervicitis, cervical or vaginal trauma, cervical carcinoma, circumvallate placenta, vasa previa, placenta previa, and abruptio placentae (Table 10-1). In some cases, however, bleeding remains unexplained even after delivery. Because you can't always determine whether the cause of the bleeding is life-threatening to the mother or fetus, evaluate all patients as follows:

● Take the blood pressure and pulse rate, bearing in mind that they may be misleadingly normal in some patients with severe hemorrhage. If there is evidence of hypotension or tachycardia, or both, the hemorrhage is probably severe and blood should be obtained promptly for cross-matching.

● Ask the patient to estimate her blood loss; then corroborate by checking for blood on her clothing, perineum, and lower extremities.

● Ask about her activity at the time bleeding began and whether uterine contractions or abdominal or back pain were associated with the onset. A quick assessment of the abdomen should note the fundal height, presence or absence of the fetal heartbeat, and fetal heart rate. Check for uterine relaxation, irritability, or tenderness, as well as contractions. Determine fetal presentation and whether the presenting part descends into the pelvis.

This initial rapid assessment will usually tell whether you're dealing with one of the two most important causes of third-trimester bleeding: placenta previa and abruptio placentae.

PLACENTA PREVIA

Implantation of the placenta low in the uterus—covering or near the internal cervical os—occurs in about one of 200 pregnancies (0.5%).[1] Midtrimester sonograms have shown a much higher incidence of placenta previa than is reported at delivery.[2, 3] Apparently the placenta moves up and away from the cervical os as the uterus grows.

Although the cause of placenta previa is unknown, several risk assessment factors have been identified: increasing maternal age, increasing parity, past cesarean delivery, and past history of placenta previa.

The condition is significant to the mother because the blood lost is hers. Before blood transfusions and cesarean delivery virtually eliminated maternal deaths from placenta previa, maternal mortality was more than 10%.[4]

Once placenta previa became safer for the mother, attention was directed at perinatal mortality, the main cause of which was prematurity. Now that expectant management[5, 6] is possible—prolonging pregnancy until fetal maturity while not endangering the mother's life—perinatal mortality has dropped from its former level of 50% to 60%, but is still much higher than in uncomplicated pregnancy.[7-10] Aggressive use of transfusion therapy may further improve perinatal outcome.[11]

Diagnosis. The diagnosis is suggested by a history of vaginal bleeding not associated with pain or uterine contraction. Typically, the woman reports discovering the blood after feeling warmth and wetness. This is the history in 80% of cases. Approximately 10% of cases are diagnosed when patients report contractions, and 10% before the onset of symptoms. This last number is rising as more placenta previa is coincidentally discovered in patients who have sonography for other reasons.

Suggestive physical findings include a soft, noncontracting uterus and a fetal presenting part high above the pelvis. (Abnormal fetal presentations are encountered in a quarter of placenta previa patients.)

TABLE 10-1

Causes of third-trimester bleeding

Abruptio placentae	Heavy "show"
Cervical carcinoma	Placenta previa
Cervical or vaginal trauma	Vasa previa
Cervicitis	Unexplained
Circumvallate placenta	

Speculum examination is safe,[5, 9] but a digital examination may cause torrential hemorrhage.[9, 12] Therefore, the presumptive diagnosis is usually confirmed by sonography. Every labor unit should have immediate access to a scanner, which has proven highly accurate for placental localization.

Management. If the placenta is shown lying low in the uterus, placenta previa is possible and the woman should be managed accordingly. Expectant management is based on the principle that the main cause of perinatal loss is prematurity and that mothers rarely die of bleeding unless they are anemic at the time, are in active labor, or have a pelvic examination. The aim is to delay delivery until the fetus is mature without increasing the mother's risk.

Traditionally, women have been kept in the hospital from the time of diagnosis until delivery. As the mean gestational age at the time of the first bleeding episode is 30 weeks,[12, 13] this could mean a long hospitalization. At Medical Center Hospital, we allow patients to return home if we're sure the environment is safe, as outlined in Table 10-2. We have managed more than 100 patients this way without maternal or fetal difficulty. But if we have any doubts about the home situation, we keep the patient in the hospital; the longest stay has been 12 weeks.

Because we know delivery will be cesarean, the only variable to consider is the time of delivery. We terminate management when the fetus is mature or the mother or fetus is in jeopardy, as detailed in Table 10-3. Occasionally patients with placenta previa have premature labor and are not bleeding. These patients are candidates for tocolytic therapy if they can be monitored carefully.

TABLE 10-2

Criteria for outpatient management of placenta previa

Premature fetus

No recent bleeding

No anemia (hematocrit 35% or more)

Patient lives within 20 minutes of hospital

Someone at home with patient

Reliable transportation at home

Telephone at home

Relatives understand patient's condition

Several problems may be encountered during cesarean. First, the placenta is often located just under the area chosen for the uterine incision. This means the surgeon must be prepared to move rapidly through the placenta and clamp the umbilical cord to minimize fetal blood loss. Second, with low implantation, contractions may not be strong enough to produce hemostasis after the placenta is removed. You should therefore anticipate postpartum hemorrhage. Ecbolic agents may be tried, but if they don't help, arterial ligation and even hysterectomy may be necessary to stop the bleeding.

Finally, morbid adherence of the placenta to the uterine wall is much more common with placenta previa than with normally implanted placentas.[7] Our service encounters two or three cases a year of placenta previa coupled with placenta accreta. This condition is best managed by hysterectomy.

Some patients with placenta previa can be delivered vaginally, but the attempt should be made only when it's time for delivery and a double setup has been prepared. As vaginal examination can provoke torrential hemorrhage, the exam must be done in an operating room with blood available, anesthesiologists in attendance, and all personnel scrubbed and ready for immediate cesarean delivery.

ABRUPTIO PLACENTAE

Premature separation of the normally implanted placenta complicates 0.5% to 2.5% of pregnancies. Once a common cause of maternal death, abruptio is rarely fatal today, because blood replacement therapy is better understood.

Pritchard studied 200 cases of abruption severe enough to have killed the fetus.[14] He confirmed that trauma and sudden decompression of an overdistended uterus can cause premature placental separation, but

---

TABLE 10-3

Reasons to terminate expectant management

Fetus is mature

Fetus is dead or has anomalies incompatible with life

Active labor begins

Excessive bleeding occurs

Other obstetric reason to terminate pregnancy
(e.g., pregnancy-induced hypertension, intra-amniotic infection, Rh isoimmunization)

---

also found that this didn't explain the majority of cases. He did find positive associations with hypertension, high parity, and past history of placental abruption. Causes specifically looked for and not encountered were short umbilical cord, inferior vena cava occlusion, and maternal folate deficiency. Other researchers have also found the association with parity, hypertension, and past history.[15, 16]

From 1977 through 1979, Medical Center Hospital had 18,220 deliveries and 137 placental abruptions, an incidence of 1:133 (0.75%). There were 36 perinatal deaths, yielding a mortality rate of 26% among those with abruptio placentae. Overall, 9.7% of our perinatal mortality was due to abruptio placentae. There are several reasons for this high rate. First, if placental separation is extensive enough—generally over 50%—the fetus will succumb to hypoxia. Second, maternal hypotension may cause hypoperfusion of the remaining placenta. Third, most placental abruptions occur before 36 weeks,[15] so many infants delivered alive die in the nursery of complications of prematurity or perinatal asphyxia.

Diagnosis. The diagnosis of placental abruption is usually clinical. A typical case is hard to miss and the findings are well known: vaginal bleeding; abdominal pain; uterine tenderness, irritability, and rigidity; fetal death; and shock.

All the findings are variable in expression. Vaginal bleeding may be scant or even absent if the hemorrhage is concealed. Rarely, pain is absent[17] or may mimic the pain associated with normal labor. Uterine tenderness may vary and rigidity may be absent. Internal fetal monitoring commonly shows an elevated uterine resting pressure. The fetus does not always die, and inability to hear the fetal heart through a stethoscope is not proof of fetal death—ultrasound is more definitive. The appearance of shock is variable. More than half of patients are hypertensive before abruption, so a "normal" blood pressure reading in these women may represent hypotension.

Management. Treatment plans hinge on whether the fetus is alive. Abruption is known to be milder if the fetus is still alive—and the prognosis is better for the mother. But you can't always tell how much of the placenta has separated and whether the fetus will be able to tolerate additional insult.

This uncertainty has led some investigators to conclude that if the fetus is alive and viable when abruption is diagnosed, the woman should be delivered at once—by cesarean, if necessary.[16, 18] Our own unpublished data do not yield the same conclusion. Of 21 stillborn fetuses, 18 were dead at dignosis in the labor room. Two grossly immature fetuses died during labor and one died during cesarean. Of the 15 nursery deaths, nine babies died of complications of prematurity, two of the complications of asphyxia, and four of other causes. Three cesareans were performed in this group, and doing more cesareans would not have produced more survivors. Of 101 surviving infants, 38 were delivered by cesarean.

Management of patients with an abruption and a live fetus, outlined in Table 10-4, includes a blood count and clotting study; cross-matching blood; giving IV fluids; monitoring urinary output, vital signs, and fetal status; and preparing for cesarean section if vaginal delivery is contraindicated.

When the woman is carrying a dead fetus in severe abruption, there are many more complications. Coagulopathy occurs in 13% to 28%,[16, 19] and is often present on admission to the labor room. Blood loss averages 2,500 mL, with minimum loss 1,000 mL. The uterus may be hypertonic and may rupture spontaneously. Hypovolemic shock can cause maternal death or produce fatal renal cortical necrosis.[16, 20] Postpartum uterine atony from uteroplacental apoplexy (Couvelaire uterus) is another complication. Fortunately, many patients with severe abruptions have a very rapid labor and delivery.[19]

Management, outlined in Table 10-5, includes IV infusion with a crystalloid solution and infusion of 2 units of blood as soon as it is available. A blood count and clotting study should be done by the laboratory, but a microhematocrit and clot observation can be performed rapidly in the labor room. Coagulopathy is diagnosed if the tube of blood doesn't clot within 8 minutes.

Fluid replacement must be monitored. Serial determinations of urinary output and hematocrit are sufficient to monitor fluid replacement in some patients. Using the Swan-Ganz catheter gives much more infor-

---

TABLE 10-4

Managing abruption with live fetus

Do CBC and urinalysis; observe clot

Cross-match 4 units of blood

Start IV fluids

Monitor urinary output

Monitor vital signs

Monitor fetal status

Consider cesarean delivery; it is definitely indicated if there is suspicion of fetal distress, heavy bleeding, failure to progress in labor rapidly, or any contraindication to labor

---

mation, especially in oliguric patients. Central venous pressure monitoring is another choice, but it doesn't give as much information. Vital signs should be recorded frequently but may not reflect the patient's true condition.

Amniotomy may or may not benefit the course of labor, but it should be done to allow insertion of an intrauterine pressure monitor—valuable to assess uterine activity. It also permits identification of the few patients who benefit from oxytocin augmentation, and it can provide early diagnosis of uterine rupture.

We used to teach that delivery should be accomplished within about 6 hours to minimize complications.[21] More vigorous transfusion therapy has lessened the need for rapid delivery, and in some cases vaginal delivery has been awaited for many hours without harmful effect to the mother.[1, 22] Cesareans are now limited to those cases of severe abruption with hemorrhage that cannot be controlled, and to those in which the cervix does not dilate.

Treatment of coagulopathy is controversial. In my view, it usually does not need to be treated and I direct management toward transfusion therapy and delivery. Coagulopathy will not improve until after delivery.[19] Generally, such conditions should be treated before a surgical in-

---

TABLE 10-5

Managing abruption when the fetus is dead

Perform CBC, urinalysis, and clotting studies; observe clot

Cross-match 6 units of blood

Start IV fluids

Infuse 2 units of blood when available

Monitor fluid administration by serial hematocrits and hourly urine output; consider balloon flotation catheter, especially if patient is oliguric

Rupture membranes and institute intrauterine pressure monitoring

Try for vaginal delivery unless labor is contraindicated

Treat coagulopathy with fresh frozen plasma or cryoprecipitate if surgery is contemplated

Consider cesarean delivery if there is excessive bleeding, contraindication to labor, or failure of cervix to dilate

Anticipate postpartum hemorrhage

cision, but in most cases episiotomy and postpartum bleeding are not reasons for coagulation therapy.

Fibrinogen has long been given to patients whose coagulopathy is caused by placental abruption.[1, 16, 20] The usual dose is 4 to 8 gm. Concern over the possibility of transmitting hepatitis B has led to use of other agents: Cryoprecipitate has been advocated, as well as fresh frozen plasma in a dose sufficient to produce clotting. Platelets are also given, but their value is questionable.

Postpartum, uterine atony, possibly complicated by coagulopathy, may be a problem. Uterine massage, high-concentration oxytocin infusion, and perhaps methylergonovine usually resolve the problem. In refractory cases, give fresh frozen plasma as well as blood (in anticipation of laparotomy). Prostaglandin analogs have stimulated uterine contractions when other drugs have failed.[23] Occasionally hysterectomy is necessary to control hemorrhage. Arterial ligation is generally unsuccessful when the patient has a coagulopathy.

The cornerstones of successful treatment of severe abruption are rapid, liberal use of blood transfusions and monitoring of its effects. These steps have improved maternal outcome even in severe abruptions. Perinatal mortality, unfortunately, is still quite high.

REFERENCES

1. Pritchard JA, MacDonald PC: *Williams Obstetrics*, ed 16. New York, Appleton-Century-Crofts, 1980, pp 487-507
2. Wexler P, Gottesfeld PW: Second trimester placenta previa: An apparently normal placentation. Obstet Gynecol 50:706, 1977
3. Rizos N, Doran TA, Miskin M, et al: Natural history of placenta previa ascertained by diagnostic ultrasound. Am J Obstet Gynecol 133:287, 1979
4. Bill AH: The treatment of placenta previa by prophylactic blood transfusion and cesarean section. Am J Obstet Gynecol 14:523, 1927
5. Macafee CHG: Placenta previa—A study of 174 cases. J Obstet Gynaecol Br Commonw 52:313, 1945
6. Johnson HW: The conservative management of some varieties of placenta previa. Am J Obstet Gynecol 50:248, 1945
7. Pedowitz P: Placenta previa: An evaluation of expectant management and the factors responsible for fetal wastage. Am J Obstet Gynecol 93:16, 1965
8. Semens JP: A second look at expectant management of placenta previa. Postgrad Med 44:207, 1968
9. Hibbard LT: Placenta previa. Am J Obstet Gynecol 104:172, 1969
10. Crenshaw C Jr, Jones DED, Parker RT: Placenta previa: A survey of 20 years experience with improved perinatal survival by expectant therapy and cesarean delivery. Obstet Gynecol Surv 28:461, 1973
11. Cotton C Jr, Read JA, Paul RH, et al: The conservative aggressive management of placenta previa. Am J Obstet Gynecol 137:687, 1980
12. Morgan J: Placenta previa: Report on a series of 538 cases. J Obstet Gynaecol Br Commonw 72:700, 1965
13. Yepes LG, Eastman NJ: The management of placenta previa. South Med J 39:291, 1946
14. Pritchard JA: Genesis of severe placental abruption. Am J Obstet Gynecol 108:22, 1970

15. Paintin DB: The epidemiology of antepartum haemorrhage. J Obstet Gynaecol Br Commonw 69:614. 1962

16. de Valera E: Abruptio placentae. Am J Obstet Gynecol 100:599. 1968

17. Notelovitz M, Bottoms SF, Dase DF, et al: Painless abruptio placentae. Obstet Gynecol 53:270. 1979

18. Knab DR: Abruptio placentae: An assessment of the time and method of delivery. Obstet Gynecol 52:625. 1978

19. Pritchard JA, Brekken AL: Clinical and laboratory studies on severe abruptio placentae. Am J Obstet Gynecol 97:681. 1967

20. Krupp PJ, Barclay DL, Roeling WM, et al: Maternal mortality—A 20-year study of Tulane Department of Obstetrics and Gynecology at Charity Hospital. Obstet Gynecol 35:823. 1970

21. Page EW, King EB, Merrill JA: Abruptio placentae: Dangers of delay in delivery. Obstet Gynecol 3:385. 1954

22. O'Driscoll K, McCarthy JR: Abruptio placentae and central venous pressure. J Obstet Gynaecol Br Commonw 73:923. 1966

23. Hayashi RH, Castillo MS, Noah ML: Management of severe postpartum hemorrhage due to uterine atony using an analogue of prostaglandin $F_{2\alpha}$. Obstet Gynecol 58:426. 1981

11

Ruptured Uterus

MARY JO O'SULLIVAN, MD

CLINICAL SIGNIFICANCE: A rare event, occurring once in every 1,000 to 3,000 deliveries, uterine rupture may be catastrophic or subtle in its manifestations. Although the chances of encountering a case are slim, the trend away from "once a section, always a section" means many more obstetricians will have to keep in mind the diffuse signs and symptoms of this entity. Hysterectomy is the usual management, although in some situations a more conservative approach is possible.

The practicing obstetrician may never encounter a case of ruptured uterus. Occurring in 0.03% to 0.08% (1:1,204 to 1:2,861) of all deliveries, it is among the rarest of obstetric emergencies (Table 11-1).[1-7] By rupture is meant complete separation of the uterine musculature through all layers, not the dehiscence that characterizes incomplete rupture. The faster you confirm the diagnosis and start treatment, the better the chances of good maternal and fetal outcome.

Since cesarean section has replaced many obstetric manipulations in the uterus and eliminated prolonged dysfunctional labors, one would expect a decrease in the incidence of traumatic rupture and an increase in scar rupture. Table 11-2 classifies the deliveries listed in Table 11-1 as pre-1960 (group A) and post-1970 (group B). It shows that the distribution of ruptures among Krishna-Menon's three categories (spontaneous, traumatic, and scar) has not changed significantly over the two time periods.[8] However, when ruptures are considered as a percentage of total deliveries, all categories show a decrease in the period since 1970. The decreases are greatest in the scar and traumatic groups. Perhaps a change in surgical technique is responsible for the downward trend in the scar group. After 1970, most abdominal deliveries would have been low segment. Before 1960, there would have been more classical sections. However, the trend toward more vaginal deliveries of pa-

TABLE 11-1

Summary of ruptured uteri studies*

| AUTHOR | TOTAL RUPTURES | TOTAL PATIENTS | INCIDENCE (%) | UTERINE SCAR | | | | TRAUMATIC | SPONTANEOUS |
				TOTAL	PREVIOUS LOW SEGMENT	CLASSICAL CESAREAN	OTHER		
Erving[2] (1930-1956)	37	96,153	0.04	20	3	15	2	15	2
Ferguson[3] (1935-1955)	84 (42)	101,108	0.04-0.08	18	5	13	—	9	15
Ware[6] (1932-1956)	40	70,837	0.06	16	2	14	—	15	9
Donnelly[1] (1948-1961)	43	118,626	0.04	15	13	—	2	15	13
Schrinsky[5] (1950-1975)	47 (34)	126,770	0.03-0.04	12	4	8	—	10	12
Mercer[4] (1971-1979)	18 (15)	51,500	0.03-0.04	6	4	1	1	5	4
Totals	269 (211)	564,994	0.04-0.05	87	31	51	5	69	55
Per cent of total ruptures				41.23%				32.70%	26.07%

( ) indicates only overt ruptures. Percentages are based upon overt ruptures only.
*Adapted from O'Sullivan, Fumia, Halsinger, et al.[11]

tients who previously had cesareans may increase the incidence of scar rupture in the future.

Numerous classifications of uterine rupture have been proposed, based on a variety of anatomic and etiologic factors. Probably the simplest is that of Krishna-Menon.[8] Spontaneous and traumatic ruptures are usually more catastrophic than the scar variety in terms of signs, symptoms, and maternal and fetal prognosis. Scar rupture, the most common type, usually is secondary to rupture of a previous cesarean scar. The distinction between traumatic and spontaneous rupture is based on cause; spontaneous rupture is unrelated to any known predisposing factor.

CAUSES

Any of the following factors may cause uterine rupture—and they may be additive:

- Trauma antecedent to the present pregnancy, including curettage; uterine perforation—either recognized or unrecognized—inflicted by a sound, curette, or similar instrument; previous uterine surgery—myomectomy; cesarean section, hysterotomy, or Strassman or similar procedure; or cornual resection.
- Obstetric factors in the present pregnancy, including excessive uterine stimulation—spontaneous or drug-induced; operative obstetrics—version, extraction, midforceps; hydrocephaly or other obstructive fetal mass; shoulder dystocia; neglected labor; excessive fundal pressure; grand multiparity; abruptio placentae; trophoblastic disease; or placenta increta-percreta.
- Other factors, such as uterine anomalies, trauma, cornual pregnancy, or unknown causes.

TABLE 11-2

Distribution of ruptures by type has remained constant over several decades

	BEFORE 1960		AFTER 1970	
TYPE OF RUPTURE	DELIVERIES (%)	RUPTURES (%)	DELIVERIES (%)	RUPTURES (%)
Scar	0.018	42.59	0.012	40.00
Traumatic	0.014	33.33	0.009	33.33
Spontaneous	0.010	24.07	0.008	26.66

DIAGNOSIS

Most ruptures occur in the lower uterine segment. Rupture of the unscarred uterus, most common during labor or delivery, is usually longitudinal in the region of the uterine vessels, and most often on the left.[9] Since the vessels are involved, often there is excessive external or concealed bleeding.

The classical symptoms are sudden tearing abdominal pain followed by relief of pain, shock, loss of fetal heart tones, cessation of contractions, tachycardia, and abdominal tenderness. But pain may be minimal. There may be some maternal restlessness, tachycardia, and retraction or ascent of the presenting part if delivery has not occurred. Fetal heart tones initially may be stable. Bleeding may be out into the broad ligament and so may remain in the retroperitoneum and concealed. These symptoms, which are not classical, contribute to delay in diagnosis. Bleeding that is intra-abdominal usually gives more obvious signs, consistent with an acute abdomen.

Since uterine contractions usually do not cease when the lower segment ruptures, spontaneous or assisted vaginal delivery may be concluded successfully. However, rupture may occur during delivery as a result of forceps injury, fundal pressure, shoulder dystocia, or difficulty with the aftercoming head. Again, bleeding may be external or concealed. And if external bleeding is attributed to concomitant cervical or vaginal lacerations, the low-segment laceration may go unrecognized until the patient has persistent unexplained bleeding and is in shock, or until she is explored for uncontrolled bleeding with the diagnosis made retrospectively.

Persistent bleeding despite a well-contracted uterus and no apparent lacerations should arouse your suspicions. In fact, you should think of the possibility of a rupture whenever a patient has any of the predisposing factors. Think rupture and you are unlikely to miss it!

A scarred uterus should alert you to the possibility of uterine rupture. Here, too, rupture is more common in the lower segment and may be very subtle. The site of rupture—the scar—is relatively avascular, so bleeding is often less than in spontaneous or traumatic rupture. Should rupture occur during labor, contractions will frequently continue. Maternal tachycardia, restlessness, and change of personality may be seen. Fetal heart tones may or may not change, depending on uteroplacental/ umbilical continuity. Irregularity over the suprapubic area or swelling and retraction of the presenting part are also clues. Lower abdominal tenderness and pain are common symptoms during labor and therefore may or may not be helpful in making the diagnosis. Hypotension is a late feature, unless the rupture extends out into the broad ligament.

While spontaneous and traumatic ruptures rarely occur except during labor, some 24% of scarred uteri may rupture before labor begins.[10]

Almost invariably, fundal ruptures are found in uteri scarred by classical cesareans or myomectomies. The presenting signs and symptoms are more obvious and also classical. Occasionally the site of rupture is occluded or compressed by a fetal part. Bleeding controlled in this way delays diagnosis. Should a fundal scar rupture during labor, continuous pain may replace the intermittent contractions of labor, followed by a tearing sensation, and then relief. Uterine contractions cease, fetal heart tones are lost, and the signs and symptoms of blood loss become obvious unless tamponade occurs.

Classical cesarean sections are unusual today, although hysterotomies are still done occasionally. When you are dealing with an immigrant population, you can't always be sure a previous cesarean was low segment. Finally, the incidence of premature delivery by cesarean section has increased. Many of these incisions start out as low segment vertical but may become classical because of a poorly developed lower uterine segment. Therefore, we have to think of the possibility of rupture in cases of abdominal pain and uterine scars, and search for other signs and symptoms to confirm or rule out the diagnosis.

Once suspicion is sufficiently aroused, prepare for immediate fluid replacement; transfusion, which may be massive; and abdominal or transvaginal exploration. Maternal death is more common following traumatic (24%) and spontaneous (11%) rupture than after scar rupture (3.07%).[11] However, much of the recent literature reports no maternal or fetal deaths.[12-14]

MANAGEMENT

Patients with previous cesarean sections who are candidates for a trial of labor must fit all the selection criteria (Table 11-3), be closely monitored during labor, and have a normoprogressive labor, ideally without oxytocin (although the latter is not totally contraindicated). Most properly selected patients will deliver vaginally without incident. When patients, physicians, and nurses are all alert to the possibility of rupture, medical personnel will intervene more often and earlier than in unscarred uteri. This will lessen blood loss and improve maternal and fetal outcomes.

After vaginal delivery of a patient who has had a previous cesarean section, a careful exam is necessary to search for a uterine defect. If this exam makes you suspect a defect or asymptomatic rupture, and the abdominal cavity is not entered, you can manage conservatively, watching carefully for any evidence of vaginal or concealed bleeding. Signs of concealed hemorrhage are tachycardia (postpartum most patients develop relative bradycardia), restlessness, hypotension, increasing fundal height, or a fundus pushed to one side despite an empty bladder. Vaginal exam may disclose fullness anteriorly (again despite an empty

TABLE 11-3

Selection criteria for trial of labor in previous cesarean patients

Only one previous low-segment transverse cesarean with no extension documented by operative note

Readily available blood, anesthesia, and operating facilities on same floor as labor suite

Previous indication no longer exists

Clinically adequate pelvis for this baby

No medical or obstetric complications

Patient acceptance and understanding of risks of abdominal and vaginal delivery

No previous uterine rupture

---

bladder) or in either parametrial region. However, if the abdominal cavity was entered or there is evidence of bleeding or hematuria, laparotomy must be carried out.

When there is suspicion of a rupture in a patient with an unscarred uterus, do a careful intrauterine exam to try to palpate the defect. Once the diagnosis of rupture is confirmed or sufficient suspicion remains, laparotomy should be done. When there is little doubt that rupture has taken place, proceed to laparotomy without examining the uterus.

The treatment of choice is total abdominal hysterectomy. Occasionally, this may have to be preceded by hypogastric artery ligation to control bleeding in the broad ligament. When hemorrhage is massive, you may also find temporary aortic compression very helpful in controlling bleeding while you are trying to obtain better visualization. Repair is rarely, if ever, indicated in a ruptured, previously intact uterus, because of increased risk of rupture the second time around.[15] However, you may consider scar repair when patients desire more children. Any subsequent delivery should be carried out by cesarean section.

Uterine rupture can be associated with very high maternal and fetal mortality and morbidity unless it is recognized and treated early enough to prevent prolonged excessive blood loss and shock secondary to uterine vessel involvement. The diagnosis should be based not only on classical signs and symptoms, but also on subtle signs of blood loss.

REFERENCES

1. Donnelly JP, Franzoni KF: Uterine rupture. A thirty year survey. Obstet Gynecol 23:774, 1964
2. Erving HW: Rupture of the uterus. Am J Obstet Gynecol 71:251, 1957

3. Ferguson RK, Reid DK: Rupture of the uterus: A twenty year report. Am J Obstet Gynecol 76:172, 1958

4. Mercer CA: *Uterine rupture during pregnancy. Annual Obstetric Gynecologic Resident's Day Symposium.* Emory University, Atlanta, June 1980

5. Schrinsky DC, Benson R: Rupture of the pregnant uterus: A review. Obstet Gynecol Surv 33:217, 1978

6. Ware HH, Jarrett AQ, Reda FA: Rupture of the gravid uterus. Am J Obstet Gynecol 76:181, 1958

7. Golan A, Sandbank O, Rubin A: Rupture of the pregnant uterus. Obstet Gynecol 56:549, 1981

8. Krishna-Menon MD: Rupture of the uterus: A review of 164 cases. J Obstet Gynaecol Br Commonw 69:18, 1962

9. Voogd LB, Wood HH, Powell DV: Ruptured uterus. Obstet Gynecol 7:70, 1956

10. Eames HH: A study of the management of pregnancies subsequent to cesarean section. Am J Obstet Gynecol 65:944, 1953

11. O'Sullivan MJ, Fumia F, Holsinger K, et al: Vaginal delivery after cesarean section. Clin Perinatol 8:131, 1981

12. Garnet JD: Uterine rupture during pregnancy. An analysis of 133 patients. Obstet Gynecol 23:898, 1964

13. Gibbs CE: Planned vaginal delivery following cesarean section. Clin Obstet Gynecol 23:507, 1980

14. McGarry JA: The management of patients previously delivered by cesarean section. J Obstet Gynaecol Br Commonw 76:137, 1969

15. Weingold AB: Rupture of the gravid uterus. Surg Gynecol Obstet 122:1233, 1966

12

Hemorrhagic Shock in Obstetrics

DENIS CAVANAGH, MD,
ROBERT A. KNUPPEL, MD, and
DONALD E. MARSDEN, MD

CLINICAL SIGNIFICANCE: The most common cause of maternal death and a frequent cause of such serious complications as acute renal failure, hemorrhagic shock is an ever-present threat throughout pregnancy.

The most frequent cause of maternal death in the US (Table 12-1), hemorrhagic shock is also responsible for such serious complications as Sheehan's syndrome, acute renal tubular necrosis, and acute renal cortical necrosis. Severe blood loss, an ever-present risk during pregnancy, may result from ruptured ectopic pregnancy, abortion, ruptured uterus, placenta previa, abruptio placentae, or postpartum hemorrhage.[4] Prompt and adequate filling of the intravascular space is necessary to preserve life. The patient's vital signs may be misleading in assessing the effect of blood loss; for example, a normal or even slightly elevated blood pressure does not preclude life-threatening hypovolemia, nor does a low pulse rate.

PATHOPHYSIOLOGY

The final event in shock is failure of tissue respiration at the cellular level as a result of reduced tissue perfusion. A number of homeostatic mechanisms are brought into play to prevent such an eventuality. When blood is lost from the vascular space and the circulating blood volume is reduced, the catecholamine level rises, causing arterioles and veins to constrict. The liberation of pressor substances helps sustain this vasoconstriction, and renal blood flow is redistributed within the kidneys to protect the medullae. Flow to the heart and brain increases, at the expense of the splanchnic, uterine, renal, muscular, and cutaneous circulations. In this early phase, which is compensated and reversible, extravascular fluid flows into the vascular compartment. Venous return and cardiac output are maintained, as the circulating volume and vascular space accommodate to each other. Tachycardia also helps maintain cardiac output. Provided bleeding is controlled, IV fluids and electrolyte solutions readily achieve homeostasis.

If the hemorrhagic process continues, however, arteriolar and capillary tone is lost and the capillary bed and vascular compartment expand. Decreased tissue perfusion and vascular stasis reduce the supply of oxygen and nutrients to the cells and the clearance of metabolites from the tissues. Initially, anaerobic metabolism compensates for hypoxia, but as the process continues, lactate and pyruvate accumulate in the tissues. Unchecked, this process leads to cellular autolysis. Metabolic acidosis, at times associated with disseminated intravascular coagulation (DIC) and stimulation of the fibrinolytic system, marks this secondary stage of late decompensation. Hepatic, renal, cardiopulmonary, or CNS failure signals irreversible hemorrhagic shock.

CLINICAL PICTURE

Shock has a reversible, primary stage with an early (warm), or compensated, phase and a late (cold), or decompensated, phase. If unchecked, it progresses to an irreversible, secondary stage. The signs and the expected response to volume replacement of each stage are outlined in Table 12-2. In the early phase, blood pressure is relatively normal and tachycardia and diaphoresis are present. The patient appears restless and anxious. This compensated phase can usually be managed easily by volume replacement.

TABLE 12-1

---

*Causes of maternal mortality in the US**

CAUSE	1975	1976	1977	1978	TOTAL
Hemorrhage†	125	110	120	89	408
Sepsis	76	71	70	61	278
Preeclampsia-eclampsia	77	83	55	62	277
All other	125	126	128	107	486
Total	403	390	373	319	1,449

*National Center for Health Statistics.
†Ruptured ectopic pregnancy, abortion, ruptured uterus, placenta previa, abruptio placentae, and postpartum hemorrhage.

TABLE 12-2

The clinical picture in hemorrhagic shock and expected response to volume replacement*

CLINICAL SIGN	PRIMARY SHOCK		SECONDARY SHOCK
	EARLY	LATE	
Mental state	Alert and anxious	Confused	Coma
General appearance	Normal and warm	Pale and cold	Cyanotic and cold
Blood pressure	Slightly hypotensive	Moderately hypotensive	Markedly hypotensive
Respiratory system	Slight tachypnea	Tachypnea	Tachypnea and cyanosis
Urinary output	30 to 60 mL/hour	<30 mL/hour	Anuria
Effect of volume challenge on:			
Blood pressure	Increased	Slightly increased	No response
Urinary output	Increased	Slightly increased	No response

*Adapted from Cavanagh. Woods. O'Connor. et al.[5]

If treatment is delayed or inadequate, the hypotensive phase ensues. This phase is also manageable in its early stages by volume replacement. But as the process evolves, treatment elicits a much less satisfactory response. Even with intensive treatment the patient may still enter the irreversible stage. However, it is often possible to reverse hemorrhagic shock very late in its evolution, and for this reason vigorous therapy is called for even if the patient appears exsanguinated.

PLAN OF ACTION FOR COMBATING SHOCK

To ensure the rapid and effective management of the patient in shock, it is imperative that medical and paramedical attendants have the proper sequence of therapeutic and diagnostic maneuvers clear in their minds. For this purpose we use the mnemonic ORDER (Table 12-3).

O—Oxygenate. Inadequate respiratory exchange is the most frequent cause of death in shock. Give 6 to 8 liters of oxygen per minute by mask,

---

TABLE 12-3

ORDER of priorities in managing the obstetric patient in shock

O—Oxygenate
Assure an airway
6 to 8 liters/minute by closed mask, nasal catheter, or
    endotracheal tube

R—Restore circulatory volume
One or more IV lines
Initially crystalloids or colloids
Where possible, blood for blood, but remember clotting factors
Initial monitoring by CVP

D—Drug therapy
Avoid vasopressors generally
Digitalize if in cardiac failure
Specific drugs for condition

E—Evaluate
Response to therapy
Basic cause
Fetal condition

R—Remedy the basic problem
Deliver fetus
Repair lacerations
Remove secundines
Ovarian and hypogastric artery ligation
Hysterectomy

---

taking care to ascertain that the airway is patent and tidal volume adequate. If in doubt about either of the latter conditions, institute intubation and positive pressure ventilation. Oxygen requirements can be monitored by arterial blood gas estimations, but in general such tests should wait until the other basic resuscitative measures are instituted.

R—Restore circulatory volume. This involves placing IV lines, which can be difficult when the patient is in shock. It is preferable to place one or more large-bore cannulas in peripheral veins. IV catheters may be inserted in the antecubital fossa, but flow rates there are limited in severe shock. The large volumes of fluid to be infused demand some form of monitoring other than the basics of pulse, blood pressure, and urine output. Arterial blood pressure is particularly unreliable as a guide to management of hemorrhage in obstetric patients, because they are well able to compensate for blood loss—particularly in abruptio placentae. A central venous catheter is ideal.[6] This may most safely be inserted via an antecubital vein, though in experienced hands the infraclavicular or supraclavicular approach is fast, simple, and safe. However, keep in mind that a complication such as pneumothorax or hemothorax may be fatal in the already compromised patient.

The initial fluid infusion will be crystalloids or colloids in most cases. But when hemorrhage is the cause of shock, blood replacement is desirable. At the time IV lines are inserted, take blood for basic hematologic testing, coagulation profile, and grouping and cross-matching. In the past, when the urgent need for transfusion precluded prior cross-matching, group O, Rh-negative blood with a low anti-A and anti-B titer was advised. This probably has no advantage over using blood of the patient's own group (for many obstetric patients this will already be known). Whenever such blood is used, it should be matched even as it is infused. Should bleeding be due to a coagulopathy, use fresh frozen plasma or fresh blood (drawn on the day of transfusion) to replace clotting factors. Platelet infusions should also be considered. With every five bags of stored blood transfused, give one bag of fresh frozen plasma to supply clotting factors.[7]

Antishock (MAST) trousers should be considered as an interim measure, especially in the management of patients requiring transport to a tertiary care facility.

Although a Swan-Ganz flotation catheter has many advantages in shock, we believe its insertion should follow the basic resuscitative measures. This avoids delaying more critical procedures, and may prevent such complications as cardiac arrhythmias in an already compromised patient. If a central line has been established, the flotation catheter may be safely inserted later, over a guide wire placed through the central line prior to its removal.[8]

D—Drug therapy. Compared with oxygenation and restoration of the circulating blood volume, drug therapy is of secondary importance. Nevertheless, several agents may prove useful. Where shock results from postpartum or postabortal hemorrhage, give IM ergonovine maleate and an IV infusion of oxytocin. Where shock is due to other causes, antibiotics, opiates, heparin, or steroids may be indicated.

Acidosis resulting from shock may be controlled by infusing 5% dextrose in saline with sodium bicarbonate added. Ringer's lactate is not appropriate in shock, as it increases the lactate load.

If cardiac competence is in doubt, especially in patients with tachycardia and a raised central venous pressure, digitalization is indicated. Vasopressors are not generally used in the treatment of hemorrhagic shock, as peripheral resistance is increased initially. Volume replacement is the critical step.

E—Evaluate. Up to this stage, the management of shock has been instituted rapidly and almost reflexly, and aimed simply at stabilizing the patient's condition. It is now essential to evaluate her response to therapy, to diagnose the basic condition that led to shock, and to consider the condition of the fetus.

Response to treatment is assessed by reviewing changes in vital signs, central venous pressure, and urinary output. Consider whether any further laboratory studies should be done or repeated. Arterial blood gas and acid-base studies, blood biochemistry, coagulation factors, and fibrin degradation product assays may be indicated. Now is the appropriate time to consider inserting a Swan-Ganz flotation catheter.

The cause of shock may be obvious or more difficult to ascertain. For instance, coagulopathies may cause hemorrhage in themselves or result from the therapy (transfusing large quantities of stored blood without replacing labile clotting factors and platelets). Abruptio placentae and placenta previa may be difficult to differentiate in some circumstances. Postpartum hemorrhage may arise from uterine atony, genital tract lacerations, retained secundines, or, less commonly, coagulopathy.

In many situations, the condition of the fetus is clearly not relevant, but in later pregnancy, when survival could be reasonably expected if delivery occurred, termination of the pregnancy may be desirable for fetal or maternal reasons. We believe that the mother's condition is the major consideration, but under some conditions immediate delivery is desirable for both mother and baby. In severe placental abruption with a live fetus, once the patient is stabilized, the best interests of both dictate immediate delivery, even by cesarean section.

R—Remedy the basic problem. Because shock is a bodily response to some other condition, it is desirable to treat the cause as soon as resuscitative measures are instituted. In certain situations the definitive therapy may need to be given before stabilization is achieved. For instance, in ruptured ectopic pregnancy, transfusion is futile unless the source of bleeding is controlled. Hence, for ruptured ectopic pregnancy, surgery should be performed once blood is cross-matched and resuscitative measures are under way. The same is true for uterine rupture.

In antepartum hemorrhage, vaginal examination with a double setup may be required. If conditions are favorable for vaginal delivery, the membranes may be ruptured; if not, cesarean section is indicated. We must emphasize that vaginal examination is hazardous when there is antepartum hemorrhage. It should be done only in the operating room with blood cross-matched and preparations made for immediate cesarean section.

In cases of continuing postpartum hemorrhage, examination under anesthesia is essential. Explore the birth canal and uterus carefully, looking for retained products of conception or lacerations. If using a speculum, look under it before concluding that all is well, because occasionally a speculum can hide bleeding from the apex of an episiotomy. Postpartum hemorrhage unresponsive to medical treatment and not due to lacerations, coagulopathies, or retained products of conception requires surgery. Medical treatment should include an oxytocin infusion, IM ergonovine maleate, and intramyometrial prostaglandin.[9]

Surgery for genital tract bleeding may be conservative or radical. In general, a ruptured uterus is best treated by hysterectomy. In selected cases where less radical surgery seems indicated, or where hysterectomy has not controlled the bleeding, hypogastric artery ligation is advisable. In pregnancy, this should include ligation of the ovarian arteries. The ureter should be identified where it crosses the common iliac artery, and then be traced throughout its pelvic course. The anterior division of the internal iliac artery is identified, gently freed from the underlying vein, and doubly ligated with No. 0 silk. The vessel is not divided. The procedure should be performed bilaterally. It is not without risk, as damage to the ureter and bleeding from the internal iliac vein are serious hazards. Hypogastric artery ligation is seldom indicated, yet may be lifesaving. We educate residents by performing sham hypogastric ligations in the course of other pelvic surgery. This affords residents an opportunity to learn the technique, and helps protect patients from dangerous attempts by the untutored "occasional" operator. As an alternative to internal iliac artery ligation, embolization of the vessels with agents such as gelatin foam has been advocated,[10] but this too is not without risk.

We must emphasize that the most experienced surgeon available should operate on these critically ill patients. A desire to be conservative should not be allowed to endanger their lives.

REFERENCES

1. National Center for Health Statistics, Department of Health, Education, and Welfare: Vital Health Stat 26:12, 1976
2. National Center for Health Statistics, Department of Health, Education, and Welfare: Vital Health Stat 28:1, 1977
3. National Center for Health Statistics, Department of Health, Education, and Welfare: Vital Health Stat 30:11, 1978
4. Cavanagh D, Knuppel RA, Copeland WJ, et al: Hemorrhagic shock in the obstetric patient. In Sakamoto S, Tojo S, Nakayama T (eds): *Proceedings of the Ninth World Congress of Gynecology and Obstetrics*, Tokyo, 1979, Aclata 25-31. Princeton, Excerpta Medica, 1979
5. Cavanagh D, Woods RE, O'Connor TCF, et al: *Obstetric Emergencies*, ed 3. New York, Harper & Row, 1982
6. O'Driscoll K, McCarthy JR: Abruptio placentae and central venous pressures. J Obstet Gynaecol Br Commonw 73:923, 1966
7. Cooksey JA, Orlina AR: Blood and blood products replacement therapy. J Reprod Med 19:233, 1977
8. Cotton DB, Benedetti TJ: Use of the Swan-Ganz catheter in obstetrics and gynecology. Obstet Gynecol 56:641, 1980
9. Takagi T, Yoshida T, Togo Y, et al: The effects of intramyometrial prostaglandin $F_{2\alpha}$ on severe postpartum hemorrhage. Prostaglandins 12:565, 1976
10. Smith DC, Wyatt JF: Embolization of the hypogastric arteries in the control of massive vaginal hemorrhage. Obstet Gynecol 49:317, 1977

13

Coagulopathy in Pregnancy

J. PATRICK LAVERY, MD

CLINICAL SIGNIFICANCE: Though fewer than 5% of pregnant patients have coagulation complications, for them the risk of mortality is significant. About a third of all maternal deaths are associated with obstetric hemorrhage, and often consumptive coagulopathy.

Coagulation disorders occur often enough in obstetrics and gynecology to oblige the physician to be prepared to take quick and decisive action in critical-care situations. Often circumstances preclude having laboratory information available that would assist clinical decision making. The ability to respond with foresight and accuracy depends on a thorough understanding of the normal coagulation mechanisms as well as the pathophysiology of the clinical conditions with which coagulation disorders are most frequently associated.

NORMAL PHYSIOLOGY OF COAGULATION

A sensitive balance between the integrity of blood vessels, the function and action of platelets, and the activation of procoagulants and fibrinolytic agents in the circulatory system must be maintained for normal coagulation. A brief outline of these significant components of coagulation follows. Detailed reviews of these systems can be found in several standard references.[1-3]

Vasoconstriction is the immediate local response to trauma, and thus blood vessels are the hemostatic system's first line of defense.[4] The blood vessel response may be potentiated by the vasoconstrictive effects of agents like thromboxane A_2, which is released by aggregating platelets. Traumatized blood vessels also activate procoagulants in the circulation by releasing substances rich in thromboplastic activity, which stimulate the extrinsic system of clotting. Several of these are found in the endothelium, and this is of consequence in pregnancy. Endothelial cells are a rich source of factor VIII, von Willebrand factor, and plasminogen activators.

Platelets. These round or oval cytoplasmic fragments measure 2 to 4 mm in diameter. When newly released from the marrow, platelets are large; with time, they decrease in size and number.

Platelets adhere to collagen and microfibrils in the vascular basement membrane, a process that depends on the polymerization of collagen and free ϵ-amino groups on collagen. For efficient platelet aggregation, calcium, fibrinogen, and other plasma factors must also be present.

Platelets contain multiple granules with active components integrally related to coagulation.[5] With aggregation, two release mechanisms occur. The first, termed release I, allows platelets to discharge adenosine triphosphate, adenosine diphosphate, serotonin, and calcium from

---

TABLE 13-1

Procoagulant factors in blood coagulation

   I. Fibrinogen
  II. Prothrombin
 III. Tissue factor
  IV. Calcium
   V. Proaccelerin
  VI. (Not used)
 VII. Proconvertin
VIII. Antihemophilic factor (AHF); antihemophilic globulin (AHG)
  IX. Plasma thromboplastin component (PTC); Christmas factor
   X. Stuart-Prower factor
  XI. Plasma thromboplastin antecedent (PTA)
 XII. Hageman factor
XIII. Fibrin-stabilizing factor

Prekallikrein—Fletcher factor

High molecular weight kinogen (HMWK)—
Fitzgerald factor
Williams factor
Flaujeac factor

dense-body granules in the cell. This step is inhibited by aspirin. Release II discharges acid hydrolases and cathepsins from the α-granules, a response that enhances clotting by potentiating platelet aggregation and vasoconstriction. Aggregating platelets, in turn, release thromboxane A_2, causing further aggregation and vasoconstriction.

FIGURE 13-1

Formation of insoluble fibrin clot

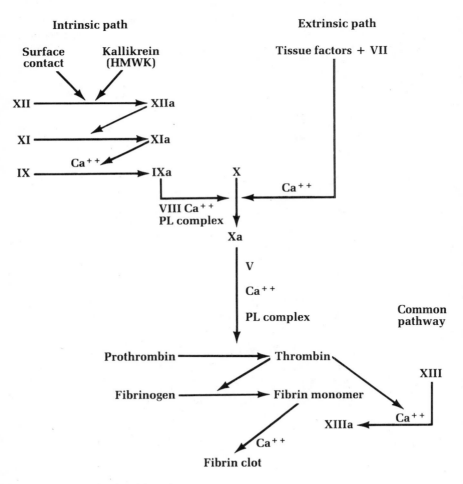

Key: PL = phospholipid; Ca++ = calcium ions.

Platelet factors 3 and 4 are liberated in the release process. Platelet factor 3, a phospholipid, is a potent catalyst for the calcium-dependent procoagulant activation of the intrinsic clotting system. Platelet factor 4, which has an antiheparin-like activity, fosters coagulation around a clot. Platelet actomyosin promotes clot retraction, decreasing the clot's permeability and maintaining hemostasis.

Coagulants. Circulating procoagulants (Table 13-1) are present in the plasma. When activated, they initiate the clotting mechanism.[6] Procoagulants form the extrinsic and intrinsic pathways that lead to a common pathway of coagulation. The arbitrary division of coagulation into two pathways makes for simplicity and correlates with laboratory assessment. In vivo, the two systems function together.

Their convergence ultimately activates thrombin, one of the most potent enzymes in the system. There is sufficient thrombin in 10 mL of blood to effect the coagulation of 2,500 mL of plasma. Formation of the insoluble fibrin clot results from the action of the common pathway (Figure 13-1). Insoluble fibrin represents the end product of the coagulation process. Platelet activation will enhance vasoconstriction, further aggregation, thrombin generation, and neutralization of endogenous heparin. The thrombus thus formed is made up of a network of insoluble fibrin and irreversibly aggregated platelets.

FIGURE 13-2

Components of the fibrinolytic system

The fragments from fibrinolytic activity are the fibrin degradation products (FDPs).

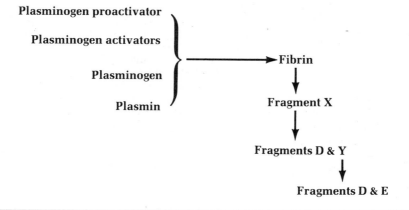

The liver is probably the place where all coagulation factors are synthesized, except for factor VII, which is synthesized in endothelial cells. The reticuloendothelial system, including the liver, participates in the removal of activated factors from the circulation.

Fibrinolysins. The coagulation mechanism is antagonized by the equally active fibrinolytic system. This system is activated by the generation of thrombin. Figure 13-2 shows the four main components of the fibrinolytic system. These components break down fibrin, releasing assayable fibrin degradation products (FDPs) into the circulation. The degradation products have anticoagulant properties, and, if present in large amounts, can render the blood incoagulable.

The tests. Hemostasis is a constant and dynamic process of clot formation and lysis. Normally, this process is extremely well balanced; imbalances can result in hemostatic disorders of considerable magnitude. The tests of coagulation function listed in Table 13-2 offer the clinician the information needed to manage a critical clotting disorder.

Whole-blood clotting is a gross guide to coagulation. The classic red-stoppered tube test by the bedside is still the best way to obtain an immediate estimate of overall coagulation factors. Clot retraction is an insensitive test of platelet function; the Ivy bleeding time is excellent for evaluating capillary integrity and platelet count and function, and can

---

TABLE 13-2

Tests to spot coagulation disorders

Tests of the coagulation system	Subject measured
Activated partial thromboplastin time	Intrinsic system and common pathway
Fibrinogen	Fibrinogen content
Ivy bleeding time	Platelet number and function; vascular integrity
Platelet count	Platelet number
Prothrombin time	Extrinsic system and common pathway, fibrinogen
Thromboplastin generation test	Intrinsic system, platelets
Whole blood (in tube)	Intrinsic system, platelets
Tests of the fibrinolytic system	**Subject measured**
Euglobulin lysis	Plasminogen activators and plasmin
Fibrin degradation products	Presence of fibrinolytic activity
Protamine paracoagulation test	Fibrin monomers, early fibrin/ fibrinogen degradation products

---

be modified for use by the bedside. The platelet count generally varies inversely with the bleeding time and may be influenced by recent aspirin ingestion.

PREGNANCY CHANGES

Pregnancy causes both quantitative and qualitative alterations in the hemostatic system.[2] The changes that pertain to the procoagulant and fibrinolytic system are listed in Table 13-3. For the most part, pregnancy results in increased coagulation factors (except XI and XIII) as well as a slight lowering of the coagulation inhibitors antithrombin III and antifactor Xa.[2]

During normal pregnancy, activation of the coagulation system increases synthesis of fibrinogen and other clotting factors so that it exceeds the rate of consumption.[2] This is why pregnancy is sometimes referred to as a hypercoagulable state. Fibrinogen synthesis may be mediated in part by hormonal changes and by increased demand for utilization locally in the uteroplacental circulation.

Factor VIII is markedly elevated during pregnancy. In contrast to the greater-than-100% increase in fibrinogen and factor VIII, factor XIII (fibrin-stabilizing factor) shows as much as a 50% decrease at term, and this may have some influence on clot stabilization and lysis during the latter part of gestation. Increased platelet factors late in pregnancy contribute to endogenous heparin resistance.

Changes in the platelet count during gestation have been reviewed by several investigators. Fenton and associates found no significant change in the courses of 44 normal pregnancies.[7] On the other hand, in a prospective study of 23 gravidas, Pitkin and White found a significant decline in platelet count from the first to the third trimester.[8] A declin-

---

TABLE 13-3

Changes in procoagulant and fibrinolytic system in pregnancy

PROCOAGULATION FACTORS	LYTIC FACTORS
I-X and XII increase	Antithrombin III decreases
XI and XIII decrease	Antifactor Xa decreases
Fibrinogen increases	Plasminogen activator decreases
Platelet adhesiveness (phospholipid factor 3) increases	
Platelet factor 4 increases	

ing platelet count appeared to be the most consistent finding of several groups who studied whole blood.[9]

There is evidence of decreased fibrinolytic activity during gestation, particularly in the third trimester. This results from an enhanced capacity to form fibrin and a diminished capacity of lytic agents to degrade this substance as pregnancy nears term. Additional factors that inhibit fibrinolysis may be present in the placenta and contribute to depression of the fibrinolytic system.[2] Fibrinolytic activity returns to normal by 1 week postpartum.

During normal labor, aberrations in laboratory parameters of coagulation may occur in up to 27% of parturients.[10] These changes generally do not have major clinical consequences.

Many conditions are characterized by disturbances in the coagulation mechanism. Those most commonly encountered in obstetrics and gynecology are listed in Table 13-4. The clinician must be alert to aberrations in coagulation even before the diagnosis is firmly established. It's imperative to obtain baseline information about coagulation/lysis activity. With placental abruption, the problem is very obvious, because of massive bleeding and the physical finding of a tense uterus. In those cases when many other concomitant medical problems require immediate attention, as with septic abortion, coagulation disturbances may easily be overlooked.

TABLE 13-4

Clinical conditions with associated coagulation disorders

Abruptio placentae

Amniotic fluid embolus

Dead fetus syndrome

Eclampsia/severe preeclampsia

Gestational sepsis/shock

Gestational trophoblastic disease

Hypovolemic shock

Incompatible blood transfusion

Massive transfusions

Placenta accreta

Saline abortion

Uterine rupture

THE THREAT OF DIC

The pathophysiology of disseminated intravascular coagulation (DIC) consists of nearly simultaneous uncontrolled activation of procoagulants and fibrinolytic enzymes in the microvasculature.[11] The process depletes platelets and procoagulants. Plasmin (fibrinolysis) is elevated, leading to further digestion of fibrin clots, which releases FDPs and inhibits polymerization.

The process may be initiated by activation of either the extrinsic or the intrinsic clotting system. The placenta is an extremely rich source of thromboplastin, and when infarct or separation damages it, the extrinsic pathway may be activated. Leukocytes may release thromboplastin and stimulate the extrinsic system, while endotoxins and immunologic vasculitis stimulate the intrinsic system. Once the DIC process begins, the consumable fraction—fibrinogen, factors V, VIII, and XIII, and platelets—may be severely depleted. The fibrinolytic mechanism is secondarily activated, leading to the elevation of fibrin split products. When fibrin is deposited on blood vessel walls, a microangiopathic hemolytic anemia may result. This is rare, but may occasionally accompany severe preeclampsia-eclampsia, when there is liver involvement. The clinical presentation is confusing and may lead to misdiagnosis until the condition becomes fully manifest.[12] This recently defined syndrome includes hemolysis (H), elevated liver enzymes (EL), and low platelet count (LP). HELLP may be confused with other clinical problems, but still is related to preeclampsia-eclampsia and requires aggressive management and delivery.[13]

Laboratory findings that confirm the presence of a coagulopathy are listed in Table 13-5. Thrombocytopenia, followed by rapid changes in other parameters, may be the first sign of a coagulopathy. Falling fibrinogen levels are an early indicator of a developing coagulopathy, as are declining antithrombin III levels. The protamine paracoagulation test,

---

TABLE 13-5

Laboratory findings in DIC

Platelet count	Decreased
Fibrinogen	Decreased
Prothrombin time	Prolonged
Partial thromboplastin time	Prolonged
Fibrin/fibrinogen degradation products	Increased
Protamine paracoagulation test	Positive

based on excessive action of thrombin on fibrinogen, points up excess clotting, another early means of detecting a developing coagulopathy. This test is positive when there is a large clot, as in deep vein thrombosis or disseminated coagulopathy in the microvasculature. The presence of FDPs persists for some 24 to 48 hours after the coagulopathy has been terminated, and is not a good indicator of active DIC. All these changes reinforce the need for early baseline values to determine developing trends before the consequences are beyond repair.

STEP-BY-STEP THERAPY

The first step in managing a coagulopathy is to stabilize the patient's clinical condition while replacing depleted coagulation factors. Many times, therapy must be initiated before the full extent of the coagulopathy is determined. It's essential to maintain stable vital signs and good urine output during the first critical 1 to 2 hours of therapy.

Institute appropriate use of blood component therapy as soon as possible. The agents supplied by the principal components are listed in Table 13-6.

Massive transfusion (greater than 3 liters), especially with whole blood, will aggravate an already disturbed coagulation system by further depleting platelets, factor V, and factor VIII. Transfusing sufficient fresh frozen plasma (FFP) will mitigate the depleting of these coagulation factors. Whole blood cannot be looked upon as a satisfactory source of platelets because 50% of platelet function will be lost within 72

TABLE 13-6

Component replacement

FACTOR	VOLUME (mL)*	SUPPLIES
Platelet concentrate	40-60	Increased count of viable platelets— by 25,000-35,000
Cryoprecipitate	30-50	Fibrinogen Factors VIII, XIII (3-10 times the equivalent volume of plasma)
Fresh frozen plasma	200	All factors except platelets; 1 gm fibrinogen
Packed RBC	200	Hematocrit 60% to 65%
Fibrinogen†	300	Increased fibrinogen (1-2 gm)

*Depends on local blood bank service.
†Not available in the US.

hours. However, whole blood that is 6 to 12 hours donor fresh is an ideal replacement. In most circumstances, this is unavailable. Fresh frozen plasma offers a satisfactory way of replacing coagulation factors, including fibrinogen. One unit of FFP should be given for each 2 units of blood after 6 units are transfused.

Pooled fibrinogen carries an extremely high risk of transmitting hepatitis. The acute administration of 4 gm of fibrinogen would raise the plasma concentration about 100 mg/dL. The same results can be achieved by administering 15 to 20 bags of cryoprecipitate, even though the content of fibrinogen in cryoprecipitate varies considerably from bag to bag.

In most ob/gyn conditions, alleviation of the primary problem, by delivery or evacuation of the septic uterus, enables the endogenous stores of platelets to restore essential requirements to the circulation and obviates the need for using pooled platelet-rich concentrates, which, like pooled fibrinogen, carry a significant hepatitis risk.

Most clinical mistakes stem from failure to appreciate the magnitude of the problem. Personal contact must be made with the blood bank, as 10 to 20 units of blood, 10 to 15 units of FFP, and 70 to 100 units of cryoprecipitate may be necessary to manage a fulminant coagulopathy. Depleted plasma volume can be ascertained with central venous or Swan-Ganz monitoring. Urinary output is critical, as renal failure is a recognized consequence of coagulation disorders.

Uterine bleeding is best controlled by evacuation of the contents. Occasionally, further bleeding may result from fibrinolytic activity at the placental site. Only very rarely is there need to employ antifibrinolytic agents such as ε-aminocaproic acid.[14]

Once delivery is accomplished, the coagulation factors will often become close to normal within 24 hours. The platelet count generally takes several days to return to laboratory norms, but bleeding will be unlikely if the count exceeds 20,000 to 30,000/cu mm.

CLINICAL CONDITIONS

On the ob/gyn service, the most common clinical problem associated with coagulation failure is abruptio placentae. The overall incidence of this condition is 1:120 deliveries (0.83%), and severe coagulopathy occurs in up to 38% of these cases.[15, 16]

With concealed abruption, the critical problem facing the clinician is a uterus that at term may hold nearly 5 liters of blood. This is close to the whole maternal volume, and active management in delivering the fetus—viable or nonviable—is of paramount importance. If the fetus is viable, early cesarean delivery appears to improve fetal survival.[14] At the time of cesarean, you may encounter a Couvelaire uterus with blood extravasated into the myometrium. Judicious use of oxytocics, prostaglandins, or ergots allows for reasonable contractility, and no further intervention is warranted.

Attempts to modify the coagulation mechanism by the use of heparin, as has been recommended, should be condemned. There is practically no occasion, especially with placental abruption, when heparin therapy is helpful in managing a fulminant coagulopathy. The one exception is with a death in utero—a complication rarely encountered today. Aggressive management and delivery, using prostaglandin induction, is the usual treatment of the dead fetus syndrome. Within 3 weeks, spontaneous labor occurs in 75% of cases.[17] If there is a developing coagulopathy in this chronic situation, the administration of low-dose heparin (1,000 units/hour) will modify the aberrations in platelets and fibrinogen and allow for orderly induction of labor. This is possibly the only instance in which heparin therapy has any role in the treatment of a coagulopathy.

Severe preeclampsia and eclampsia have been associated with coagulation abnormalities, but in most cases the problem is not severe. Pritchard and co-workers found thrombocytopenia (fewer than 150,000 platelets/cu mm) in 29% of a series of 95 eclamptics.[18] However, only 3% had a serious condition (<50,000/cu mm). Other investigators have noted changes in platelet count as early as the second trimester in patients destined to develop severe preeclampsia, and believe that this may be an early and critical feature of the disorder.[19] The cause of these changes is unclear. It has also been suggested that mild chronic DIC may exist with preeclampsia and form the basis for placental insufficiency and subsequent growth retardation.[20]

In several cases of such impending gestosis, Goodlin and Holdt noted significant thrombocytopenia unassociated with either an immune disorder or a subsequent fulminant coagulopathy.[21] Therefore, while fulminant coagulopathy is unlikely with the preeclampsia-eclampsia syndrome, you should be aware of this possibility. Roberts and May reported a 2.6% incidence of this clinical finding among severe preeclamptics.[22] When a coagulopathy is present in the preeclampsia-eclampsia syndrome, delivery is the necessary treatment. Even with appropriate component replacement, thrombocytopenia may take several days to resolve, but rarely requires platelet transfusion.

REFERENCES

1. Henry JB, ed: *Todd-Sanford-Davidsohn Clinical Diagnosis and Management by Laboratory Methods*, ed 16. Philadelphia, WB Saunders, 1979

2. Hathaway WE, Bonnar J: *Perinatal Coagulation*. New York, Grune & Stratton, 1978

3. Graeff H, Kuhn W: *Coagulation disorders in Obstetrics*, vol 13 of Friedman EA, ed: *Major Problems in Obstetrics and Gynecology Series*. Philadelphia, WB Saunders, 1980

4. Davey FR: Blood vessels and hemostasis. In Henry JB, ed: *Todd-Sanford-Davidsohn Clinical Diagnosis and Management by Laboratory Methods*, ed 16. Philadelphia, WB Saunders, 1979, p 1101

5. Davey FR: Platelets and platelet disorders. Ibid, p 1109

6. Davey FR: Blood coagulation and its disorders. Ibid, p 1131

7. Fenton V, Saunders K, Cavill I: The platelet count in pregnancy. J Clin Pathol 30:68, 1977

8. Pitkin RM, Witte DL: Platelet and leukocyte counts in pregnancy. JAMA 242:2696, 1979

9. Sejeny SA, Eastham RD, Baker SR: Platelet counts during normal pregnancy. J Clin Pathol 28:812, 1975

10. Arocha Piñango CL, Linares J, Cova A, et al: Intravascular coagulation in obstetrics: Serial dilution protamine sulfate test throughout labor. Am J Obstet Gynecol 124:18, 1976

11. Bonnar J, McNichol GP, Douglas AS: Fibrinolytic enzyme system and pregnancy. Br Med J 3:387, 1969

12. Killam AP, Dillard SH, Patton RC, et al: Pregnancy-induced hypertension complicated by acute liver disease and disseminated intravascular coagulation. Am J Obstet Gynecol 123:823, 1975

13. Weinstein L: Syndrome of hemolysis, elevated liver enzymes and low platelet count. Am J Obstet Gynecol 142:159, 1982

14. Beller FK, Glas H, Roemer H: Fibrinolysis as the cause of obstetrical hemorrhage. Am J Obstet Gynecol 82:620, 1961

15. Knab DR: Abruptio placentae. Obstet Gynecol 52:625, 1978

16. Kitay DZ: Bleeding disorders in pregnancy. Contemp Ob/Gyn 7(1):87, January 1976

17. Tricomi V, Kohl SG: Fetal death in utero. Am J Obstet Gynecol 74:1092, 1957

18. Pritchard JA, Cunningham FG, Mason RA: Coagulation changes in eclampsia. Am J Obstet Gynecol 124:855, 1976

19. Redman CWG, Bonnar J, Beilin L: Early platelet consumption in pre-eclampsia. Br Med J 1:467, 1978

20. Trudinger BJ: Platelets and intrauterine growth retardation in preeclampsia. Br J Obstet Gynecol 83:284, 1976

21. Goodlin RC, Holdt D: Impending gestosis. Obstet Gynecol 58:743, 1981

22. Roberts JM, May WJ: Consumptive coagulopathy in severe preeclampsia. Obstet Gynecol 48:163, 1976

14

Fetal Bradycardia

EDWARD J. QUILLIGAN, MD

CLINICAL SIGNIFICANCE: Decreased oxygenation of the fetus is often signaled by bradycardia. Continuous fetal heart rate (FHR) monitoring, backed up by scalp blood sampling when available, will help determine whether to wait or deliver. When pH is unknown, deliver when the FHR pattern shows severe variable or late decelerations.

There is ample evidence that bradycardia is frequently associated with decreased oxygenation of the fetus.[1, 2] But which episodes of bradycardia are associated with how much hypoxia, and what is the best way to manage suspected hypoxia? In general, the following conditions indicate increased fetal hypoxia: baseline tachycardia, when the mother has no fever; decreased FHR variability, when the mother hasn't been given drugs; and meconium staining of the amniotic fluid.

BASIC GUIDELINES

Benson and others found a high false-negative rate for the traditional indicator of fetal distress—any auscultated heart rate decrease below 100 beats per minute (bpm), lasting beyond a uterine contraction.[3] Hon placed the diagnosis of fetal distress on a firmer footing when he described the periodic changes in FHR associated with uterine contractions.[4] He classified decelerations as early, late, or variable—according to their onset in relation to the onset of the uterine contraction—and characterized their waveforms. Early and late decelerations are reverse images of the contraction waveform, with a slow decrease and recovery, and variable deceleration has a rapid descent and recovery. When this analysis is used, head compression seems associated with early deceleration, uteroplacental insufficiency with late deceleration, and umbilical cord compression with variable deceleration (Figure 14-1).

Caldeyro-Barcia's group in Montevideo combined early and early variable decelerations into the type I dip, and late plus late variable decelerations into the type II dip.[5] Late decelerations, severe variable decelerations, and type II dips are potentially ominous because these patterns have been associated with a decrease in fetal arterial oxygen tension. The clinical significance of these patterns is modified by the baseline FHR, the variability of FHR, and meconium staining.

MANAGING SPECIFIC CASES OF BRADYCARDIA

The studies of Haverkamp and co-workers raised doubts about the value of continuous fetal heart rate monitoring for predicting the baby's condition.[6, 7] But we find the technique valuable, especially when backed up with blood sampling.

FIGURE 14-1

---

*Classifying FHR decelerations**

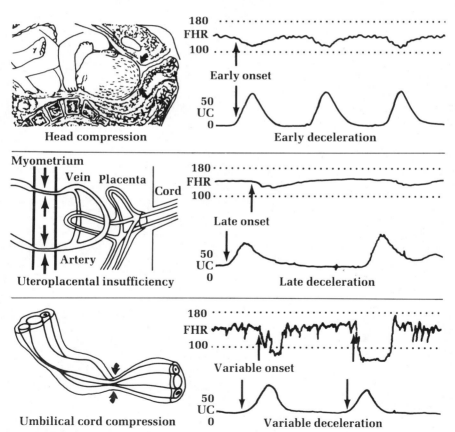

Head compression — Early deceleration

Uteroplacental insufficiency — Late deceleration

Umbilical cord compression — Variable deceleration

*Adapted from Hon.[4]

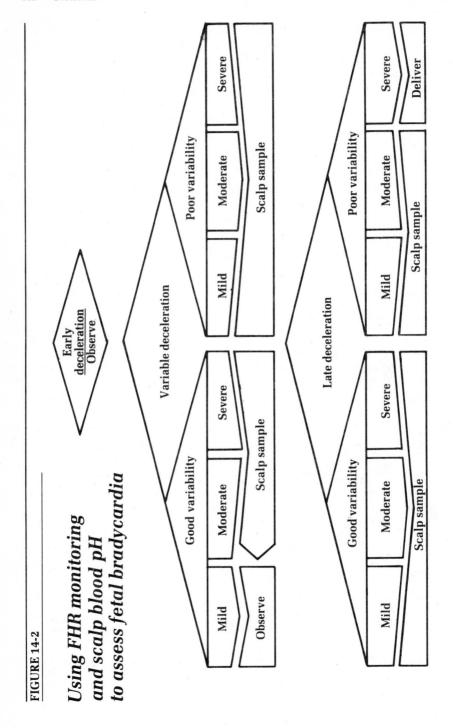

FIGURE 14-2

Using FHR monitoring and scalp blood pH to assess fetal bradycardia

When fetal scalp blood sampling facilities are available, follow the monitoring protocol shown in Figure 14-2. When ominous patterns are present, give the mother 100% oxygen by mask and change her position to right or left lateral (or dorsal), depending on the position she was in when the deceleration was picked up. Correct any factors that may be responsible for reduced uterine blood flow. If the mother is receiving oxytocin and the uterine contractions are too frequent, stop the drug. If she becomes hypotensive following conduction anesthesia, give 500 to 1,000 mL lactated Ringer's solution, put her in a lateral position, and give 25 mg ephedrine if the blood pressure remains low.

If a normal pattern results, carefully observe the patient for further changes, but obtain a fetal scalp sample if the deceleration pattern persists. If the pattern is one of severe late deceleration (FHR <80 bpm) without variability, proceed to immediate delivery.

If the scalp sample indicates pH is greater than 7.25, continue to observe unless the FHR pattern worsens—for example, if mild late decelerations become moderate late decelerations. Take another sample 30 minutes later, unless the FHR has returned to normal. If a more ominous pattern develops, obtain scalp blood immediately and deliver the infant if the pH has decreased.

If the pH is 7.20 to 7.25, take another scalp sample in 15 minutes and deliver the baby if the pH is going down. If the initial pH is less than 7.20, deliver immediately. Sampling is useful if the FHR pattern is unclear or if there is no variability, even without ominous decelerations.

When scalp sampling is not available or not feasible, you must follow a different protocol, depending on whether fetal monitoring is external (Figure 14-3) or internal (Figure 14-4). When the pattern is ominous, internal fetal monitoring with a scalp electrode is always preferable but occasionally impractical if the cervix is not dilated. When mild or moderate late deceleration with poor variability, thick meconium, or baseline tachycardia is present, a 30-minute observation period is recommended. During this time, prepare for delivery by cesarean section.

The differences between the two approaches outlined in Figures 14-3 and 14-4 reflect the fact that FHR variability cannot yet be accurately assessed using only an external transducer. A general rule to follow is to err on the side of overdiagnosing fetal distress when the FHR pattern is confusing and scalp sampling is not feasible.

Sometimes, the fetus develops a bradycardia that lasts more than 2 minutes and that begins like a variable deceleration but does not return to baseline. In such cases, move to the delivery/section room and be prepared for an emergency delivery unless the FHR returns to normal within 5 minutes. Three or more decelerations of this type call for delivery. Although the baby is usually well at the time of delivery, there have been some deaths.

FIGURE 14-3

*Using FHR monitoring with
an external transducer
to assess fetal bradycardia*

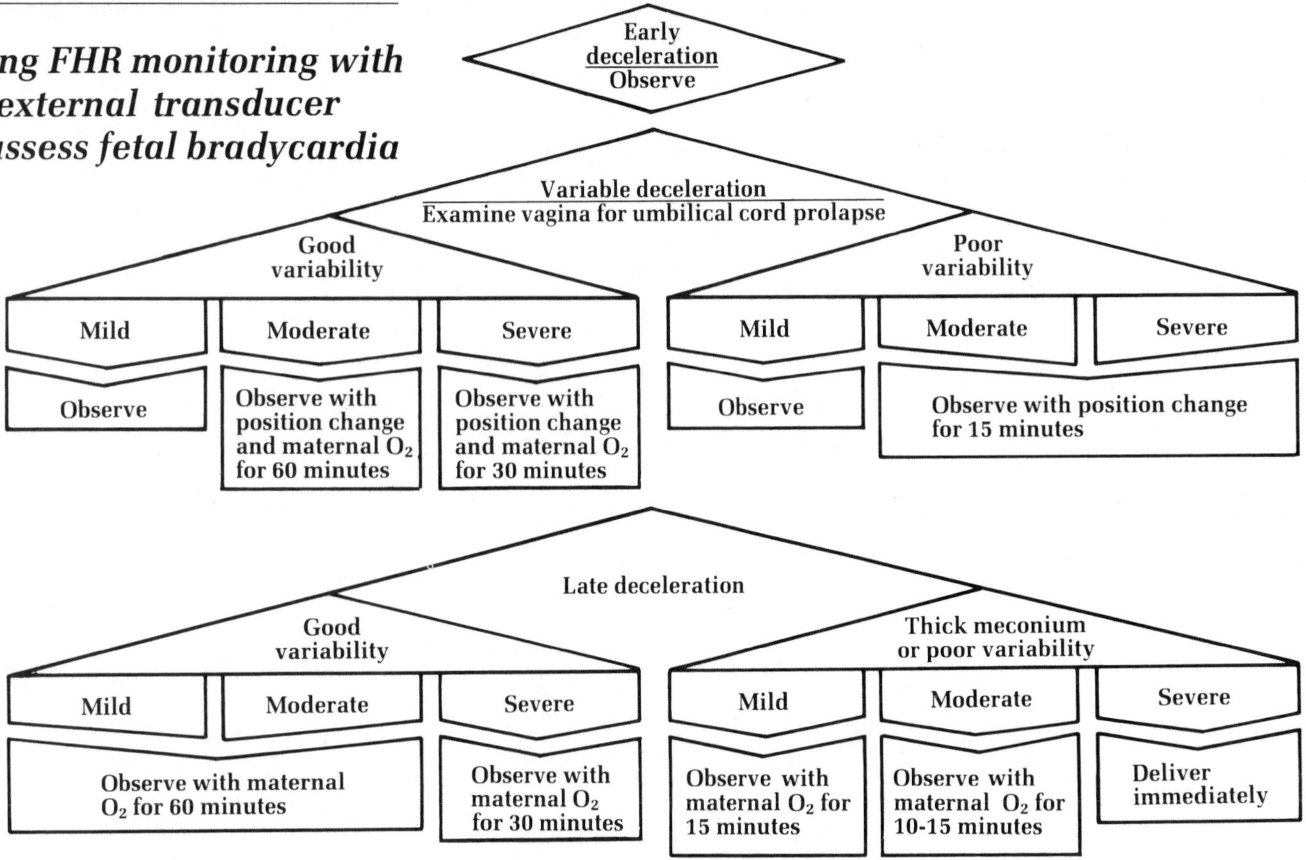

Early deceleration
Observe

Variable deceleration
Examine vagina for umbilical cord prolapse

Good variability

Mild — Observe

Moderate — Observe with position change and maternal O_2 for 60 minutes

Severe — Observe with position change and maternal O_2 for 30 minutes

Poor variability

Mild — Observe

Moderate — Observe with position change for 15 minutes

Severe

Late deceleration

Good variability

Mild — Observe with maternal O_2 for 60 minutes

Moderate

Severe — Observe with maternal O_2 for 30 minutes

Thick meconium or poor variability

Mild — Observe with maternal O_2 for 15 minutes

Moderate — Observe with maternal O_2 for 10-15 minutes

Severe — Deliver immediately

FIGURE 14-4

Using FHR monitoring with a scalp electrode to assess fetal bradycardia

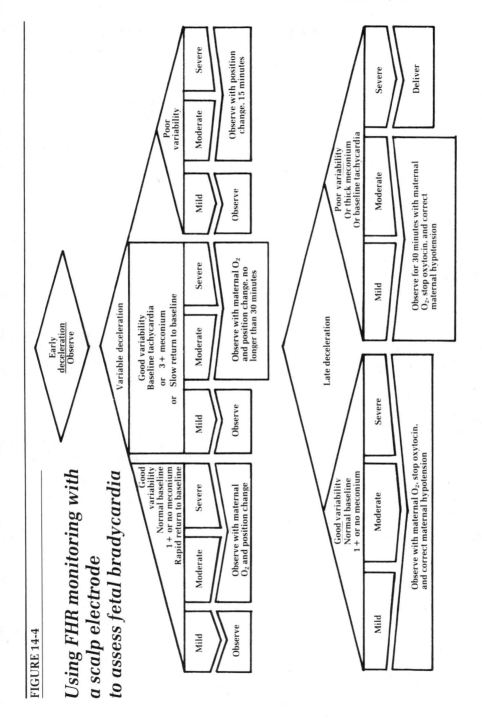

For prolonged bradycardia following paracervical block anesthesia, give the mother oxygen to breathe (100% at 5 liters/minute). Don't begin delivery until the FHR has returned to normal for 15 to 20 minutes.

Continuous baseline bradycardia (<100 bpm) occasionally occurs with fetal heart block. You can distinguish this pattern from a maternal heart rate that is being picked up through a dead fetus if you record fetal and maternal ECGs or count maternal and fetal rates simultaneously. If a true fetal heart block is present, as demonstrated by lack of P waves in the fetal ECG, don't treat until after delivery. Occasionally, the fetus will develop a terminal baseline bradycardia associated with a flat FHR. In such a case, you should deliver immediately.

REFERENCES

1. Myers RE, Mueller-Heubach E, Adamsons K: Predictability of the state of fetal oxygenation from a quantitative analysis of the components of late deceleration. Am J Obstet Gynecol 115:1083, 1973

2. Kubli FW, Hon EH, Khazin AF, et al: Observations on fetal heart rate and pH in the human fetus during labor. Am J Obstet Gynecol 104:1190, 1969

3. Benson RC, Shubeck F, Deutschberger J, et al: Fetal heart rate as a predictor of fetal distress. A report from the collaborative project. Obstet Gynecol 32:259, 1968

4. Hon EH: Observations on pathologic fetal bradycardia. Am J Obstet Gynecol 77:1084, 1959

5. Schwarcz RL, Belizan JM, Cifuerites JR, et al: Fetal and maternal monitoring in spontaneous labors and in elective inductions. Am J Obstet Gynecol 120:356, 1974

6. Haverkamp AD, Thompson HE, McFee JG, et al: The evaluation of continuous fetal heart rate monitoring in high risk pregnancy. Am J Obstet Gynecol 125:310, 1976

7. Haverkamp AD, Orleans M, Langendoerfer S, et al: A controlled trial of the differential effects of intrapartum monitoring. Am J Obstet Gynecol 134:399, 1979

15

Fetal and Neonatal Anemias

MARTIN L. GIMOVSKY, MD, and
BARRY S. SCHIFRIN, MD

CLINICAL SIGNIFICANCE: Up to 5% of term and 20% of preterm babies are anemic at birth. Often FHR patterns are the first clue to the condition. In severe anemia, FHR may show a sinusoidal pattern that reverts to normal after uterine transfusion. Less severe anemia may be manifested by baseline tachycardia and late decelerations.

Though anemia may be life-threatening to the fetus or newborn, obvious clues to its presence are few. Generally it is suspected only in cases of maternal Rh isoimmunization. Indicators of fetal anemia are rare. Many hydropic fetuses have an accompanying polyhydramnios, but usually this is not severe. Rarely, the mother of the hydropic fetus will manifest "pseudotoxemia" or "mirror syndrome," characterized by modest hypertension and generalized edema. Until recently, the less common causes have not been amenable to antenatal diagnosis (Table 15-1). We tend to dismiss most vaginal hemorrhage as maternal in origin, and it therefore is rarely a useful clue.

Diagnosing anemia in utero was once a formidable task. Today, ultrasound, electronic fetal monitoring, and fetal blood and tissue sampling have enhanced antenatal detection of anemia as well as of anomalies, intrauterine growth retardation (IUGR), and asphyxia.

The consequences of fetal anemia depend on rate of blood loss as well as underlying cause. Acute blood loss during labor and delivery may produce shock, myocardial infarction, and perinatal death. If chronic, anemia may lead to the syndrome of hydrops fetalis, with extramedullary hematopoiesis, IUGR, and death. In twin-twin transfusion syndrome, one infant may have polycythemia, plethora, and congestive heart failure while the other has severe anemia and IUGR.

Hemolytic anemias due to Rh disease or infection cause excessive production of bilirubin, which may overwhelm the mother's placental transport or the newborn's limited metabolic capabilities. Debilitating kernicterus results. Although maternal hemoglobinopathy dramatically increases fetal wastage, these babies are rarely anemic. Mothers with a structural problem in hemoglobin synthesis, such as homozygous α-thalassemia, don't have anemic babies, but impaired oxygen release results in fetal hydrops, distress, and stillbirth, or early neonatal death.[1]

TABLE 15-1

Causes of fetal/neonatal anemia

Blood loss
Amniocentesis
Cephalohematoma
Cesarean section
External version
Intrafetal hemorrhage: CNS, pulmonary, visceral
Placenta previa or abruptio placentae
Twin-twin transfusion
Umbilical cord
    Rupture
    Varix
    Aneurysm or hematoma

Hemolysis
Immune
    Isoimmune
        Rh, ABO, minor groups
        Drugs
    Autoimmune
        Viral, ?collagen vascular diseases
Nonimmune
    α-Chain structural anomalies
    α-Thalassemia
    Coarctation of the aorta
    Hemangioma
    Large-vessel thrombi
    RBC enzyme deficiencies
    RBC membrane disorders
    Renal artery stenosis
    Sepsis
    Syphilis
    ?CMV, rubella, herpes
    ?Hypersplenism

Hypoplasia
Congenital hypoplasia

DIAGNOSING FETAL ANEMIA

How useful a particular surveillance technique is depends on the type and severity of the anemia. In severe anemia, the fetal heart rate tracing may demonstrate a sinusoidal pattern. This poorly understood pattern may signal numerous conditions, but finding it should spur efforts to rule out anemia. If a diagnosis of fetal anemia is made, the prognosis is grave unless treatment is begun promptly.[2] The sinusoidal pattern may revert to a normal FHR pattern following successful completion of intrauterine transfusion.

Less severe anemia may show up as baseline tachycardia and late decelerations. Indeed, these FHR patterns may be the first clue to the condition. Acute fetal exsanguination produces abrupt, prolonged decelerations, punctuated by transient acceleration.

During labor, even severely anemic babies may have a normal pH at the outset; but as labor progresses, deterioration may be rapid. Fetal scalp sampling not only provides clues to fetal acid-base status but also permits hematocrit determination to confirm the diagnosis.

Ultrasound may help document the source of acute hemorrhage by locating both cord and placenta. Premature separation of the placenta is difficult to pick up, even sonographically. Ultrasound is far more useful in identifying chronic anemia and its consequences—the hydropic fetus. Effusions and dilation of the umbilical vein are early signs of incipient hydrops visible on ultrasound. M-mode scanning of the fetal heart provides insight into cardiac dynamics, severity of the hemodynamic problem, and potential for recovery.[3]

When erythroblastosis fetalis is suspected, the most widely employed diagnostic technique is the study of amniotic bilirubin levels. Understanding the relationship between hemolysis, ΔOD, and neonatal survival is the keystone.[4] Rh problems account for 90% to 95% of all isoimmune fetal hemolytic anemias. Other blood group antigens, such as Kell and Duffy, occasionally cause severe anemia in the hydropic fetus. Because of the prevalence of the Rh problem and the infrequency of the others, all are managed as Rh incompatibility. It should be noted that the original management schemes, which emphasized timing of the intrauterine transfusion and delivery, were developed before the L/S ratio and real-time ultrasound became available.

Direct visualization and study of the midtrimester fetus represents one of the frontiers of prenatal diagnosis. Blood samples from the placenta obtained by direct aspiration through the fetoscope have already been applied to the prenatal detection of severe hemoglobinopathies. Sickle cell disorders may be identified by separation of hemoglobins S (HbS) and A (HbA) on carboxymethyl cellulose columns. The diagnosis of β-thalassemia depends on quantitative differences in β-chain production after incubation of the sample with tritiated leucine.[5]

TESTS OF FETOMATERNAL TRANSFUSION

The Apt test. In 1953, Apt and Downey described a method of differentiating adult from fetal hemoglobin (HbF), based on the differing resistance of HbF and HbA to denaturation with alkali.[6] In an alkaline solution (0.25 N sodium hydroxide), adult hemoglobin changes from pink to brown-yellow over a 2-minute interval, while fetal hemoglobin remains pink. We recommend an Apt test, when practical, in all cases of third-trimester bleeding.

Kleihauer-Betke test. This test may be performed on a fixed blood smear to differentiate HbA from HbF.[7] When a citrate-phosphate buffer (pH 3.3 to 3.4) is washed over the slide, it elutes HbA, leaving red cell ghosts, while RBCs containing HbF remain intact. The technique permits a quantitative assessment of fetomaternal hemorrhage.

Clayton and colleagues used the Kleihauer-Betke test to show a correlation between evidence of fetal hemoglobin and poor fetal outcome in women with third-trimester bleeding.[8] Detection of fetal bleeding mandates intensive fetal surveillance and, in many cases, prompt delivery. When the test fails to detect any fetal hemoglobin, a more conservative approach may be taken with glucocorticoids to hasten lung maturation and tocolysis when indicated.

BLOOD LOSS DURING LABOR

The blood volume of the term infant is approximately 80 to 100 mL/kg, or 240 to 300 mL. At delivery, the average maternal blood loss is 500 mL—about twice the entire fetal volume. At cesarean section, maternal blood loss is approximately 1,000 to 1,500 mL. When the indication for intervention is third-trimester bleeding, maternal blood loss is likely to be greater. Thus, maternal bleeding may obscure significant fetal blood loss. In the adult, loss of 30% of the total circulating blood volume (about 1,500 mL in the gravida at term) may precipitate shock.[9] In the fetus, the same degree of hemorrhage would amount to only 72 mL of blood. Even at the relatively low pressures in the fetal cardiovascular system, such a loss may occur in a relatively short time.

The rupture of a normal umbilical cord, with cord entanglement, a precipitous delivery, or an unattended birth may result in serious fetal hemorrhage. Abnormalities of the cord and vessels—varices, aneurysms, velamentous insertion, communications between succenturiate lobes, short cord, and vasa previa—may produce the same adverse results.[10, 11] Unfortunately, these abnormalities are unlikely to be recognized antepartum. If you suspect vasa previa, examine the membranes by amnioscopy at double setup before rupture of membranes.

Cesarean section poses potential hematologic hazards to the fetus.[12] An anterior placenta may be lacerated when the uterus is incised. Expeditious clamping of the cord, even before the baby is delivered, may prevent blood loss. During vaginal delivery, the timing of cord clamping may also have a considerable effect on the baby's blood volume. Usher and colleagues found that a 5-minute delay in cord clamping, with the baby held at the level of the introitus, increased newborn blood volume by 61%, compared with those clamped immediately.[13] About 25% of the total transfusion occurred within 15 seconds, and 50% within 1 minute, but fully half the increase occurred well after the time when the cord is usually clamped. If the baby is held above the mother before clamping, neonatal blood volume may be significantly reduced. At delivery, take care to avoid stretching the cord. Clamping should be done immediately when the fetus is plethoric or anemic as well as at cesarean section. The effect of early clamping when the fetus is premature has not yet been settled. Bear in mind that the second monozygous twin may hemorrhage through the unclamped cord of the delivered twin. When delivering monozygous twins, clamp or ligate both ends of the severed cord promptly.

Fetal bleeding may accompany any form of placenta previa, producing an incidence of newborn anemia as high as 30%. Cotton and colleagues reported that fetal anemia was 10 times as frequent when cesarean was done during an acute hemorrhage as when elective cesarean was done before a second episode of bleeding.[14] Hemorrhage from placental abruption, whether the hemorrhage is concealed or overt, may occasionally include fetal blood. Among neonates who survived abruption, Golditch and Boyce found a 4% incidence of anemia.[15]

AMNIOCENTESIS AND VERSION

The fetal viscera or the umbilical vessels may be lacerated during amniocentesis.[16] The procedure may also initiate retroplacental bleeding, causing premature separation of the placenta. Using ultrasound with amniocentesis has dramatically lessened fetomaternal bleeding that results in isoimmunization. As in third-trimester bleeding, the Apt test helps identify the source of hemoglobin when amniocentesis is complicated by a bloody tap. If the test suggests the source of the blood is maternal, and if there is the potential for isoimmunization, give RhoGAM. If the source is fetal, electronic fetal monitoring and real-time B-scan are necessary. Immediate delivery may sometimes be required; the fetus may already have exsanguinated.

External cephalic version used to be considered a cause of cord laceration, premature placental separation, or fetomaternal bleeding in up to 25% of the procedures. These problems may have been caused by excessive force or by the use of adjuvant general anesthesia. Newer techniques, involving tocolytic agents and total avoidance of anesthesia, have lessened the risk of fetomaternal bleeding. Van Dorsten and colleagues reported only a 4% incidence (1:25) of positive Kleihauer-Betke (K-B) tests following version.[17] A follow-up report, on over 100 patients, found less than a 1% incidence of positive K-B tests.[18]

TRAUMA DURING DELIVERY

Internal or external bleeding may be produced by injury of the fetus during delivery. The head is one of the most common sites of injury. The cephalohematoma is frequently associated with midforceps procedures (incidences as high as 33%) but complicates normal deliveries as well. In fact, these injuries occur in approximately 1% of all deliveries—most frequently among male infants of primigravidas. The bleeding is subperiosteal and does not cross suture lines. Birth trauma may

---

TABLE 15-2

Differential diagnosis in hydrops fetalis

Cardiac
Atrial myxoma
A-V malformation
Cardiac anomalies
Dysrhythmias
  Atrial tachycardia
  Heart block
Premature closure of ductus venosus
Premature closure of foramen ovale

Hypoproteinemia
Hepatic
Renal

Infection
Cytomegalovirus
Syphilis
Toxoplasmosis

Other
Achondroplasia
Chagas' disease
Choriocarcinoma
Cystic adenomatoid malformation of the lung
Diabetes
Diaphragmatic hernia
Gaucher's disease
Neuroblastoma
Parabiosis
Pulmonary lymphangiectasis
Sacral teratoma

also cause intracranial or intrapulmonary bleeding, or bleeding secondary to ruptured viscera. Such bleeds, especially adrenal, may pose a difficult diagnostic problem. Abdominal distention and shock or anemia may be clues to intra-abdominal injury. The liver is the organ most frequently injured. Ultrasound scanning of the neonatal abdomen may prove helpful. Real-time ultrasound scanning of the neonate's brain is a useful tool in diagnosing intracranial hemorrhage (ICH).[19]

Breech deliveries, whether by the vaginal route or cesarean section, as well as fetal macrosomia, low birth weight, and difficult or precipitous deliveries are all associated with an increased risk of ICH. In the term infant, ICH has received only scant attention, but the risk may be greater than previously appreciated. Maternal drugs, such as aspirin, warfarin, phenytoin, and barbiturates may predispose to nontraumatic fetal bleeding.[20] We have seen two patients receiving phenytoin for seizure disorders whose fetuses had significant hemorrhages after scalp sampling.[21] In the first patient, we controlled the bleeding by applying a silver clip through a vaginal endoscope. In the second case, the bleeding point was difficult to isolate, hemostatic agents failed to control bleeding, and cesarean section was necessary. Acute blood loss and potential for glial laceration from scalp sampling have been reported. Traumatic removal of scalp electrodes has also resulted in significant hemorrhage. Hydrops fetalis, which may accompany chronic anemia, has a wide spectrum of causes (Table 15-2).

Fetus-to-fetus transfusion, which may affect up to 15% of all monochorionic twins, carries potential risks for both twins. Differences in hemoglobin greater than 5 gm/dL are considered diagnostic of twin-twin transfusion syndrome. Their other problems include asymmetrical growth retardation and the risk of distress and death in utero. Serial ultrasound evaluation of growth has been increasingly employed in multiple gestations to make this diagnosis antepartum.

IMMUNE HEMOLYSIS

Isoimmunization, produced by Rh antibody and resulting in the syndrome of erythroblastosis fetalis, is the classic example of fetal and neonatal anemia. Although fetal cells can be demonstrated in the maternal circulation as early as 3 months' gestation, the greatest transfer of red cells occurs in the third trimester, especially during labor and delivery. In most cases, the transfusion is slight, but in approximately 1% of pregnancies more than 40 mL enters the maternal circulation. In the case of Rh incompatibility, Queenan estimated that as little as 0.25 mL of RBCs may represent sufficient antigen to elicit an antibody response.[4] While this amount is unlikely to cause a primary immune response, repeated exposure to even relatively small amounts of antigen can elicit an amnestic response.

In a first Rh-incompatible pregnancy, the risk of sensitization is 1% or less, according to Zipursky, et al.[22] Up to 7.5% of mothers who fail to develop antibodies during the first pregnancy will do so within 6 months postpartum; another 7.5% will develop antibodies during the second pregnancy.

The immune response of the Rh-negative mother to the challenge of Rh-positive fetal red cells includes production of IgG (7 S) antibodies. These cross the placenta, bind to fetal RBC surfaces, and initiate attachments to monocytes and macrophages. Complement plays a role in this interaction by opsonizing cells. With hemolysis, unconjugated bilirubin is released and cleared by the placenta. Compensatory hemopoiesis, primarily extramedullary, may supplement RBC production. The newborn's ability to clear bilirubin is limited. Unconjugated (and lipid-soluble) bilirubin above 20 mg/dL in a term infant may exceed the plasma binding capacity, leading to deposit of bilirubin in the CNS. To avert kernicterus, bilirubin is removed by exchange transfusions.

A milder form of hemolytic disease is seen with ABO incompatibility (Table 15-3). Unlike Rh isoimmunization, this commonly develops in first pregnancies and is especially likely to affect a fetus that has A or B blood and a group O mother. The spontaneously occurring anti-A and anti-B antibodies of group O mothers are also of the IgG (7 S) class. The anti-A antibodies of group B mothers as well as the anti-B antibodies of group A mothers, which are predominantly of the IgM (19 S) class, do not cross the placenta. Lesser amounts of these antibodies belong to the IgA and IgG classes. However, even an IgG antibody response to ABO

TABLE 15-3

Comparison of Rh and ABO incompatibility

	Rh	ABO
Mother	Negative	Type O
Infant	Positive	A or B
Antibody	IgG	IgG, IgM, IgA
Risk in first pregnancy	5%	40% to 50%
Severity increases in later pregnancies	Usually	Rarely
Anemia	Severe	Mild
Coombs test	3 to 4 +	0 to 1 +
Hydrops	Frequent	Rare

incompatibility does not greatly reduce RBC survival, because the affected fetus has fewer A and B antigenic sites on the RBC surfaces than in Rh disease. Minor blood group antigens, responsible for approximately 2% of isoimmunization cases, vary tremendously in their immunogenicity. For example, 50% of Rh-negative individuals would be expected to be sensitized from a Kell antigen challenge, while fewer than 0.05% will be sensitized by Duffy or Kidd antigens. Hemolysis in utero elevates bilirubin pigments in amniotic fluid, and the amount of bilirubin present predicts neonatal outcome.

Do serial amniocenteses to follow the hemolytic process and to determine whether intervention is needed. Ultrasound helps delineate the anatomic changes that accompany severe hemolysis, pericardial and pleural effusions, fetal ascites, placental enlargement, scalp edema, and polyhydramnios. In addition, ultrasound is invaluable when intrauterine transfusion is indicated.

When certain drugs bind with maternal proteins and function as haptens, a less common form of immune hemolytic anemia may result. α-Methyldopa, L-dopa, mefenamic acid, insulin, quinine, certain sulfonamides, and antihistamines have been implicated.

NONIMMUNE HEMOLYSIS

Infection may cause hemolysis of normal fetal RBCs. Abnormal RBCs and membrane and enzyme defects may cause the hemolytic process to accelerate.

Malaria is the most common cause of hemolytic anemia, worldwide. When RBCs are parasitized by *Plasmodium falciparum*, their osmotic fragility increases, with consequent decrease in survival. Other congenital infections, such as *Clostridium*, toxoplasmosis, syphilis, cytomegalovirus, rubella, herpes, influenza, and Epstein-Barr and Coxsackie viruses, have been linked to hemolytic anemia. Autoimmunity may play a role.

Hemolysis of normal RBCs may be purely mechanical. Turbulent flow may generate forces strong enough to destroy red cells, a phenomenon seen in coarctation of the aorta and diseases of the microcirculation. Finally, hemolytic-uremic syndrome may destroy red cells.

RARE ANEMIAS

Abnormal RBC membranes may result in a nonimmune hemolytic fetal anemia. Hereditary spherocytosis and glucose 6-phosphate dehydrogenase (G6PD) deficiency are examples. Although hemolysis accompanies G6PD deficiency, several studies support the theory that the condition predisposes to neonatal hyperbilirubinemia.

Other membrane defects—elliptocytosis and stomatocytosis—rarely result in severe neonatal anemia but, as in G6PD deficiency, hyperbilirubinemia is a more common indication for exchange transfusion than is the anemia.

Two forms of thalassemia may cause neonatal anemia. Homozygous α-thalassemia may produce fetal hypoxia in utero. Infants are stillborn or hydropic and moribund. Heterozygous α-thalassemia and homozygous β-thalassemia may produce anemia, but heterozygous β-thalassemia has not been found to do so.

Fetal and neonatal RBCs are especially sensitive to the toxic effects of drugs that are oxidizing agents, a vulnerability ascribed to a relative deficiency of glutathione peroxidase, which is necessary to metabolize hydrogen peroxide.[23] Metabolically, these cells resemble G6PD-deficient RBCs. Vitamin E deficiency has also been causally related to hemolytic anemia on the basis of peroxidation of the lipid components of the red cell membrane. Water-soluble, vitamin K-derived sulfonamides,

---

FIGURE 15-1

Simple laboratory tests in the initial differential diagnosis of neonatal anemia

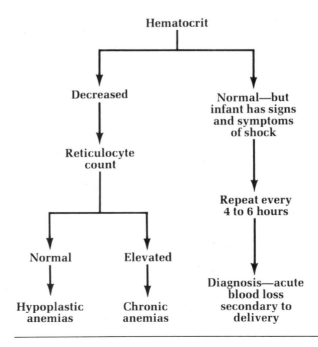

and drugs known to trigger hemolysis in G6PD-deficient individuals, should be avoided during the perinatal period. Once the diagnosis has been made, proceed either to elective abortion or to intensive fetal surveillance.

EVALUATING THE ANEMIC NEWBORN

Begin by reviewing the history of the antecedent pregnancies and the physical findings on the neonatal exams. Most newborn anemias follow blood loss or hemolysis. Whether the blood loss is acute or chronic, or whether one of various causes of hemolysis is implicated, may be inferred from clinical findings and simple laboratory assays: hematocrit, reticulocyte count, Coombs test, and evaluation of the peripheral blood smear (Figure 15-1).

A low hematocrit is the sine qua non for diagnosing anemia. The critical value at which this diagnosis is made depends on gestational age. The hematocrit requires several hours to equilibrate following an acute episode of bleeding, and may not reflect the severity of acute hemorrhage for several hours.

At sea level, 95% of term infants will have a cord blood hemoglobin between 13.7 and 20.1 gm/dL, with a mean of 16.8 gm/dL. Prematurity reduces the level. At 28 weeks, female infants have a mean value of 13.6 gm/dL. Mean RBC values during pregnancy are a function of gestational age as well as sex (Table 15-4).

TABLE 15-4

*Mean red cell values during gestation**

GESTATIONAL AGE (weeks)	HEMOGLOBIN (gm%)	HEMATOCRIT (%)	MEAN CELL VOLUME (μm^3)	RETICULOCYTES (%)
12	8-10	33	180	5-8
16	10	35	140	2-4
20	11	37	135	1
24	14	40	123	1
28	14.5	45	120	0.5
34	15	47	118	0.2
Term cord	16.8	53	107	3-7
Day 1	18.4	58	108	3-7

*Adapted from Oski FA: Hematologic problems. In Avery GB (ed): *Neonatology: Pathophysiology and Management of the Newborn*. Philadelphia, JB Lippincott, 1975, p 380.

The reticulocyte count, corrected for hematocrit, is a functional measurement of RBC production. Elevated values are seen in chronic anemia; decreased values in hypoplastic anemia. Normal values in conjunction with a decreased hematocrit suggest acute blood loss. If the acute loss is recent, the hematocrit and the reticulocyte count may both be normal. Here the clinical signs of pallor, shock, oliguria, and cyanosis may be the only findings.

The Coombs test demonstrates the presence or absence of certain IgG antibodies that cross the placenta and nondestructively attach to the surface of fetal red cells. When such cells are mixed with anti-IgG antibodies, they agglutinate (positive Coombs test). Rh and other minor

---

FIGURE 15-2

*Work-up of Coombs negative anemia**

The presence or absence of jaundice (hyperbilirubinemia) plays a pivotal role in the work-up.

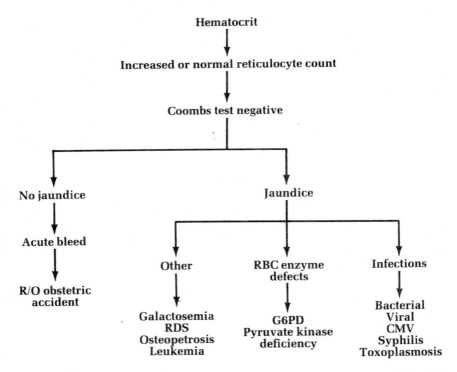

*Adapted from Oski FA, Narman JL: *Hematologic Problems in the Newborn*, ed 2. Philadelphia, WB Saunders Co. 1972.

TABLE 15-5

Signs of anemia

FETAL	NEONATAL
Anomalies	Failure to thrive
Hydrops fetalis	Pallor
IUGR	RDS
Sinusoidal FHR pattern	Sepsis
Positive stress test	Shock
Tachycardia	

blood group antigens such as Kell and Duffy will elicit the necessary IgG response and carry the potential for causing erythroblastosis fetalis.

The peripheral smear should be examined by a physician experienced in the hematology of all types of anemia, especially when reticulocyte counts are normal or elevated and the Coombs test is negative (Figure 15-2).[24] Anemias with characteristic peripheral smears include spherocytosis, elliptocytosis, stomatocytosis, and pyknocytosis. Microcytic and hypochromic cells usually reflect iron deficiency and chronic blood loss, but may also provide clues to hemoglobinopathies (especially thalassemia). If the peripheral smear shows normochromic and normocytic RBCs, proceed to comprehensive physical and laboratory examination and consultation. Determining whether jaundice is present will help you make the diagnosis.

To sum up, the signs of fetal and neonatal anemia are inherently similar and related to the pathophysiologic accompaniments of the anemic state (Table 15-5). The newer modalities—electronic fetal monitoring, ultrasound, and fetal blood sampling—in conjunction with simple laboratory tests to determine the source and cause of bleeding are helping us improve the outcomes in these high-risk situations.

REFERENCES

1. Hunt JA, Lehman H: Hemoglobin Barts: A fetal hemoglobin without chains. Nature 184:872, 1959
2. Rochard F, Schifrin BS, Goupil F, et al: Nonstressed fetal heart rate monitoring in the antepartum period. Am J Obstet Gynecol 126:699, 1976
3. DeVore G, Donnestein M, Klunman C, et al: Fetal echocardiography: The diagnosis and significance of a pericardial effusion using real-time M-Mode echocardiography. Presented at Society of Perinatal Obstetricians Annual Meeting, 1982
4. Queenan JT: *Modern Management of the Rh Problem*, ed 2. New York, Harper & Row, 1977

5. DeVore GR, Mahoney MJ, Hobbins JC: Antenatal diagnosis of hemoglobinopathies, hemophilia, and Von Willebrand's disease. Fetal blood analysis. Clin Obstet Gynaecol 7(1):41, 1980

6. Apt L, Downey W: Melena neonatorum: The swallowed blood syndrome. J Pediatr 47:6, 1955

7. Kleihauer E, Braun H, Betke K: Demonstration von fetalem Hämoglobin in den Erythrocyten eines Blutausstrichs. Klin Wochenschr 35:637, 1957

8. Clayton E, Pryor J, Wierdsma J, et al: Fetal and maternal components in third trimester obstetric hemorrhage. Obstet Gynecol 24:56, 1964

9. Guyton A: Textbook of Medical Physiology, ed 6. Philadelphia, WB Saunders, 1981, p 333

10. Vajo T, Caspi E: Antepartum bleeding due to injury of velamentous placental vesse s. Obstet Gynecol 20:671, 1962

11. Carp H, Mashiach M, Serr D: Vasa previa: A major complication and its management. Obstet Gynecol 53:273, 1979

12. Sisson T, Knutson S, Kendal N: The blood volume of infants. IV. Infants born by cesarean section. Am J Obstet Gynecol 117:351, 1973

13. Usher R, Shepard M, Lind J: The blood volume of the newborn infant and placental transfusion. Acta Pediatr 52:497, 1963

14. Cotton DB, Read JA, Paul RH, et al: The conservative aggressive management of placenta praevia. Am J Obstet Gynecol 137:687, 1980

15. Golditch IM, Boyce NE: Management of abruptio placentae. JAMA 212:288, 1970

16. Esley C: Laceration of the fetal spleen during amniocentesis. Am J Obstet Gynecol 116:582, 1973

17. Van Dorsten JP, Schifrin BS, Wallace RL: Randomized control trial of external cephalic version with tocolysis in late pregnancy. Am J Obstet Gynecol 141:427, 1981

18. Wallace RL, Eglington G, Gimovsky ML, et al: External cephalic version under tocolysis—A followup report. Am J Obstet Gynecol, in press

19. Lebed M, Schifrin BS, Waffman F, et al: Real time B-scanning in the diagnosis of neonatal intracranial hemorrhage. Am J Obstet Gynecol 140:525, 1981

20. Srinirasen G, Seeler R, Tiruvury A, et al: Maternal anticonvulsant therapy and hemorrhagic disease of the newborn. Obstet Gynecol 59:250, 1982

21. Gimovsky ML, Petrie RH: Fetal hemorrhage after scalp sampling in gravidae exposed to analeptic drugs. Submitted

22. Zipursky A, Hull A, White FD, et al: Fetal erythrocytes in the maternal circulation. Lancet 1:451, 1959

23. Gron R, Braoci R, Rudolph M: Hydrogen peroxide toxicity and detoxification in the erythrocytes of newborn infants. Blood 29:481, 1967

24. Oski FA, Narman JL: Hematologic Problems in the Newborn, ed 2. Philadelphia, WB Saunders, 1972

16

Shoulder Dystocia

LESTER T. HIBBARD, MD

CLINICAL SIGNIFICANCE: With an incidence of 1:1,000 births (1:50 among babies weighing over 4,000 gm), shoulder dystocia is an uncommon obstetric complication. But it is a major source of infant morbidity, causing brachial plexus injuries and cerebral hypoxia. Confronted with this unexpected problem, the clinician must decide quickly among several rarely practiced maneuvers.

Few obstetricians are skilled in the difficult manipulations required to resolve shoulder dystocia. This potentially disastrous complication of delivery is difficult to predict and seldom fully anticipated.

A common scenario for shoulder dystocia is attempted spontaneous or vacuum delivery of a multiparous patient under local or pudendal block anesthesia. Because her previous parturitions were successful and labor has progressed normally so far, the fetus's large size is discounted. By the time help arrives, the fetus is likely to be compromised.

The shoulders of an average fetus, with a bisacromial diameter of 12.4 cm, are just small enough to fit comfortably through the widest diameter of the average pelvic inlet. Unusually broad shoulders will fit if there is sufficient room for a degree of adduction and flexion. Most adults can hunch their shoulders to reduce the diameter by a quarter to a third (Figure 16-1). The more flexible fetus should do as well or better.

But in shoulder dystocia, neither shoulder has a chance to adduct and flex. The shoulders are trapped in an extended and abducted position, overriding the brim of the pelvis and immobilized by traction of the soft tissues of the lower birth canal, which clutch the infant's neck like a tight turtleneck sweater (Figure 16-2). Further traction risks brachial plexus injury.[1] Undue delay risks hypoxic brain damage. The bulky fetus fills the pelvis, hampering efforts to expedite delivery by vaginal maneuvers. After you've ruled out other obstetric complications that mimic shoulder dystocia, such as distended bladder, fecal impaction, contraction ring, fetal anomalies, a short umbilical cord, and pelvic tumors, a successful delivery depends on decisive and concerted action.

To manage shoulder dystocia adequately, the obstetrician requires help.[2] Frequently, more anesthesia is needed. Also, someone must apply effective fundal pressure at the proper moment. (The chance of injuring the uterus by fundal pressure is far less than the chance of injuring the fetus by undue traction). After delivery, additional help may be necessary to resuscitate the infant and to manage postpartum hemorrhage caused by atony, obstetric trauma, or both.

STEPS FOR MANAGING SHOULDER DYSTOCIA

A truly adequate episiotomy is essential, to eliminate interference from the soft tissues of the lower birth canal. An episioproctotomy provides a maximum of space, entails less blood loss, and is more easily repaired than a wide mediolateral episiotomy.

The key to successful delivery is any maneuver that results in the release and subsequent flexion and adduction of the anterior shoulder. Of the several possible maneuvers, no one is clearly superior.

Flexion-adduction. This maneuver is simple, rapid, and requires minimal dexterity. The anterior shoulder must be pushed, pried, or carried posteriorly until it is released from the pubic bone.[3] This can sometimes be accomplished by external pressure of the fist directed against the lower abdomen at the point of impaction or internal digital pressure

---

FIGURE 16-1

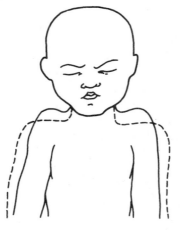

The more flexible fetus may be able to flex its shoulders to reduce the diameter.

---

against the shoulders.[4] A second, more effective method is to press an open palm against the fetal neck, pushing both backward and upward to displace the torso and carry the anterior shoulder toward the chest. This adducts and frees the entrapped anterior shoulder (Figure 16-2).[5]

Both these maneuvers are considerably more effective if combined with sturdy fundal pressure immediately following displacement of the anterior shoulder and continued while a judicious amount of lateral traction releases the posterior shoulder. Applying fundal pressure before the release of the anterior shoulder not only is ineffective, but also can increase adduction, impaction, and the risk of brachial plexus injuries. When the shoulder cannot be dislodged, fundal pressure should not be used.

A third flexion-adduction maneuver uses the pubic bone as a fulcrum while leverage is applied to the anterior shoulder. Because there is usually not enough room to insert a hand for this purpose, Chavis has introduced an ingenious device that serves as a sort of obstetric shoehorn (Figure 16-3).[6] When inserted between the shoulder and pubic bone, it acts as both a lever and an inclined plane, permitting the shoulder to slip free. (The device is not yet available commercially.)

Many physicians routinely utilize the dubious combination of lateral flexion and traction for the birth of shoulders. In the absence of dystocia, the degree of traction applied is harmless. But if the shoulders are trapped, traction can be disastrous, particularly if panic has set in.

Rotation maneuvers. Occasionally, manual rotation will release the anterior shoulder into an oblique position, to take advantage of the largest diameter of the bony pelvic inlet. Or continued rotation can bring it down into the hollow of the sacrum.[3] If this effort fails, more elaborate maneuvers will become necessary.

A popular method is to extract the posterior arm and then rotate the arm and shoulder forward.[7] The anterior shoulder follows, rotating into the hollow of the sacrum, adducting and flexing enough so delivery can be completed with a combination of traction and fundal pressure. Although release of the posterior shoulder is frequently successful, it is a difficult maneuver, potentially traumatic to both mother and baby, and time-consuming.

A more elegant and more complicated method of rotation involves a coordinated backward internal rotation of the trunk.[8] While this maneuver is undoubtedly effective, it must be learned well if it is to be dependable in a moment of crisis.

Miscellaneous maneuvers. Although the shoulder diameter can be reduced by deliberate fracture of the clavicle, this should not be considered as a primary procedure. It is often surprisingly difficult to achieve,

---

FIGURE 16-2

Step-by-step method to free the trapped shoulders

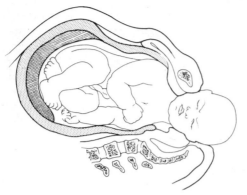

The soft tissues of the lower birth canal clutch the infant's neck like a tight turtleneck sweater.

Firm pressure against the infant's jaw and neck, in a posterior and upward direction, will release the anterior shoulder.

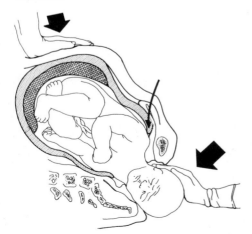

As the anterior shoulder slips free, an assistant applies strong fundal pressure, while the pressure against the jaw and neck is shifted slightly, toward the rectum.

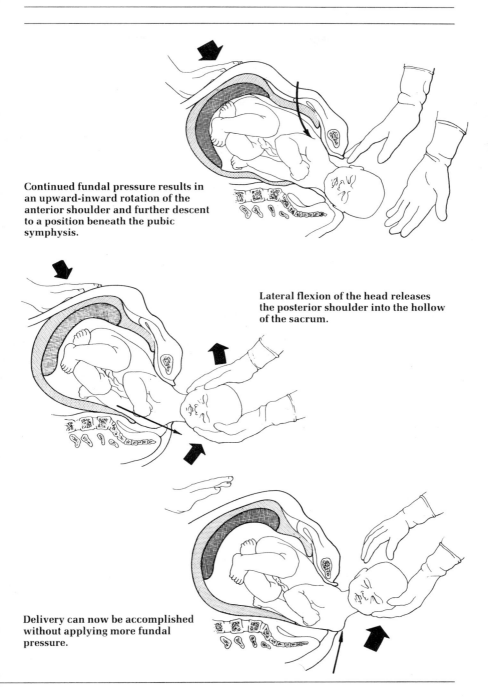

Continued fundal pressure results in an upward-inward rotation of the anterior shoulder and further descent to a position beneath the pubic symphysis.

Lateral flexion of the head releases the posterior shoulder into the hollow of the sacrum.

Delivery can now be accomplished without applying more fundal pressure.

risks injury to the subclavian vein, and may not accomplish its purpose without additional manipulations. If the fetus is dead, cleidotomy can also be considered, after other maneuvers have failed.

Symphysiotomy, to enlarge the bony pelvis, is a practical, effective procedure in places—such as Africa—where it is accepted practice for cephalopelvic disproportion. But this is not a simple operation and cannot be recommended to an inexperienced operator.

ANTICIPATING THE PROBLEM

An abdominal delivery is the only hope of preventing shoulder dystocia for those infants considered to be at high risk. Cesarean section for mac-

---

FIGURE 16-3

Simple and direct— the obstetric shoehorn

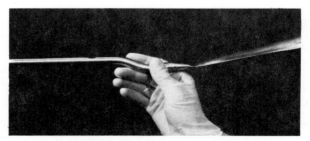

A stainless steel device that serves as an obstetric shoehorn acts as both a lever and an inclined plane, permitting the shoulder to slip free. It has an indented handle, a slipper-like insert, and a cylindrical intermediate segment connecting handle and insert. The insert has a convex surface converging toward a flattened surface on the intermediate segment.

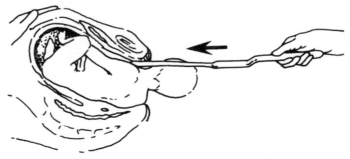

For more detail on this device, see Chavis.[6]

---

rosomic infants (4,500 gm), for pelvises suspected of being inadequate, and for abnormal progress of labor reduces the incidence of shoulder dystocia.

There are no reliable criteria to identify every case. However, the complication can often be anticipated, based on past obstetric history, on maternal obesity or diabetes mellitus, and on clinical assessment of the fetus, pelvis, labor pattern, or the need to interfere in a prolonged second stage of labor when the head fails to descend. In these cases, advance preparations will not avoid dystocia, but may reduce both the difficulties and the adverse consequences.

In short, there is no sure way to avoid shoulder dystocia and no clearly superior method of effecting delivery. Be prepared to act quickly and decisively. A generous episiotomy is necessary and supplementary anesthesia is often needed. The judicious use of fundal pressure to replace strong traction can be extremely helpful. You should not avoid it because of fear that the uterus will be ruptured. Since timely delivery is essential, try only a limited number of maneuvers. Begin with a simple manipulation and, if necessary, proceed without delay to a more complicated method. The most familiar maneuvers are usually the best.

REFERENCES

1. Morris WIC: Shoulder dystocia. J Obstet Gynaecol Br Emp 62:302, 1955
2. Dignam WJ: Difficulties in delivery, including shoulder dystocia and malpresentations of the fetus. Clin Obstet Gynecol 19:577, 1976
3. Rubin A: A management of shoulder dystocia. JAMA 189:835, 1964
4. Heery RD: A method to relieve shoulder dystocia in vertex presentation. Obstet Gynecol 22:360, 1963
5. Hibbard LT: Shoulder dystocia. Obstet Gynecol 34:424, 1969
6. Chavis WM: A new instrument for the management of shoulder dystocia. Int J Gynaecol Obstet 16:231, 1978-79
7. Benedetti T: Managing shoulder dystocia. Contemp Ob/Gyn 14(3):33, September 1979
8. Woods CE: A principle of physics as applicable to shoulder delivery. Am J Obstet Gynecol 45:796, 1943

17
Neonatal Distress

JOHN W. SCANLON, MD

CLINICAL SIGNIFICANCE: Up to 10% of newborns may be compromised in some way at birth. The prompt, expert care that can save lives and prevent neurologic handicaps is not difficult and requires minimal equipment. But anticipation and preparation are key.

Conditions that interrupt the placenta's capacity for supplying oxygen and removing carbon dioxide and hydrogen ions can cause fetal hypoxemia, hypercapnia, or acidosis. Biochemically, this is perinatal asphyxia. Placental insufficiency may be chronic if the mother has severe hypertension, subacute with preeclampsia or acute with abruption.

PERINATAL ASPHYXIA

Breathing difficulties can also begin at birth if, for example, maternally administered anesthetics diminish the neonate's respiration. Perinatal asphyxia is serious by itself and can aggravate kernicterus, necrotizing enterocolitis, or encephalopathy.

Whatever the cause of the asphyxia, the baby's homeostasis is violently altered as it attempts to maintain perfusion of the heart and central nervous system. The major goals when resuscitating an asphyxiated baby are removing carbon dioxide by establishing adequate ventilation, oxygenating tissues by raising Pa_{O_2}, and decreasing intracellular hydrogen ion concentration (raising the pH).

A number of excellent reviews deal with management of the acutely asphyxiated neonate.[1-5] What follows is based on our experience at Columbia Hospital for Women, Washington, D.C.[6]

Equipment. The equipment needed for neonatal resuscitation is not extensive (Table 17-1), but must be in perfect working order. Before each resuscitation, check the laryngoscope bulb and battery, heaters, face masks, endotracheal tubes, and suction and oxygen systems. We install an 80-mL mucus trap in line to gather a gastric or tracheal specimen during resuscitation. Later, if needed, this material may be analyzed for surfactant content, neutrophil count, and fetal and maternal blood.

Delivery room personnel should be assigned to collect basic patient data, and one person should be responsible for recording all resuscitative efforts (see Figure 17-1).

Procedures. Aspirate the oropharynx with a bulb syringe as soon as the head is expelled. A DeLee trap is mandatory when amniotic fluid is meconium-stained. Obtain a doubly clamped segment of umbilical cord for blood gas measurements to document the extent of intrauterine asphyxia. This step is clinically and medicolegally important.

Whoever takes the infant from the obstetrician should be gowned but need not wear gloves. The infant is received in a warm, absorbent blanket, transferred immediately to a warming table, and placed in a head-down position, with a blanket roll under the shoulders to extend the neck slightly. If the infant's head is turned to one side, secretions will be easier to remove because they will accumulate in the corner of the mouth. The optimal time for cord clamping has not been determined. Transfer of an asphyxiated infant to an experienced resuscitator, therefore, should take precedence over arbitrary policy about the time of cord clamping.

TABLE 17-1

Basic equipment for resuscitation

Laryngoscope with No. 0 or 1 Miller blades

Straight endotracheal tubes

Infant stethoscope

Overhead heating unit

Bulb syringe

Sideport suction catheters (5 to 10 French)

Doppler flow probe and newborn sphygmomanometer

Umbilical venous catheter set

Butterfly needles (23 and 25 gauge)

Neonatal intracatheters (23 and 25 gauge)

Sodium bicarbonate (neonatal dilution)

Albumin (25%)

Dextrose (5% in water)

Epinephrine (1:10,000 dilution)

All delivery room personnel should be familiar with the Apgar scoring system, which is simply a measure of neonatal vital signs and primitive neurologic capacity. The Apgar scores should be ascertained immediately and serially during resuscitation.[7, 8] If the Apgar score is 8 or above, keeping the baby warm may be all that is necessary. After a high-risk delivery, however, the baby must not be dismissed from care just because 1- and 5-minute Apgar scores are normal. Such a baby must be watched until it seems clear that problems are unlikely.

If the baby is mildly depressed (Apgar of 5 to 7), it may need only 100% oxygen by free-flow mask or general stimulation. Usually, positive pressure ventilation (PPV) is unnecessary because such infants are breathing spontaneously.

FIGURE 17-1

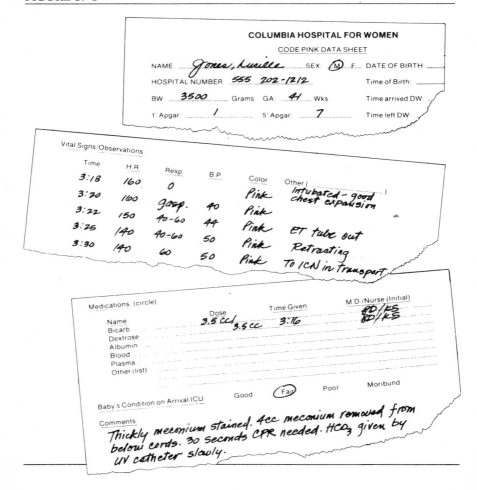

Some positive pressure ventilators must be pumped. Just holding such a device across the airway without rhythmically squeezing the bag will asphyxiate the baby. We strongly recommend having two oxygen delivery systems in each resuscitation area: one attached to the manual ventilator, the other to a free-flow delivery system. Don't use blast insufflation pressures.

When a baby is moderately depressed (Apgar of 3 or 4), provide 100% oxygen by intermittent PPV, initially by bag and mask. If bradycardia— FHR under 100 beats/minute (bpm)—does not promptly reverse with intermittent PPV, begin intermittent mechanical ventilation using an endotracheal tube.

We find 100% oxygen beneficial for asphyxia, because a rising arterial Po_2 is the major determinant of adequate neonatal pulmonary blood flow. Exposing an asphyxiated baby briefly to 100% oxygen does not increase the risk of oxygen toxicity.

The most important indication of adequate ventilation is movement of the baby's chest wall with each breath during mechanical ventilation. If it does not move, you should determine whether the airway is clogged, the trachea obstructed, your technique poor, or your equipment broken. The problem must be corrected immediately.

The severely compromised neonate (Apgar of 1 to 2) needs aggressive resuscitation, initially with bag and mask and then by endotracheal ventilation with 100% oxygen. If the pulse is persistently below 100 bpm (or below 60 at any time), closed-chest cardiac massage must be done. Two skilled resuscitators must be present, one for ventilation and one for cardiac massage. Cardiac massage is performed by placing two fingers in the middle of the infant's sternum and compressing this halfway to the spinal column (cycled rates between 60 and 80 times per minute are optimal).

If closed-chest massage is not effective, try intracardiac epinephrine (0.1 mg diluted to 1 mL). To administer, insert a 21-gauge needle below the costal margin to the left of the xiphoid, angling the needle upward and slightly toward the midline. Dark ventricular blood wells into the syringe when the needle enters the ventricle.

If cardiac massage is necessary, assume severe metabolic acidosis. Administer dilute sodium bicarbonate (2 mEq/kg estimated weight) slowly into the umbilical vein. Bicarbonate, epinephrine, and colloids are the main medications used in the delivery room. The prime emphasis in newborn resuscitation should be directed toward reversing cardiorespiratory dysfunction, providing adequate ventilation, and ensuring thermal homeostasis.

Keeping the baby warm is especially important. Proper drying and wrapping at the time of birth will preserve the infant's thermal environment and an overhead radiant warmer will reduce heat loss. Unfortunately, vigorous resuscitative efforts frequently block the output from the overhead warmer. Therefore, make sure the infant is dry and expose only the part of the body necessary for observation or hands-on care.

For adequate resuscitation and stabilization, the baby's peripheral vascular perfusion must be maintained. Capillary filling time is a useful measure of cutaneous blood flow. Press on the infant's skin and see how long it takes for the blanched area to resume its previous color. Normally, this should take only 3 to 4 seconds.

Blood pressure measurements taken with a Doppler pulse flow detector are also valuable. Apply the pressure cuff above the pulse to be measured and lower pressure until you hear the pulse. This value approximates the systolic blood pressure, which you can compare with norms for various birth weights.[9]

Practical guides for artificial mechanical ventilation and endotracheal tube insertion are available,[1, 2, 4] but there is no substitute for direct training, using dummies and live newborn animals, and periodic review of the procedures.[10] Personnel who rarely perform resuscitations may be unsure of invasive techniques, even with periodic review. This is particularly true of endotracheal intubation, which may be risky for the inexperienced to do. Bag and mask techniques can provide excellent oxygenation and ventilation for a relatively long time. Remember, chest movement is the hallmark of adequate ventilation, and a pulse rate over 100 bpm suggests oxygenation at least of myocardial tissue. The long-term neurologic outcome for even severely asphyxiated neonates is surprisingly good, although the onset of seizures, hypotonia, or hypertonia in the immediate neonatal period is worrisome.[11]

CARDIOVASCULAR COLLAPSE

The baby's intravascular volume must be expanded to maintain tissue perfusion when there is acute blood loss or asphyxial shock. Shock from blood loss may occur with vasa previa and also in fetomaternal or fetofetal transfusions. The pathophysiology of hypotension with low peripheral perfusion includes asphyxia.

The neurovascular response to asphyxia is to maintain myocardial and CNS perfusion by reducing blood flow to the peripheral vessels. The umbilical vessels are under limited sympathetic control. During asphyxia, there is relatively more blood than normal in the placenta. Following birth, and after acidosis has been corrected, the neonate's blood volume may be insufficient when the peripheral vessels fill. The infant will be pale, blood pressure may be substantially lowered, and capillary filling time may be prolonged. Immediate volume replacement is necessary.

When there is a high risk of neonatal shock—if an Apt test has revealed fetal hemoglobin or if the baby is delivered before 30 weeks' gestation—have Rh-negative blood available that has been cross-matched with the mother's. For acute cases, the dose is 10 mL fresh blood per kilogram of estimated birth weight. If blood is not available, give salt-poor albumin, 1 gm/kg estimated birth weight as a 5% solution. If the baby has lost blood and no maternally cross-matched blood is available, use heparinized blood from the placenta. The dose of heparin is 1 unit/mL blood drawn.

Intrauterine asphyxia severe enough to produce myocardial ischemia with congestive heart failure may cause systemic hypotension and peripheral hypoperfusion. In these cases, volume expansion is not beneficial, but measures to control congestive heart failure and the administration of a positive inotropic agent (isoproterenol) may be. Infants in this type of shock will have hepatomegaly, a myocardial ischemic pattern on ECG, and the ubiquitous association of hypoglycemia. The blood sugar can be checked with a reagent strip (Dextrostix). Because diagnosis is difficult in the delivery room, assume that neonatal shock is hypovolemic and treat immediately by volume expansion.

MECONIUM ASPIRATION

Whenever there is meconium in the amniotic fluid, have a skilled neonatal resuscitator present at delivery, because the newborn may be asphyxiated. More important, aspiration of meconium can start a downward spiral of pneumonia, ventilatory insufficiency, hypoxemia, acidosis, brain damage, and death. Gregory and co-workers showed that PPV or respiratory stimulation at birth will impel meconium into the lung's periphery.[12] This thick, viscid material must be removed before the infant's first breath. Furthermore, almost 10% of infants with meconium in their airways have none in their mouths or oropharynges. If every baby with thick meconium-stained amniotic fluid had direct laryngoscopy and tracheal suction, death and morbidity from the meconium aspiration syndrome would be reduced almost to zero.

To remove the meconium, carefully suction the oropharynx with a DeLee catheter as soon as the head is free. After completing delivery, pass the infant promptly to the resuscitator, who can examine the trachea with a laryngoscope. Any tracheal meconium should be removed by direct suction using a large-bore (10 to 12 French) catheter, which usually requires at least 100 cm H_2O pressure. Occasionally, if there are large chunks of meconium, direct laryngoscopy with the use of a large-bore endotracheal tube and mouth-to-tube suction may be necessary.

HYDROPS FETALIS

Fluid accumulation due to Rh disease is becoming rare, but hydrops from other causes still occurs. The fatality rate approaches 100%, yet infants, if properly managed, can survive with an excellent prognosis.[13, 14]

Careful, expert ventilatory control is the first step in caring for the hydropic baby. Two people skilled in resuscitation are needed in the delivery room: one to intubate and manage the ventilation, the other to maintain tissue perfusion and adequate colloid oncotic pressure as the extensive anasarca is decreased. Be sure 100 mL of maternally cross-matched Rh-negative blood are available in the delivery room whenever there is even a hint that a hydropic infant is to be delivered. The person responsible for maintaining perfusion should catheterize the umbilical vein and perform an abdominal paracentesis. As blood is transfused into the vein in 10-mL aliquots, an equal volume of abdominal ascitic fluid is removed through a 22-gauge intracatheter inserted in the left peritoneal gutter or through a 22-gauge butterfly needle placed in a more anterior abdominal location.

Because the major pathophysiologic deficit in hydrops fetalis is low serum protein,[15] simultaneously removing ascitic fluid and replacing blood in isovolumetric amounts maintains adequate tissue oxygenation and colloid oncotic pressure. The procedure must be done carefully, however: Removing ascitic fluid too rapidly may precipitate shock and infusing blood too quickly may aggravate congestive heart failure. When sufficient fluid is removed to allow adequate pulmonary ventilation, the baby can be transferred to the NICU for an immediate exchange transfusion. A diligent search for the etiology of hydrops is essential. Take a blood sample before the transfusion, and examine the placenta, because vascular anomalies can produce hydrops.

WHAT TO TELL THE MOTHER

The senior member of the neonatal team should succinctly but compassionately tell the mother what has been done and what the prognosis is. If possible, let her see the baby in the transport incubator. Show her where the NICU is located and tell her which physicians and nurses will care for her baby. Inform her if transfer of the infant to a tertiary center is contemplated. Such communication is an integral part of the resuscitative procedure.

In summary, the techniques of neonatal resuscitation are simple and straightforward. The keys to success are an obstetrician who anticipates all potential problems and other personnel in the delivery room ready to begin resuscitative efforts promptly and continue them until the baby can breathe on its own.

REFERENCES

1. Akamatsu TJ: Management of the newborn, including resuscitation. Clin Obstet Gynecol 2:673, 1975
2. Fisher DE, Paton JB: Resuscitation of the newborn infant. In Klaus MH, Fanaroff AA (eds): *Care of the High-Risk Neonate*, ed 2. Philadelphia, WB Saunders, 1979

3. Gluck L (ed): *Intrauterine Asphyxia and the Developing Brain*. Chicago, Year Book Medical Publishers, 1977

4. Gregory GA: Cardio-pulmonary resuscitation of the newborn. In Shnider SM, Moya FP (eds): *The Anesthesiologist, Mother and Newborn*. Baltimore, Williams & Wilkins, 1974

5. Volpe JJ: Perinatal-hypoxic ischemic brain injury. Pediatr Clin North Am 23:383, 1976

6. Daze AM, Scanlon JW: *Code Pink: A System of Neonatal Resuscitation*. Baltimore, University Park Press, 1981

7. Apgar VA: Proposal for a new method of evaluation in the infant. Curr Res Anesth Analg 32:260, 1953

8. Scanlon JW: How is the baby: The Apgar score revisited. Clin Pediatr 12:61, 1973

9. Scanlon JW, Nelson T, Grylack LJ, et al: *A System of Newborn Physical Examination*. Baltimore, University Park Press, 1979

10. Harkavy KL: Learning the technical skills for resuscitation. In Daze AM, Scanlon JW (eds): *Code Pink: A System of Neonatal Resuscitation*. Baltimore, University Park Press, 1981

11. Grylack LJ: The outcome for asphyxiated babies. In Daze AM, Scanlon JW (eds): *Code Pink: A System of Neonatal Resuscitation*. Baltimore, University Park Press, 1981

12. Gregory GA, Goodings C, Phibbs RH, et al: Meconium aspiration in infants: A prospective study. J Pediatr 85:848, 1974

13. Oh W, Arbit J, Blonsky ER, et al: Neurologic and psychometric follow-up study of erythroblastotic infants requiring intrauterine transfusions. Obstet Gynecol 100:330, 1971

14. Scanlon JW, Muirhead DM: Hydrops fetalis due to anti-Kell isoimmune disease: Survival with longterm outcome. J Pediatr 88:484, 1976

15. Phibbs RH, Johnson R, Tooley WH: Cardiorespiratory status of erythroblastotic newborn infants. Pediatrics 53:13, 1974

18

Postpartum Hemorrhage

ROBERT H. HAYASHI, MD

CLINICAL SIGNIFICANCE: Although severe hemorrhage occurs in only 0.5% of cases, the overall incidence is about 4%. To avoid significant maternal morbidity and even death, prompt recognition and correction are necessary.

Still a major contributor to maternal mortality, postpartum hemorrhage (PPH) complicates approximately 4% of deliveries on most large obstetric services.[1] However, hemorrhage severe enough to cause the signs and symptoms of hypovolemic shock—generally more than 1,000 mL of blood loss—has an incidence of only 0.5%.

The bleeding may be brisk or slow, but it is continuous. When bleeding is slow, treatment is frequently delayed because the amount of blood lost is at first underestimated.

WHAT CAUSES PPH

Uterine atony. This condition is responsible for most serious PPH (76% to 81%).[2, 3] We recently reviewed our experience, over a 1-year period, with 20 patients who had severe PPH due to uterine atony. Over half had multiple predisposing factors (Table 18-1).[4] Preeclampsia and precipitous labor were the most frequent single factors. The majority of patients with preeclampsia were receiving prophylactic magnesium sulfate; none of those with precipitous labor had a placental abruption.

Genital tract trauma. Trauma during delivery is the second most common cause. Vaginal and cervical lacerations occur not only with operative vaginal deliveries, but with spontaneous delivery as well. Neglected lacerations can cause substantial blood loss through slow vaginal bleeding over many hours. When a low cervical transverse uterine incision is lacerated during delivery of the head at cesarean section, a large amount of blood may be lost, especially when the cervical branches of the uterine arteries are severed.

Spontaneous uterine rupture is rare—1:1,900 deliveries. The clinical picture depends on whether the fetus is extruded into the abdominal cavity or delivered vaginally. With the former, massive bleeding and shock are the usual findings; the latter may result in persistent or intermittent vaginal bleeding.

Improper management of the third stage of labor can cause uterine inversion, particularly when the placenta is implanted in the fundus and not completely separated and the uterus is atonic. In this situation, bleeding is brisk. In the inverted position, the uterus exerts a pulling pressure on peritoneal structures, which can elicit a vasovagal response.[5] The resulting vasodilation increases bleeding and the risk of hypovolemic shock.

Retained placental tissue. Retention is associated with PPH, both acute and delayed (24 hours after delivery). Placental fragments were found in about half of patients with delayed PPH at curettage, but the incidence of delayed PPH is less than 1%.[6, 7] A partial placenta accreta can occur with placenta previa—or when the placenta is implanted low in the uterus—and requires hypogastric artery ligation or hysterectomy to control bleeding.[8] Hysterectomy is the procedure of choice.

Routine manual exploration of the uterus following the third stage of labor has been recommended to minimize PPH due to retained placental fragments (occurring once in 3,000 explorations in one study).[9] However, in another study of delayed PPH, 20% of the patients had had routine uterine explorations immediately postpartum; despite this, two

---

TABLE 18-1

Factors that predispose to uterine atony

Chorioamnionitis

Dystocic labor (cesarean section)

General anesthesia

Grand multiparity

Low placental implantation or previa

Overdistended uterus (twins, polyhydramnios, macrosomia— over 4,500 gm)

Precipitous labor

Preeclampsia

Prolonged labor (vaginal delivery)

of four delivered by cesarean had retained placental fragments. Techniques for uterine exploration are obviously not infallible.

Peripartal coagulopathies. These hold a high risk for PPH but fortunately are rare. Patients with acquired coagulation problems such as thrombotic thrombocytopenic purpura, or amniotic fluid embolism or abruptio placentae, or those with idiopathic thrombocytopenic purpura or von Willebrand's disease may develop PPH because of inability to form a clot in the placental vascular bed.

Patients with von Willebrand's disease are likely to have a decreased bleeding diathesis because pregnancy elevates factor VIII levels. But they are susceptible to both immediate and delayed PPH.[10] Acquired postpartum factor VIII deficiency due to an inhibitor is rare (27 reported cases); the entity is associated with delayed PPH.[11]

STEPWISE APPROACH TO TREATMENT

Awareness that hemorrhage is associated with high maternal mortality is the first step toward good management. Patients with uterine atony, genital tract trauma, retained placental fragments, and coagulopathy are at particular risk, as are those with a history of significant PPH.

Patients at risk should be screened for anemia and atypical blood antibodies (particularly after receiving a transfusion), to make sure type-specific blood is on hand. You might consider autologous blood banking antepartum.

The approach to PPH produced by uterine atony involves a stepwise progression, with standard medical therapy instituted first, then presurgical therapy if bleeding does not subside, and finally operation for hemorrhage unresponsive to the first two treatment steps (Table 18-2).

Standard therapy. An estimated blood loss of 1,000 mL is the signal to begin treatment. Treatment is also indicated if the uterus does not contract and if there is no appreciable slowing of the bleeding.

Management of PPH due to uterine atony begins by making sure the uterus is empty, using manual exploration. If retained placental tissue is found, perform curettage, using a large "elephant" curette. Try to be thorough, but remember a too vigorous procedure can result in uterine synechiae (Asherman's syndrome). Bleeding that worsens as the curettage proceeds may signal placenta accreta, uterine rupture, or both, and mandates laparotomy. Ultrasound may be useful in documenting the presence and absence of intrauterine placental fragments before and after curettage.[12]

Once the uterus is empty, administer a rapid, continuous infusion of dilute oxytocin (40 to 80 units in 1 liter of normal saline). Oxytocin given as an undiluted IV bolus can produce cardiac arrest or aggravate the hypotension.[13] If the uterus remains atonic during the oxytocin infusion, ergonovine maleate or methylergonovine, 0.2 mg, may be given IM or as an IV bolus. The ergot drugs are contraindicated in the treatment of hypertension, since their pressor effect may dangerously elevate blood pressure.

TABLE 18-2

Steps to take when postpartum hemorrhage is due to uterine atony

Step 1. Standard therapy

1. Manual uterine exploration. If retained placental fragments present, remove by curettage. Once uterus is empty, start:
2. IV dilute oxytocin infusion. Give 40 to 80 units/liter of normal saline. If uterus remains atonic during infusion, start:
3. Ergonovine maleate. Give 0.2 mg IV or IM. (Ergot drugs are contraindicated in hypertension.) After drugs are given, start:
4. Bimanual uterine massage. Take care not to lacerate broad ligaments.

Response should occur within 5 to 15 minutes. If uterus does not contract and bleeding does not stop, institute:

Step 2. Presurgical therapy

1. Obtain hematocrit. This serves as baseline.
2. Insert uterine packing. Check for continued bleeding by monitoring vital signs, obtaining hematocrit every hour.

Response should be seen in 1 hour. If bleeding does not stop, consider surgery. Alternative presurgical therapies are embolization with gelatin foam, use of a gravity suit, or use of PGF_{2_α} analogs.

Step 3. Surgical therapy

This is last resort when uterine bleeding is unresponsive to steps 1 and 2. Choice of procedure depends on patient's condition and desire to retain reproductive potential. Perform manual aortic compression in all patients once the abdomen is open, but before the corrective procedure is begun, to cut down on blood loss.

1. Hypogastric artery ligation. Cuts down pulse pressure of vessels that perfuse the uterus and allows a clot to form. May be ineffective if uterus is very atonic. The patient will continue to bleed from collateral circulation around the uterine artery. If so, perform:
2. Uterine artery ligation. If bleeding continues, perform:
3. Ovarian artery ligation. If bleeding continues, perform:
4. Hysterectomy. This is indicated when above procedures do not stop bleeding and when the patient wants sterilization.

Vigorous bimanual uterine massage (not so vigorous as to lacerate the broad ligaments) often promotes uterine tone and the abatement of PPH. These conservative measures are successful in the majority of patients. Expect a response within 5 to 15 minutes after administration of the drugs. If the bleeding does not subside and uterine tone does not increase within 15 minutes, institute the next stage of therapy.

Vaginal lacerations should be repaired with good exposure and meticulous technique, applying the principles of hemostasis and tissue approximation without dead space. Most important is placing the first suture well above the apex of the laceration. A running locked suture is the most hemostatic. Cervical lacerations need not be sutured unless they are bleeding. Management of puerperal uterine inversion is covered well by Donald.[5]

When PPH is associated with a coagulopathy, the coagulation defect should be corrected by administration of appropriate blood products.

Presurgical therapy. Packing the cavity to control uterine hemorrhage remains controversial. Most modern textbooks don't recommend it because it can give a false sense of security that bleeding is under control, thus delaying more definitive therapy. Nevertheless, it is still standard therapy. Recently several investigators reported favorable results using uterine packing to control PPH.[3, 14] When uterine packing is used, take vital signs every 15 minutes and obtain hematocrits at least once an hour. Packing should stop bleeding within 1 hour. If it does not, consider surgical intervention.

Other presurgical therapies are less frequently used. There have been reports of success in managing pelvic hemorrhage by selective transcatheter arterial embolization with hemostatic materials (gelatin foam, powder, pledgets, or silicone rubber).[15]

A recent, exciting, and very effective advance in treating uterine atony is the use of prostaglandin $F_{2\alpha}$ analogs. The 15-methyl analog is more potent and acts longer than the parent compound. In two clinical trials of 20 and 16 patients each, an IM injection of 15-methyl-PG was more than 90% effective in controlling severe PPH unresponsive to standard therapy.[4, 16] Interestingly, a few patients who were treatment failures in each of these studies had severe chorioamnionitis complicating the clinical picture. Intramyometrial injection of prostaglandin $F_{2\alpha}$ has also been successful in PPH due to uterine atony.[17] However, the PG analog has not been approved by the FDA for this indication.

Surgical therapies. Operative intervention is a last resort, to be employed when all other treatment has failed to control PPH. At surgery, compress the abdominal aorta manually to cut down blood loss before the corrective procedure is begun. External aortic compression, using a cushioned block placed transabdominally against the vertebrae, may also be used during medical therapy to minimize blood loss while waiting for the uterotonic drugs to act.[18]

Uncontrolled severe PPH requires a decision on whether to proceed with a hysterectomy or to attempt to preserve childbearing potential. If the patient wants sterilization and her condition is fairly stable, do an abdominal hysterectomy. If speed is essential because her condition is precarious, you can quickly do a supracervical procedure.

If preservation of the uterus is a goal, or the patient's condition is so precarious that a hysterectomy might cause severe stress, a bilateral hypogastric artery ligation will decrease pulse pressure distal to the ligation and promote local hemostasis.[19] If this procedure does not control bleeding, the uterine artery may be ligated. If bleeding still continues, the ovarian artery may be ligated in the infundibular ligaments.[20] Should none of these procedures control bleeding, a hysterectomy will be required.

It has been well documented that patients can become pregnant and maintain the pregnancy after a hypogastric or uterine artery ligation. The effect of ovarian artery ligation is less well known. Any patient who has once had a PPH is at high risk for this complication in the future.

REFERENCES

1. Gibbs CE, Locke WE: Maternal deaths in Texas, 1969-73. Report of 501 consecutive maternal deaths from the Texas Medical Association Committee on Maternal Death. Am J Obstet Gynecol 126:687, 1976

2. Weeks LR, O'Toole DM: Postpartum hemorrhage: A five year study of Queen of Angels Hospital. Am J Obstet Gynecol 71:45, 1956

3. Hester JD: Postpartum hemorrhage and reevaluation of uterine packing. Obstet Gynecol 45:501, 1975

4. Hayashi RH, Castillo MS, Noah ML: Management of severe postpartum hemorrhage due to uterine atony using an analogue of prostaglandin $F_{2\alpha}$. Obstet Gynecol 58:426, 1981

5. Donald I: In *Practical Obstetric Problems*. London, Lloyd-Luke, 1979, pp 804-811

6. Paydar M, Ostourzadeh M: Late postpartum hemorrhage. Int J Gynaecol Obstet 12:141, 1974

7. Thorsteinsson VT, Kempers RD: Delayed postpartum hemorrhage. Am J Obstet Gynecol 107:555, 1970

8. Pedowitz P: Placenta previa: An evaluation of expectant management and the factors responsible for fetal wastage. Am J Obstet Gynecol 93:16, 1965

9. Hawkins RJ: Exploration of the uterus following delivery. Am J Obstet Gynecol 69:1094, 1955

10. Noller KL, Bowie EJ, Kempers RD, et al: Von Willebrand's disease in pregnancy. Obstet Gynecol 41:865, 1973

11. Michiels JJ, Bosch LJ, van der Plas PM, et al: Factor VIII inhibitor postpartum. Scand J Haematol 20:97, 1978

12. Lee CY, Madrazo B, Drukker BH: Ultrasonic evaluation of the postpartum uterus in the management of postpartum bleeding. Obstet Gynecol 58:227, 1981

13. Weis FR Jr, Markello R, Mo B, et al: Cardiovascular effects of oxytocin. Obstet Gynecol 46:211, 1975

14. Druckar M, Wallach RC: Uterine packing: A reappraisal. Mt Sinai J Med 46:191, 1979

15. Heaston DK, Mineau DE, Brown BJ, et al: Transcatheter arterial embolization for control of persistent massive puerperal hemorrhage after bilateral surgical hypogastric artery ligation. AJR 133:152, 1979

16. Toppozada M, El-Bossaty M, El-Rahman HA, et al: Control of intractable atonic postpartum hemorrhage by 15-methyl prostaglandin $F_{2\alpha}$. Obstet Gynecol 58:327, 1981

17. Takagi S, Yoshida T, Togo Y, et al: The effects of intramyometrial injection of prostaglandin $F_{2\alpha}$ on severe postpartum hemorrhage. Prostaglandins 12:565, 1976

18. Pelligra R, Sandberg EC: Control of intractable abdominal bleeding by external counterpressure. JAMA 241:708, 1979

19. Burchell RC, Olson G: Internal iliac artery ligation: Aortograms. Am J Obstet Gynecol 94:117, 1966

20. O'Leary JL, O'Leary JA: Uterine artery ligation in control of intractable postpartum hemorrhage. Am J Obstet Gynecol 94:920, 1966

19

Genital Tract Birth Trauma

BRUCE A. WORK JR., MD

CLINICAL SIGNIFICANCE: Although fewer than 5% of vaginal deliveries result in severe injury, all produce at least minimal trauma. Planning the delivery is the prime safeguard, along with careful inspection of the genital tract after the third stage is complete. Patients should be observed for at least an hour postpartum for evidence of acute hypovolemia or hemorrhage.

Birth trauma is the only aspect of a spontaneous delivery that absolutely requires a physician. If necessary, the parturient can deliver herself of both infant and placenta; she can massage the uterus to help it contract after delivery of the placenta; and she can nurse her baby to stimulate endogenous oxytocin secretion and, consequently, uterine contractions. However, she cannot perform a thorough and careful inspection of the birth canal. Any injury, from superficial lacerations to uterine rupture, can result in morbidity, even mortality, if it is not diagnosed and appropriately treated.

PERINEAL LACERATIONS

Postpartum inspection of the genital tract begins with the perineum. The term "laceration" should be reserved for trauma to patients who have had no episiotomy, while "extension" is used to describe the traumatic end point of an episiotomy that extends beyond the original incision. There is a significant difference in the degree of force required to produce each of these conditions. Far more pressure is required to produce a laceration that begins at the vaginal mucosa and goes through the rectal mucosa than is required simply to extend an episiotomy, cut to the level of the anal sphincter, through the sphincter and across the rectal mucosa.

A carefully planned and executed episiotomy is the best way to prevent perineal laceration (Figure 19-1). If one does occur, remember it may well involve deeper structures: the pelvis, pelvic diaphragm, and vagina. Carefully inspect perineal lacerations before commencing repair, to ascertain the degree to which the pelvic diaphragm, anal sphincter, and rectal mucosa are involved. Whenever the perineal laceration is accompanied by a vaginal laceration, the repair procedure should be coordinated—begin suturing in the vagina and finish in the perineal skin.

Lacerations of the pelvic floor are divided into degrees as follows:
- First degree—epithelial separation only
- Second degree—involvement of subepithelial tissue but no major support structures
- Third degree—tear through the anal sphincter
- Fourth degree—tear of the rectal mucosa.

FIGURE 19-1

A carefully planned and executed episiotomy is the best way to prevent laceration

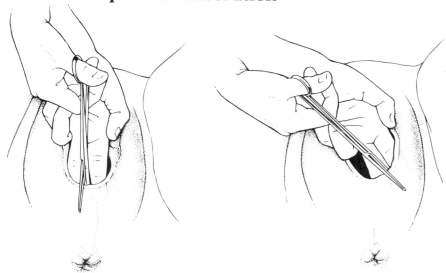

Incise the perineum in the midline, from the posterior fourchette toward the anus, until the sphincter is visible (left) or from the midline of the fourchette toward the ischial tuberosity (right).

Periurethral lacerations should be repaired if they are bleeding. Interrupted 3-0 chromic catgut is appropriate for repair of such simple lacerations. Be careful to protect the urethra. The patient with extensive periurethral lacerations may require drainage of the bladder for several days because edema and pain make urination difficult.

Labial lacerations are often superficial and require little repair, unless they are bleeding. Use 3-0 absorbable interrupted sutures. Just as with episiotomy repair, careful attention to reapproximation of pelvic diaphragm tissue will help prevent relaxation of the pelvic floor later. A 2-0 absorbable suture provides better support of these tissues during healing than does 3-0. Be careful to approximate the bulbocavernosus muscle, if it has separated, to assure satisfactory sexual function.

VAGINAL LACERATIONS

The vagina can tear at any level—extensions of episiotomies, tears secondary to forceps use, and those over the ischial spines, with or without the application of forceps (Figure 19-2). Look for hematoma formation over the ischial spines; incision and drainage, with control of bleeding, are necessary if a hematoma is expanding.

Hematomas caused by genital tract injury take several forms, both superficially and higher in the birth canal (Figure 19-3). They are most common in the lateral vaginal wall in the area of the ischial spines, where they are often associated with forceps delivery. Inspect the tract thoroughly, lest a hematoma go unobserved.

A hematoma of the vagina or perineum of 3 cm or less that does not enlarge in 5 minutes requires no further therapy. Hematomas that continue to enlarge despite pressure must be opened. Try to isolate the bleeding point to achieve hemostasis. If the source cannot be identified, careful packing is required. Hemostatic agents such as bovine collagen may be useful for oozing surfaces.

Hematomas higher in the pelvis generally appear after the immediate postpartum examination. Signs and symptoms of significant intra-abdominal blood loss accompany pelvic or broad ligament hematomas (Figure 19-4). Do paracentesis, examination under anesthesia, and laparotomy to diagnose and manage them. Finally, a late-developing hematoma below the pelvic diaphragm may represent delayed postpartum hemorrhage. Infrequently, a patient requiring more than average postpartum analgesia will have such a hematoma. Gentle rectal or vaginal examination will define this entity. Drainage is often required.

Upper vaginal lacerations, often associated with forceps deliveries, can occur at any site but are found most frequently in the posterior fornix; less often in the lateral fornix. They are often difficult to see, so careful inspection is essential. Repair requires adequate exposure and appropriate instruments. You will need assistance for retraction. Long

FIGURE 19-2

Lacerations of the pelvic floor and vagina are divided into degrees

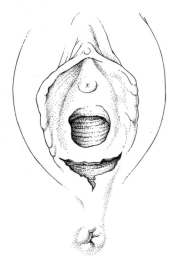

A. First degree: perineal laceration.

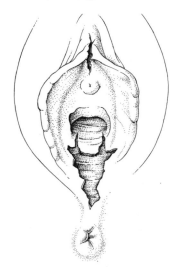

B. Second degree: perineal lacerations plus a tear of the clitoris.

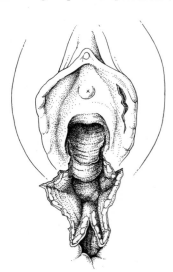

C. Third degree: perineal laceration and labial tear.

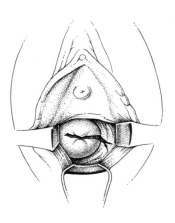

D. High vaginal laceration.

instruments make repair easier. I find the Heaney needle holder particularly helpful, because its curved blades make "end-on" suturing possible. Use 3-0 absorbable sutures.

CERVICAL LACERATIONS

Most lacerations on the cervix that can be identified warrant suturing. Retraction of the vagina and traction on the cervix allow adequate exposure to permit approximation with 3-0 absorbable suture.

UTERINE LACERATION

Following any operative delivery, inspect the uterus carefully. Signs of laceration include a palpable defect, a mass in the area of the broad ligament (Figure 19-4), and shock that is out of proportion to visible blood loss and a well-contracted uterus. If the cause of bleeding cannot be detected, examination under adequate anesthesia is necessary.[1]

Garnet reported that 30% to 35% of cesarean sections are performed for prior cesarean section.[2] Of the 60% of uterine ruptures that occur before labor, 55% are in prior scars and 42% of those are "silent."[3]

FIGURE 19-3

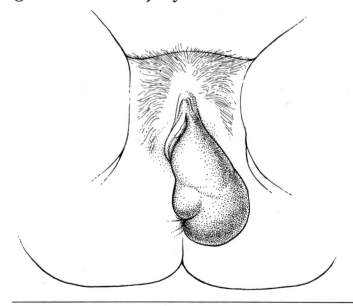

Labial hematoma caused by genital tract injury

Rupture of the uterus must be considered during all stages of labor and postpartum. It may be spontaneous (13.5%), traumatic (31.6%), or occur at the site of a prior scar (54.9%). The chance that a rupture is due to a classical scar has decreased because fewer classical incisions are made. Classical scars are 10 times as likely to rupture as low transverse. Dehiscences confound the issue, as they are often relatively benign events. Dehiscence follows cesarean section in 1:99 cases.

Antepartum signs and symptoms include pain and tenderness, which may be minimal; shock, with maternal tachycardia; alteration in fetal heart rate; maternal anxiety; vaginal bleeding; and cessation of contractions. Postpartum signs include bleeding and shock with a well-contracted uterus and no lacerations after reinspection of the birth canal.

Rigorous review of favorable and unfavorable factors is essential for a patient who has had a previous cesarean and is considering a trial of labor. She must be informed of the risks and of the likelihood of satisfactory vaginal delivery: 64% to 70% of trials of labor in such patients will result in a vaginal delivery. Informed consent is essential. The operating team, including anesthesiologist and surgeon, must be prepared for immediate surgery and immediate replacement of a large volume of blood. There must be no contraindication to labor, such as cephalopelvic disproportion, no unknown prior scar or classical scar, and no proscription of vaginal delivery by a prior obstetrician.

If you suspect that rupture has occurred, rapidly perform a laparotomy and replace blood lost. Once you have determined the type of rupture, you'll be able to decide how to manage it.

FIGURE 19-4

Broad ligament hematoma with rupture of the uterus

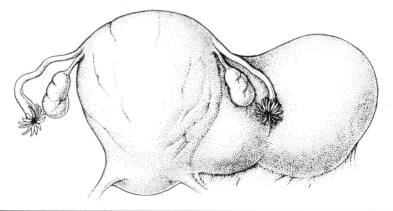

Not all cases of uterine rupture mandate hysterectomy. However, most ruptures in the active segment do. A relatively clean rupture in the lower segment, which involves no major vessels and little bleeding, can probably be managed conservatively. Pay meticulous attention to technique to avoid ureteral injury, particularly if repair requires suturing lateral portions of the uterus.

Careful inspection of the birth canal after delivery and appropriate repair of soft tissue injury should maintain the integrity and function of the female genital tract. Omission of this important step can lead to morbidity, even mortality.

REFERENCES

1. O'Sullivan MJ: Ruptured uterus: Still a challenge. Contemp Ob/Gyn 18(1):145, July 1981

2. Garnet JO: Uterine rupture during pregnancy. Obstet Gynecol 23:898, 1964

3. Horowitz BJ, Edelstein SW, Lippman L: Once a cesarean . . . always a cesarean. Obstet Gynecol Surv 36:592, 1981

4. Lawrence RB: Rupture of the transverse uterine scar after lower segment cesarean section. J Obstet Gynaecol Br Emp 56:1024, 1949

20

Postpartum Endometritis

PHILIP B. MEAD, MD

CLINICAL SIGNIFICANCE: A 0.9% to 3.9% risk following vaginal delivery, and a 10% (and, in certain populations, up to 50%) risk following cesarean section, make postpartum endometritis the commonest post-abdominal-surgery infection in women. With 450,000 US women per year having cesareans, postpartum endometritis results in considerable morbidity and discomfort, although it is rarely fatal.

Inadequately treated, postpartum endometritis may progress to endomyometritis, pelvic cellulitis, pelvic abscess, or septic pelvic thrombophlebitis. Early symptoms include a fever that is greater than 100.4°F and uterine tenderness, with or without foul lochia. The uterus is frequently subinvoluted.

The US Joint Committee on Maternal Welfare's definition of standard puerperal morbidity—a temperature of 100.4°F in any two of the first 10 days postpartum, exclusive of the first 24 hours—probably is no longer useful in the modern hospital setting. Because patients are being discharged earlier now, these criteria can no longer be fully applied. Moreover, many patients with infection respond to antibiotic therapy so rapidly that they do not meet the temperature requirements for standard morbidity.

PREDISPOSING FACTORS

Incidence is overwhelmingly related to the route of delivery. Following vaginal delivery, incidences range from 0.9% to 3.9%; the higher rates are found on services caring for indigent patients. Following cesarean section, the incidence on most private services is approximately 10%; it is as high as 50% or more on large teaching services caring for indigent patients.

Although prolonged membrane rupture, midforceps delivery, anemia, and maternal soft tissue trauma are commonly mentioned as predisposing factors following vaginal delivery, these events—not identified in most patients who develop infections—are probably *relative* risk factors. Predisposing factors following cesarean section include duration of rupture of membranes and labor, duration of internal fetal monitoring, antepartum or postpartum anemia, number of vaginal examinations, obesity, and presence of meconium. Sophisticated statistical procedures like discriminate or regression analysis have failed to settle the question of which of these events relate most directly to subsequent endometritis. In general, patients undergoing elective repeat sections or primary sections before onset of labor and membrane rupture are at low risk of developing postpartum endometritis, whereas patients undergoing cesarean following prolonged labor, prolonged rupture of membranes, or prolonged internal fetal monitoring are at high risk.

RESPONSIBLE ORGANISMS

Organisms normally found in the vaginal flora are the usual causes of endometritis. They include gram-negative aerobic bacilli (*Escherichia coli* most commonly, but occasionally *Klebsiella* species, *Enterobacter* species, or *Proteus mirabilis*); anaerobic bacteria (especially peptostreptococci, but occasionally *Bacteroides fragilis* and other anaerobes); and enterococci (*Streptococcus faecalis*). Group B β-hemolytic streptococcal endometritis occurs infrequently and is often self-limited, although severe infections, including meningitis, and death have been reported. Group A β-hemolytic streptococcal endometritis, the dreaded "childbed fever" of Semmelweis and Oliver Wendell Holmes, is fortunately rare. Its onset is often florid and the lochia is usually not foul. *Clostridium perfringens*, a rare cause of puerperal infection, produces a characteristic clinical picture. In severe cases, massive intravascular hemolysis causes jaundice, mahogany-colored urine, and extreme degrees of anemia in an incredibly short time—within hours. Such hemolysis frequently results in acute renal failure secondary to lower nephron nephrosis. *Clostridium tetani* endometritis is rare, with fewer than 150 cases reported. Mortality is high, however.

Platt et al reported that the commonest cause of postpartum fever following vaginal delivery at Boston City Hospital was *Mycoplasma hominis* infection, defined by a fourfold or greater rise in mycoplasmacidal antibody titer.[1] The clinical significance of this is unclear since most patients did not have physical findings compatible with endometritis.

Similarly, *Chlamydia trachomatis* has been linked to puerperal infection. Women with antepartum *C. trachomatis* vaginal colonization or infection who deliver vaginally have a five- to sixfold increased risk of intrapartum fever and late postpartum endometritis (48 hours to 6 weeks postpartum). However, the therapeutic implications of these data are still unclear.

The difficulty of obtaining meaningful culture specimens is a stumbling block in the precise bacteriologic evaluation of the patient with endometritis. Although numerous transcervical techniques have been tried,[2] no practical way has been found to obtain uncontaminated endometrial cultures. Gibbs, O'Dell, et al, using a transcervical culture technique designed to avoid contamination, found no difference between the bacterial flora of the endometrial cavity in patients with endometritis and those who were not infected.[3] Transabdominal needle aspiration of the endometrial cavity avoids the problem of lower tract contamination, but is not a practical approach in routine patient care. Blood cultures can be helpful, but are positive in fewer than 1% of patients delivered vaginally, and in fewer than 5% of those delivered by section.

MAKING THE DIAGNOSIS

Remember that postpartum endometritis is a rare occurrence following vaginal delivery in a nonindigent patient. Accordingly, assiduously rule out other causes of fever in such patients before accepting postpartum endometritis as the entity to be treated. Failure to heed this warning occasionally results in delayed and inappropriate treatment of other, potentially life-threatening disorders.

The differential diagnosis of postpartum endometritis includes urinary tract infection, mastitis, appendicitis, subgluteal or retropsoas synergistic bacterial infection, infectious mononucleosis or other viral disease, septic pelvic thrombophlebitis, and right ovarian vein syndrome.

OBTAINING CULTURES

Once a working diagnosis of postpartum endometritis has been made, do a pelvic examination on an appropriate examining table. Using a sterile speculum, visualize the cervix, swab it with povidone-iodine, and take a transcervical swab for aerobic culture. If the culture report shows group A β-hemolytic streptococci, you can assume that this is the responsible pathogen, as it is never part of the normal vaginal flora. This finding has major epidemiologic as well as therapeutic implications. If group B β-hemolytic streptococci are isolated, they may or may not be the cause, as these organisms are found in as many as 35% of normal gravidas. However, a culture of group B streptococci from the vagina has obvious neonatal implications. The finding of *Clostridium perfringens* in the absence of the typical clostridial syndrome probably suggests that the organism represents only normal flora (*C. perfringens* is found in the vaginal flora of approximately 5% of normal patients). A heavy growth or pure culture of *C. perfringens* should alert you to explore further. With these exceptions, isolation of other bacteria is not helpful, since it is impossible to differentiate between infection and contamination with normal flora. We therefore do not obtain anaerobic cultures.

In patients who delivered vaginally, you can gently insert an empty sponge forceps into the uterine cavity when you do the speculum exam for aerobic culture. This procedure will occasionally break up a "lochial block," establishing free drainage, and will itself lyse the fever. Most obstetricians prefer not to perform this procedure after cesarean section, for fear of disrupting the uterine incision.

If the patient is initially moderately to severely ill, or if she has failed to respond to presumably appropriate therapy, it is worthwhile to obtain both aerobic and anaerobic blood cultures. Obtain additional cultures, up to a total of three sets, coincident with fever spikes.

ANTIMICROBIAL THERAPY

For patients with mild endometritis, antimicrobial therapy depends to some extent on susceptibility patterns of the common gram-negative aerobic bacilli in your hospital. In general, we have chosen to treat patients with mild postpartum endometritis with ampicillin 2 gm by intermittent IV administration initially, followed by 1.5 gm IV every 4 hours, or with cefoxitin 1 gm IV every 4 hours. Continue therapy until the patient has been afebrile and without significant uterine tenderness for approximately 3 days.

The value of discharging the patient on an additional course of oral antibiotics to complete a 7- to 10-day course has never been scientifically documented. The rare patient with group A β-hemolytic streptococcal infection should, however, be treated for a total of 10 days.

It is difficult to distinguish patients with mild infections from those whose infections are severe. However, most experienced clinicians are able to make this useful distinction, based on patterns of pulse and fever, general systemic toxicity, and clinical course. If patients appear to have severe endometritis or endometritis associated with possible pelvic abscess or septic pelvic thrombophlebitis, the question is whether to cover for *Bacteroides fragilis*. While most studies find that only 15% to 20% of patients with postcesarean endometritis require such coverage for cure, including this coverage in the antibiotic regimen decreases initial therapeutic failures from 36% down to 14% or less. Moreover, review of the recent literature suggests that pelvic abscess and septic pelvic thrombophlebitis did not develop when patients were given an initial regimen effective against *B. fragilis*, whereas 7% of patients who were not on such a regimen developed one or both of these serious complications, and wound abscesses occurred twice as often.

Based on this experience, we treat patients with severe postpartum endometritis (or those suspected of having associated septic pelvic thrombophlebitis or pelvic abscess) with a regimen of clindamycin 600 mg IV every 6 hours and tobramycin 1.0 to 1.5 mg/kg IV every 8 hours. Clindamycin covers all anaerobes, and tobramycin covers most gram-negative aerobic bacilli. This regimen does not cover enterococci.

Patients receiving clindamycin, as well as other antibiotics, should be monitored closely for the development of diarrhea. Discontinue clindamycin if the patient has five or more stools per day. Usually, discontinuing the antibiotic is all that is necessary to treat either the diarrheal syndrome or the syndrome of pseudomembranous enterocolitis. Serious cases of pseudomembranous enterocolitis can be effectively managed with oral vancomycin or bacitracin.

Before starting aminoglycoside antibiotics such as tobramycin or gentamicin, take a careful history and do appropriate laboratory studies. If you find any renal compromise, or if the patient is seriously ill, it is extremely important to test serum aminoglycoside levels to ensure that toxic levels have not developed and that optimal therapeutic levels are being achieved. Draw peak and trough aminoglycoside levels only after the first three to five doses have been given, as it takes the drug this long to equilibrate. Obtain peak levels either 1 hour after an IM dose, or from the opposite arm ½ hour after an IV dose. Obtain trough levels just before the next dose. Peak levels of tobramycin or gentamicin should be 4 to 10 μg/mL, and trough levels less than 2 μg/mL. Obtain a serum creatinine every other day during therapy. Other antibiotics effective against B. fragilis include chloramphenicol, metronidazole, cefoxitin, piperacillin, and carbenicillin.

If fever persists, the failure of apparently appropriate antibiotic therapy can often be ascribed to failure to diagnose a pelvic or wound abscess. Search diligently for a hidden abscess by bimanual examination and examination of the abdominal wound. If you strongly suspect an abscess but cannot find it by physical examination, turn to ultrasonography, computed tomography (CT scanning), or gallium-67 scanning.

If there are no localizing signs or symptoms, begin with a gallium scan to try to identify and locate the general anatomic position of the abscess. CT scanning or ultrasound is the most precise way to locate and characterize the mass. Once you have located the abscess, you are ready to decide on the best technique for draining it.

Patients who remain febrile, with hectic fever spikes and plateau tachycardia, even though an abscess has been ruled out, may have septic pelvic thrombophlebitis. This clinical picture, associated with an arterial oxygen tension below 80 mm Hg in the nonsmoker, is strongly suggestive, although this is primarily a diagnosis of exclusion. If the diagnosis is correct, full IV heparin anticoagulation will result in rapid lysis of the fever, usually within 48 hours. Most infectious disease experts recommend instituting or continuing antimicrobial therapy, including coverage for B. fragilis.

A variant of septic pelvic thrombophlebitis is the so-called puerperal ovarian vein syndrome, a condition usually characterized by lower abdominal pain, fever, and a typical right paraumbilical abdominal mass. Brown and Munsick have provided an excellent review of this condition.[4] Treatment is the same for both conditions.

EPIDEMIOLOGY

The isolation of group A β-hemolytic streptococci from a patient with postpartum endometritis is potentially significant. Cases are usually sporadic, but serious epidemics of group A streptococcal puerperal sepsis do occur even in this era of effective antibiotics. The rapidity with which such an epidemic can develop demands unusual vigilance.

When group A β-hemolytic streptococci are isolated from a patient with postpartum endometritis, all patients with a clinical diagnosis of endometritis should have lochial cultures taken for group A streptococci. (Many services take such cultures routinely.) If a second patient is found with a positive culture, be concerned about a possible epidemic. Take the following steps: Notify local health authorities; employ strict isolation of all infected patients; institute a cohort nursery system; culture all professional and support hospital staff and relieve from duty any who are colonized; culture all newborns for group A streptococci; reduce numbers of visitors; stress adherence to aseptic technique, especially handwashing; save positive group A streptococcal cultures (for specific serotyping).

REFERENCES

1. Platt R, Lin JL, Warren JW, et al: Infection with *Mycoplasma hominis* in postpartum fever. Lancet 2:1217, 1980

2. Knuppel RA, Scerbo JC, Dzink J, et al: Quantitative transcervical uterine cultures with a new device. Obstet Gynecol 57:243, 1981

3. Gibbs RS, O'Dell TN, MacGregor RR, et al: Puerperal endometritis. A prospective microbiologic study. Am J Obstet Gynecol 121:919, 1975

4. Brown TK, Munsick RA: Puerperal ovarian vein thrombophlebitis: A syndrome. Am J Obstet Gynecol 109:263, 1971

SUGGESTED READING

- Biello DR, Levitt RG, Melson GL: The roles of gallium-67 scintigraphy, ultrasonography, and computed tomography in the detection of abdominal abscess. Semin Nucl Med 9(1):58, 1979
- Collins CG, Ayers WB: Suppurative pelvic thrombophlebitis. III. Surgical technique. Surgery 30:319, 1951
- Cunningham FG, Hauth JC, Strong JD, et al: Infectious morbidity following cesarean section. Comparison of two treatment regimens. Obstet Gynecol 52:656, 1978
- DiZerega G, Yonekura L, Roy S, et al: A comparison of clindamycin-gentamicin and penicillin-gentamicin in the treatment of post-cesarean section endomyometritis. Am J Obstet Gynecol 134:238, 1979
- Gibbs RS, Jones PM, Wilder CJ: Antibiotic therapy of endometritis following cesarean section: Treatment successes and failures. Obstet Gynecol 52:31, 1978

- Gibbs RS, Rodgers PJ, Castaneda YS, et al: Endometritis following vaginal delivery. Obstet Gynecol 56:555, 1980
- Gibbs RS, Weinstein AJ: Puerperal infection in the antibiotic era. Obstet Gynecol 124:769, 1976
- Josey WE, Cook CC: Septic pelvic thrombophlebitis: Report of 17 patients treated with heparin. Obstet Gynecol 35:891, 1970
- Ledger WJ, Gee CL, Pollin PA, et al: A new approach to patients with suspected anaerobic postpartum pelvic infections. Transabdominal uterine aspiration for culture and metronidazole for treatment. Am J Obstet Gynecol 126:1, 1976
- Mariona FG, Ismail MA: *Clostridium perfringens* septicemia following cesarean section. Obstet Gynecol 56:518, 1980
- Monif GRG, Hempling RE: Antibiotic therapy for the *Bacteroidaceae* in post-cesarean section infections. Obstet Gynecol 57:177, 1981
- Rehu M, Nilsson CG: Risk factors for febrile morbidity associated with cesarean section. Obstet Gynecol 56:269, 1980
- Sweet RL, Ledger WJ: Puerperal infectious morbidity: A two-year review. Am J Obstet Gynecol 117:1093, 1973
- Wager GP, Martin DH, Koutsky L, et al: Puerperal infectious morbidity: Relationship to route of delivery and to antepartum *Chlamydia trachomatis* infection. Am J Obstet Gynecol 138:1028, 1980

21

Septic Shock

PATRICK DUFF, MD

CLINICAL SIGNIFICANCE: An infrequent but life-threatening complication after pelvic surgery, septic shock occurs in fewer
than 1% of patients with infection at the operative site.
Nevertheless, mortality remains alarmingly high. Management of this acute surgical and medical emergency requires a thorough grasp of the pathophysiologic derangements that overwhelming bacterial infection precipitates.

Sepsis is the third most common cause of shock, a circulatory disorder
in which decreased cardiac output and tissue perfusion induce tissue
hypoxia and acidosis. Only hemorrhage and myocardial infarction are
more frequent causes. The principal pathogens responsible for septic
shock are the aerobic gram-negative coliform organisms that produce
endotoxin. In most large clinical series, *Escherichia coli* is implicated
in over 50% of cases and the *Klebsiella-Enterobacter-Serratia* group,
Proteus species, and *Pseudomonas aeruginosa* in about 30%. The remaining cases of septic shock result from atypical organisms such as
viruses, rickettsiae, fungi, gram-positive aerobic bacteria, and gram-
negative anaerobes.[1]

Septic shock occurs almost exclusively in hospitalized patients. The
microorganisms responsible usually are part of the patient's endogenous flora or are acquired from the hospital environment. The coliform
organisms are particularly likely to cause nosocomial infections. Medical patients at increased risk for septic shock include those at an advanced age, those with chronic illnesses such as diabetes mellitus or
cirrhosis, disseminated malignant diseases such as leukemia and lym-
phoma, and immunodeficiency disorders. Patients who are receiving
immunosuppressive drugs, cytotoxic agents, and parenteral hyperalimentation also may be unusually susceptible to bacteremia.[2]

Surgical procedures that clearly increase risk include operations on
the biliary, urinary, and genital tracts. Infection now is the most com-

mon complication of pelvic surgery. The incidence of endomyometritis following cesarean section may be as high as 85% in certain patient populations. Of these patients, 10% to 25% may develop bacteremia as a consequence of their primary operative site infection, and 0.5% to 1% of them may develop overt septic shock.[3]

FIGURE 21-1

Clinical manifestations of septic shock

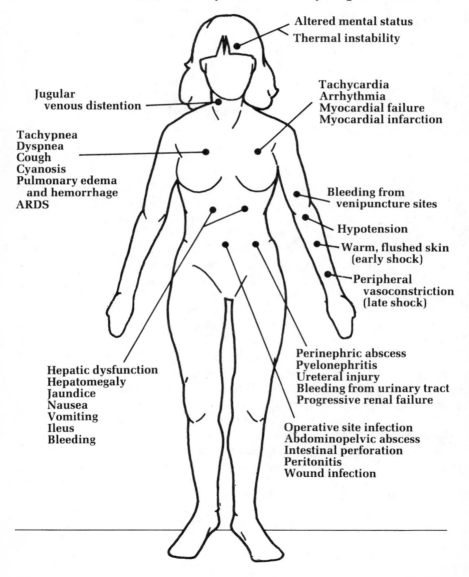

Altered mental status
Thermal instability

Tachycardia
Arrhythmia
Myocardial failure
Myocardial infarction

Jugular
venous distention

Tachypnea
Dyspnea
Cough
Cyanosis
Pulmonary edema
  and hemorrhage
ARDS

Bleeding from
  venipuncture sites

Hypotension

Warm, flushed skin
  (early shock)

Peripheral
  vasoconstriction
  (late shock)

Perinephric abscess
Pyelonephritis
Ureteral injury
Bleeding from urinary tract
Progressive renal failure

Hepatic dysfunction
Hepatomegaly
Jaundice
Nausea
Vomiting
Ileus
Bleeding

Operative site infection
Abdominopelvic abscess
Intestinal perforation
Peritonitis
Wound infection

Because septic shock usually occurs in debilitated patients, the prognosis is markedly affected by the underlying illness. In most large series, the mortality associated with bacteremia is 40%; once clinical shock develops, the proportion of fatalities increases to 50% to 80%.[2]

CLINICAL MANIFESTATIONS

Restlessness, confusion, disorientation, and impaired intellect and judgment are some of the early warning signs. Other early signs include transient hypothermia followed by hyperthermia, flushing, and peripheral vasodilation.[4]

The most prominent pathophysiologic alterations affect the cardiovascular system. A transitory increase in cardiac output and decrease in peripheral resistance invariably are followed by intense vasoconstriction associated with diminished cardiac output and blood pressure, and decreased perfusion of vital organs. Diminished tissue perfusion may lead to impaired myocardial performance manifested by tachycardia, arrhythmia, myocardial ischemia and even infarction, distention of the jugular veins, pulmonary edema, and hepatic congestion.[5]

The pulmonary system may be the primary focus of infection leading to septic shock or a principal target organ of the shock state. Evaluation may reveal tachypnea, dyspnea, stridor, cyanosis, and pulmonary consolidation and edema.[6]

Abdominopelvic examination also may show major abnormalities. There may be evidence of underlying hepatobiliary disease such as cholecystitis or ascending cholangitis, wound infection, or evisceration. Peritonitis may occur in association with intra-abdominal processes such as perforated viscus, appendicitis, diverticulitis, or inflammatory bowel disease. Palpating enlarged or tender pelvic viscera or a pelvic mass may suggest diagnoses such as septic abortion, intra-amniotic infection, endomyometritis, or abdominopelvic abscess.

Signs of pyelonephritis, oliguria, anuria, jaundice, nausea, and vomiting also help to determine the site of infection and identify organs compromised by shock. Hemorrhage from the gastrointestinal, urinary, or genital tract and bleeding from venipuncture sites may indicate a coagulopathy is developing. Figure 21-1 summarizes these principal manifestations of septic shock.

MAKING THE DIAGNOSIS

Disorders to consider in making the diagnosis include acute pulmonary embolus, cardiogenic shock, cardiac tamponade, dissecting aortic aneurysm, severe hemorrhagic pancreatitis, and diabetic ketoacidosis. It should be possible to distinguish between septic shock and these other entities on the basis of history, physical examination, and a limited number of laboratory tests (Table 21-1).

In the early stage of septic shock, the white blood cell count may be low, owing to sequestration of leukocytes in the reticuloendothelial system. As septicemia evolves, however, leukocytosis is usually prominent with a distinct shift to the left. If acute blood loss accompanies sepsis, the hematocrit may be low, or it may be elevated because of decreased circulating plasma volume and resultant hemoconcentration. A diminished platelet count, a decreased fibrinogen level, and an elevated level of fibrin degradation products are the earliest and most sensitive indicators of disseminated intravascular coagulation.[1]

Arterial blood gases alter significantly as septic shock develops. The patient may display a transient respiratory alkalosis as a result of hyperventilation induced by endotoxin. This is quickly followed by a metabolic acidosis, as increased anaerobic metabolism increases plasma levels of lactic acid.[4] Broder, Peretz, and co-workers showed that lactate levels correspond to severity of circulatory failure in the shock state and confirmed that patients with the highest lactate levels have the worst prognosis.[7, 8] Respiratory failure also contributes to severe metabolic derangements in septic shock; patients with end-stage shock may have both a metabolic and a respiratory acidosis, manifested by decreased arterial pH, $HCO_3{}^-$, and Po_2 and increased Pco_2.[8]

Septic shock will also alter renal function. With the onset of oliguria, creatinine clearance will decrease and blood urea nitrogen and creatinine levels will increase.

TABLE 21-1

Laboratory tests for evaluating the patient with septic shock

Abdominal films

Arterial blood gases, lactate
    and pyruvate levels

Chest radiograph

Coagulation profile
    Fibrin degradation products
    Fibrinogen
    Partial thromboplastin time
    Prothrombin time
    Thrombin time

Cultures of urine, blood,
    operative site wound

Electrocardiogram

Electrolytes

Excretory urogram

Hematologic parameters
    Hematocrit
    Platelet count
    White cell count

Parameters of renal function
    Blood urea nitrogen
    Creatinine
    Creatinine clearance
    Urine electrolytes
    Urine specific gravity

Microbiologic studies are an essential step in establishing the diagnosis and determining the origin of infection. Obtain an aliquot of urine by catheterization for microscopic examination and bacteriologic culture, and do sputum cultures in patients with symptoms suggestive of primary pulmonic infection. Both aerobic and anaerobic blood cultures should be performed, since bacteremias in ob/gyn patients are frequently due to multiple pathogens. Blood specimens should be evaluated for fungal growth, especially in patients receiving parenteral hyperalimentation or immunosuppressive drugs. Evaluate operative site cultures and wound cultures to isolate the responsible organism.

FIGURE 21-2

Chest x-ray of a 20-year-old woman with ARDS.

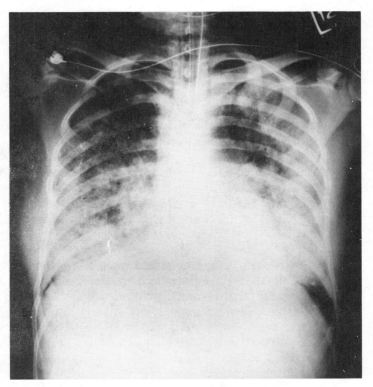

Note the characteristic diffuse bilateral infiltrates, reflecting extensive intra-alveolar and interstitial edema.

Radiographic studies also may be helpful. A chest x-ray will reveal any primary pulmonic infection and may help detect septic pulmonary emboli, cardiomegaly, pulmonary edema, and shock lung (Figure 21-2). Pulmonic changes consistent with shock lung can have a severe adverse effect on the prognosis and must be identified promptly.

If you suspect bowel obstruction, perforated viscus, or abdominopelvic abscess, obtain abdominal films. In selected instances, computerized tomography and ultrasonography may help delineate an abscess (Figures 21-3 and 21-4). Do excretory urography to rule out perinephric abscess, ruptured renal pelvis, ureteral fistula, or ureteral injury.

Seriously ill patients with septic shock must also have their cardiovascular systems evaluated precisely.[5, 9] Standard electrocardiography detects evidence of myocardial ischemia and alterations in cardiac rhythm, and echocardiography evaluates possible valvular dysfunc-

---

FIGURE 21-3

CT scan of a pelvis at the level of the ischium

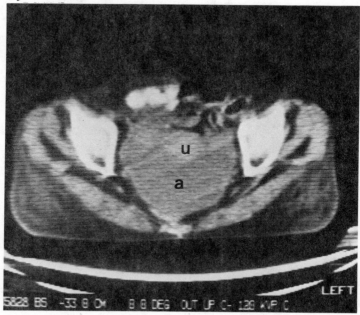

u = normal-size uterus; a = large pelvic abscess.

---

tion. Swan-Ganz catheter studies are invaluable in assessing adequacy of venous return, pulmonary artery pressure, left atrial filling pressure, and cardiac output.

TREATING INFECTION

The initial objective of therapy is to eliminate the underlying source of infection. This may require surgery to drain an abdominopelvic abscess, remove infected products of conception, or extirpate grossly contaminated pelvic organs. Surgical intervention may, in fact, be the single most important step in stabilizing the critically ill patient.

Treatment of life-threatening septicemia also requires broad-spectrum antibiotics directed against the pathogens most likely to be present at the infection site. In obstetrics and gynecology, the major organisms responsible for bacteremia and soft tissue pelvic infections are the aero-

---

FIGURE 21-4

Pelvic sonogram demonstrating a right tubo-ovarian abscess

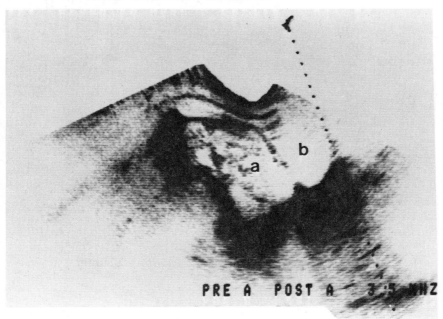

PRE A   POST A   3.5 MHZ

This is a longitudinal section, 2 cm to the right of the midline. a = abscess; b = bladder.

---

bic gram-negative rods, group B streptococci, anaerobic streptococci, and members of the *Bacteroides* family. Although it is not the only acceptable regimen, effective coverage against all these potential pelvic pathogens is provided by a combination of penicillin (5 million units every 6 hours), tobramycin or gentamicin (3 to 5 mg/kg/day in divided doses), and clindamycin (600 mg every 6 hours). Initiate therapy promptly once appropriate cultures have been obtained.

Each of these antibiotics has potentially serious side effects. In very high doses, penicillin may cause CNS impairment, including generalized seizures. Gentamicin and the other aminoglycosides may be both ototoxic and nephrotoxic. In seriously ill patients, particularly those with evidence of renal dysfunction, aminoglycoside dosage should be determined by measuring actual drug levels in the serum. Ototoxicity appears to be associated with excessive peak serum levels, and nephrotoxicity with high trough levels. Risk of toxicity is minimized when peak serum levels are maintained in the range of 4 to 10 μg/mL and trough levels are kept under 2 μg/mL.[1]

Clindamycin's most worrisome side effect is pseudomembranous enterocolitis. Although rare, this disorder may cause major morbidity, even death. It is characterized by destruction of the normal anaerobic colonic flora and overgrowth of a resistant strain of *Clostridium, C. difficile*. Demonstration of grayish-white plaques on the colonic mucosa during sigmoidoscopic examination confirms the diagnosis.[10]

Simple drug-induced types of diarrhea may stop when the antibiotic is discontinued, but pseudomembranous enterocolitis requires treatment with vancomycin, 500 mg orally every 6 hours, until the diarrhea resolves. Relapses may occur after vancomycin has been discontinued.

In certain unique situations you may need different antibiotic combinations from those outlined above. Immunosuppressed patients with neutropenia may need carbenicillin or ticarcillin in conjunction with amikacin for resistant *Pseudomonas* infections. Antifungal agents such as amphotericin may be necessary to eliminate fungal septicemia in a patient receiving parenteral hyperalimentation or in an immunosuppressed patient infected by an opportunistic invader. Substitute a semisynthetic penicillin for aqueous penicillin G when *Staphylococcus aureus* is isolated from the bloodstream. Specialized antimicrobial therapy with pentamidine or trimethoprim-sulfamethoxazole may be needed to manage *Pneumocystis carinii* infections in patients who have been severely immunocompromised.[4, 11]

CORRECTING HEMODYNAMIC ABNORMALITIES

The septic patient should be closely monitored throughout the period of resuscitation. If possible, insert a Swan-Ganz catheter to evaluate cardiac function, or position a central venous pressure catheter to provide information about filling pressure of the heart. Insert an arterial line for continuous assessment of blood pressure and arterial oxygenation. Place a urethral catheter to monitor urine output and insert a large-bore IV catheter to replace fluids and give medications.

The next goal of therapy is to gradually restore effective circulating blood volume. For acute blood loss, administer packed red cells or whole blood. If there has been no blood loss, correct plasma volume loss by infusing isotonic crystalloids such as normal saline or colloid solutions such as plasma protein fraction (Plasmanate) or albumin.

Restoration of intravascular volume should be guided by careful measurements of pulmonary artery wedge pressure (PAWP). Optimally, PAWP should be maintained at 10 to 12 mm Hg; lower levels do not provide adequate filling pressures for the heart, while higher ones may overload the cardiovascular system and cause pulmonary edema.[1] One well-defined, safe way to restore fluids is to give a bolus of 5 to 20 mL/minute for 10 minutes, then observe the change in PAWP. If PAWP increases more than 7 mm Hg above the patient's baseline, stop the infusion temporarily. If PAWP does not rise more than 3 mm Hg above baseline, give a second fluid challenge and reapply the "seven-three" rule. If CVP is used as a guideline, the upper and lower decision points are 5 cm H_2O and 2 cm H_2O.[12]

As fluid replacement begins, apply antishock trousers to improve cardiac function quickly. Pneumatic trousers mobilize blood that has pooled in the lower extremities and lower abdomen, returning it to the heart-brain-lung circulation and preventing myocardial and cerebral ischemia. The trousers are a temporary measure only, and should be gradually deflated as IV fluid therapy re-establishes normal perfusion pressure.[13]

If fluid replacement does not restore adequate tissue perfusion, persistent vasoconstriction may be alleviated by administration of dopamine, an agent with unique pharmacologic properties that make it invaluable in the management of septic shock.[14] In low doses, dopamine has a weak betamimetic effect on the heart, increasing myocardial contractility and heart rate without causing a disproportionate increase in myocardial oxygen consumption. The drug also stimulates special dopaminergic receptors in the renal, mesenteric, coronary, and cerebral vasculature to induce vasodilation. Unlike pure β-stimulants, dopamine causes vasoconstriction in skeletal muscle. Its net effect, then, is to preserve renal, splanchnic, coronary, and cerebral blood flow.

Dopamine's actions are uniquely dose-dependent. In doses that exceed 15 to 20 μg/kg/minute, its principal effect is to stimulate α-receptors. The vasoconstriction that ensues also occurs with conventional vasopressors such as metaraminol and ephedrine. The ultimate result of this vasoconstriction is a transient increase in cardiac output followed by a sustained decrease in tissue perfusion, clearly undesirable in the shock state.[14]

If overt congestive heart failure complicates septic shock, digitalization is indicated. This may be accomplished with a loading dose of 0.75 mg of digoxin in three divided doses, 4 to 6 hours apart, followed by a daily maintenance dose calculated to provide a serum digoxin level of 0.5 to 2.5 ng/mL. Digoxin dosage must be adjusted if renal function is impaired; usual maintenance doses will be 0.125 to 0.375 mg/day.[15]

Many investigators also advocate glucocorticoids for septic shock. Although there is controversy about the value of corticosteroids, several recent laboratory and clinical studies have demonstrated that they improve both circulatory hemodynamics and survival.[16] To be of benefit, the hormones must be administered in pharmacologic doses very early in the evolution of the shock state. Shumer advocates 30 mg/kg methylprednisolone or 3 mg/kg dexamethasone at the time resuscitation is initiated. The infusion may be repeated in 4 hours, if necessary.[17]

In pharmacologic doses, corticosteroids appear to have several valuable effects on the pathophysiologic derangements caused by sepsis. They increase cardiac output by exerting a positive inotropic effect on the heart. They dilate the peripheral and cerebral vasculature and improve tissue perfusion. They also promote gluconeogenesis, thus enhancing the availability of glucose to the CNS.[16, 18] Most important, glucocorticoids inhibit the intense inflammatory reaction mediated by complement cascade and leukocyte aggregation. Accordingly, their net effect at the ultrastructural level is to stabilize lysosomal membranes and preserve the integrity of capillary endothelium, thus preventing cellular autolysis and transudation of intravascular fluid into the interstitial spaces.[18, 19] This latter effect is particularly important in preventing serious immunologic injury to the pulmonary vasculature.

SUPPORTING THE RESPIRATORY SYSTEM

The most common cause of death in septic shock is respiratory failure due to adult respiratory distress syndrome (ARDS), or shock lung. Some 25% to 50% of patients with septic shock will develop ARDS. The mortality in septic shock complicated by respiratory failure may be as high as 90%, almost twice that in septic shock without ARDS.[6]

A major objective in managing the critically ill patient is *prevention* of respiratory failure. Patients with septicemia and shock are, by definition, hypoxic and acidotic and require immediate oxygen therapy with a nasal cannula or face mask. Monitor arterial blood gases frequently to detect early onset of respiratory failure. Avoid fluid overload. Most important, at the earliest sign of decreased pulmonary compliance, institute mechanical ventilation with a volume-cycled respirator to prevent irreversible hypoxic damage to the pulmonary vasculature.

ADDITIONAL SUPPORTIVE MEASURES

Wide fluctuations in temperature may aggravate existing cardiovascular dysfunction and should be kept to a minimum. Coagulation abnormalities should be identified promptly and corrected with cryoprecipitate, fresh frozen plasma, fresh whole blood, or platelets. Only rarely will heparin be necessary. Immunosuppressed patients, especially those with infections due to *Pseudomonas* organisms, may benefit from transfusion of white blood cells.[20] Table 21-2 summarizes the critical steps in management of the patient with septic shock.

TABLE 21-2

Treatment of septic shock

A. **Correct hemodynamic abnormalities**
  1. Establish reliable methods for physiologic monitoring
  2. Restore intravascular volume
  3. Consider use of antishock trousers as an adjunct to fluid replacement
  4. Improve perfusion of vital organs by administering dopamine
      a. 5-mL ampoule—40 mg/mL (total 200 mg)
      b. Dilute 2 ampoules in 250 mL sterile saline or 5% dextrose to give a concentration of 1,600 μg/mL
      c. Begin infusion at 2 μg/kg/minute
      d. Titrate dosage to achieve adequate tissue perfusion
  5. Digitalize patient if overt congestive heart failure develops
  6. Administer pharmacologic doses of glucocorticoids
      a. Methylprednisolone (30 mg/kg) or dexamethasone (3 mg/kg)
      b. Administer as IV bolus at the time fluid replacement is initiated. Repeat in 4 hours, if necessary

B. **Treat underlying infection**
  1. Initially, administer antibiotics covering entire range of potential pelvic pathogens
  2. Surgery, if indicated

C. **Support respiratory system**
  1. Administer oxygen
  2. Monitor arterial blood gases frequently to detect onset of respiratory failure
  3. Early use of mechanical ventilation with volume-cycled respirator

D. **Restore body temperature to normal**

E. **Correct coagulation abnormalities**

F. **Administer white cell transfusions** to severely immunosuppressed patients with *Pseudomonas* septicemia

---

FUTURE DIRECTIONS

Several experimental modalities may soon be more widely used in clinical management of septic shock. McCabe and associates showed that the prognosis of patients with gram-negative bacteremia improves when they develop antibodies against certain common antigens shared by the Enterobacteriaceae.[21] This raises the intriguing possibility of passively immunizing debilitated hospitalized patients before septicemia develops.

Several investigators have observed high prostaglandin levels in the circulation of experimental animals given endotoxin. Cefalo and co-workers suggested that increased prostaglandins may be responsible for constriction of the pulmonary vasculature and pulmonary hypertension, pulmonary edema, and respiratory failure. They showed that increases in prostaglandins and subsequent pulmonary injury can be prevented by treating the animals with indomethacin or ibuprofen.[22] Rao and associates found that prior treatment with aspirin ameliorates platelet aggregation in the small vessels of the kidneys and lungs, thereby minimizing stasis, microembolization, and release of inflammatory mediators such as prostaglandins and complement.[23] Antiplatelet drugs and prostaglandin inhibitors should now have clinical trials.

Finally, there is impressive evidence that the stress of sepsis triggers the release of endogenous β-endorphin into the circulation along with ACTH. In experimental animals, endorphin profoundly depresses the cardiovascular system, leading to decreased heart rate and hypotension. Faden and Holaday showed that the narcotic antagonist naloxone can reverse this hypotensive effect.[24] There are also recent reports of successful use of naloxone in treating patients with seemingly irreversible circulatory collapse.[25] More clinical research is needed to establish the value of naloxone in treating septic shock.

REFERENCES

1. Eskridge RA: Septic shock. Crit Care Q 2:55, 1980
2. Freid MA, Vosti KL: The importance of underlying disease in patients with gram-negative bacteremia. Arch Intern Med 121:418, 1968
3. DePalma RT, Leveno KJ, Cunningham FG, et al: Identification and management of women at high-risk for pelvic infection following cesarean section. Obstet Gynecol 55:185S, 1980
4. Barnett JA, Sanford JP: Bacterial shock. JAMA 209:1514, 1969
5. Motsay GJ, Dietzman RH, Ersek RA, et al: Hemodynamic alterations and results of treatment in patients with gram-negative septic shock. Surgery 67:577, 1970
6. Kaplan RL, Sahn SA, Petty TL: Incidence and outcome of the respiratory distress syndrome in gram-negative sepsis. Arch Intern Med 139:867, 1979
7. Broder G, Weil MH: Excess lactate: An index of reversibility of shock in human patients. Science 143:1457, 1964
8. Peretz DI, McGregor M, Dossetor JB: Lactic acidosis: A clinically significant aspect of shock. Can Med Assoc J 90:673, 1964

9. Weil MH, Nishijima H: Cardiac output in bacterial shock. Am J Med 64:920, 1978

10. Bartlett JG, Chang TW, Gurwith M, et al: Antibiotic-associated pseudomembranous colitis due to toxin-producing clostridia. N Engl J Med 298:531, 1978

11. Christy JH: Treatment of gram-negative shock. Am J Med 50:77, 1971

12. Shubin H, Weil MH, Carlson RW: Bacterial shock. Am Heart J 94:112, 1977

13. Waeckerle JF: Antishock garments. Crit Care Q 2:15, 1980

14. Goldberg LI: Dopamine—Clinical uses of an endogenous catecholamine. N Engl J Med 291:707, 1974

15. Doherty JE: Digitalis glycosides. Ann Intern Med 79:229, 1973

16. Sambhi MP, Weil MH, Udhoji VN: Acute pharmacodynamic effects of glucocorticoids. Circulation 31:523, 1965

17. Shumer W: Steroids in the treatment of clinical septic shock. Ann Surg 184:333, 1976

18. Emerson TE Jr, Raymond RM: Methylprednisolone in the prevention of cerebral hemodynamic and metabolic disorders during endotoxin shock in the dog. Surg Gynecol Obstet 48:361, 1979

19. Hammerschmidt DE, White JG, Craddock PR, et al: Corticosteroids inhibit complement-induced granulocyte aggregation. J Clin Invest 63:798, 1979

20. Graw RG, Herzig G, Perry S, et al: Normal granulocyte transfusion therapy. N Engl J Med 287:367, 1972

21. McCabe WR, Kreger BE, Johns M: Type-specific and cross-reactive antibodies in gram-negative bacteremia. N Engl J Med 287:261, 1972

22. Cefalo RC, Lewis PE, O'Brien WF, et al: The role of prostaglandins in endotoxemia. Am J Obstet Gynecol 137:53, 1980

23. Rao PS, Cavanagh D, Lamont WG: Endotoxic shock in the primate: Effects of aspirin and dipyridamole administration. Am J Obstet Gynecol 140:914, 1981

24. Faden AI, Holaday JW: Opiate antagonists: A role in the treatment of hypovolemic shock. Science 205:317, 1979

25. Peters WP, Friedman PA, Johnson MW, et al: Pressor effect of naloxone in septic shock. Lancet 1:529, 1981

22

Sudden Sensorium Derangements

CHARLES E. GIBBS, MD

CLINICAL SIGNIFICANCE: Sudden, severe CNS disturbances in the pregnant woman require prompt attention to the underlying cause, if maternal and perinatal morbidity and mortality are to be held to a minimum.

Convulsions and other sudden disturbances of the sensorium present acute, dramatic emergencies in pregnancy. Except for eclampsia, these conditions are not obstetric in origin; however, their severity and frequency may be influenced by gestation. The obstetrician, as the patient's principal physician, is therefore usually the one to make the diagnosis and plan treatment.

CONVULSIONS

Eclampsia is the CNS emergency most frequently encountered in obstetrics. Convulsions are almost always preceded by a preeclamptic syndrome of headache, epigastric pain, and visual disturbances, and may occur before, during, or after delivery. Convulsions first appearing more than 48 hours after delivery are unlikely to be eclamptic in origin and should be evaluated with this in mind.[1]

The convulsions of eclampsia are tonic-clonic and associated with loss of consciousness accompanied by hypertension, edema, and proteinuria. Untreated, they may occur as frequently as every 30 to 40 minutes. Pulmonary edema and oliguria/anuria are potential complications, especially in older women who have underlying chronic cardiorenal disease.

Epilepsy rarely makes a first appearance in pregnancy. But a woman whose disease has been under control may have a convulsion during early pregnancy because nausea and vomiting and more rapid clearance of antiepileptic drugs may reduce the effectiveness of anticonvulsant therapy.[1] Note that the recommended therapy for eclamptic convulsions will generally terminate an epileptic seizure, too.

Other causes of convulsions are drug abuse (withdrawal as well as ingestion), intracranial trauma, vascular disorders, infection, and tumor. The cause of the seizures may be apparent from the history and physical exam, but identifying the cause sometimes requires extensive investigation.

Treatment is directed toward stopping the attack and preventing sequelae. These are cardinal points: *Prevent injury* by inserting a soft mouth gag between the patient's teeth and placing her on the floor (or using side rails on the bed); *prevent hypoxia* by stopping the convulsion, deterring aspiration, and administering 100% oxygen by face mask; and *institute drug therapy*. If the patient has not yet delivered, the regimen is magnesium sulfate 2 to 4 gm in a 10% solution, administered over a 3- to 5-minute period, followed by 10 gm IM in a 50% solution (5 gm in each buttock) (Table 22-1).[1]

For a postpartum convulsion, give IV diazepam 10 mg over a 3- to 5-minute period. This regimen is effective in 80% to 90% of cases. An additional 5 to 10 mg may occasionally be necessary.

Sometimes anticonvulsant drugs cause respiratory depression severe enough to require tracheal intubation and assisted ventilation. Hypotension also may occur, and should be treated by intravenous volume expanders. All pregnant women who have one or more convulsions should be hospitalized until the cause is identified, the convulsions stopped, and adequate treatment instituted.[2]

OTHER DISTURBANCES OF THE SENSORIUM

Extreme lethargy, stupor, and coma are infrequently encountered obstetric emergencies. For differential diagnosis, metabolic causes to be ruled out include diabetes, electrolyte disturbances, and hepatic and

---

TABLE 22-1

Drug therapy for eclamptic convulsions

During pregnancy
Magnesium sulfate 2 to 4 gm IV in a 10% solution given over a 3- to 5-minute period, followed by 10 gm IM in a 50% solution (5 gm in each buttock)

Postpartum
Diazepam 10 mg IV over a 3- to 5-minute period; an occasional patient will require an additional 5 to 10 mg

renal failure. Cerebral oxygen deprivation may be due to hypothermia, hyperpyrexia, cardiorespiratory illness, or poisoning. Intracranial lesions resulting in coma can be infectious, neoplastic, traumatic, or vascular in origin.[2] Some cases may be puzzling, but the diagnosis most often is apparent from history and physical examination, and results of blood chemistries and urinalysis. As several of these conditions are discussed elsewhere in this volume, this chapter will be confined below to ischemic and hemorrhagic intracranial disorders.

Ischemic disorders. Arterial obstruction can be due to atheromatous plaques, thrombosis, emboli from the left side of the heart, or paradoxical emboli from venous channels that gain entrance to the arteries through a patent foramen ovale. Vascular disorders in younger persons are increasingly being reported. The possibility of a relationship between middle cerebral artery thrombosis, oral contraception, and pregnancy should be considered. And transient cerebral ischemic attacks in relatively young people (average age, 38) have been associated with mitral valve prolapse.[3] These patients had no evidence of arteriosclerotic cerebrovascular disease, were not hypertensive, had no coagulation defects, and had not been taking oral contraceptives.

Venous thrombosis of both the large collecting sinuses and other intracranial veins is also being reported in a younger age group. This condition appears to occur more frequently in some parts of the world than in others, with the US at the low end of the incidence scale compared with India and the more Westernized nations like Japan.[4-7]

TABLE 22-2

*Deaths due to stroke: Clinical and pathologic diagnosis**

	NO.	AUTOPSIES
Cerebral hemorrhage with severe hypertension	11	7
Postpartum vascular thrombosis	7	4
Intracranial hemorrhage with vascular malformation	4	4
Embolism	2	2
Uncertain	5	0
Total	29	17

*Texas, 1969-1970; data from Gibbs.[8]

The ischemic vascular disorders may be seen throughout pregnancy, but a particularly favored time is in the first 2 weeks postpartum. The disorders show great variability in their clinical presentation, but very mild symptoms such as weakness, headache, confusion, slight fever, malaise, and nausea are not unusual. Initial erroneous diagnoses include drug abuse, meningitis, hysteria, influenza, and postpartum psychosis. When hemiplegia, convulsions, and coma are present, the diagnosis is less likely to be in error.

Angiography confirms ischemic cerebral vascular disease, sometimes preceded by a CT scan. Treatment, usually medical, employs drugs that reduce edema and prevent convulsions. Occasionally embolectomy or thrombectomy may be indicated.

Intracranial hemorrhage. Intracranial hemorrhage may be a direct complication of hypertension—the latter often occurring as an acute vasospastic illness (preeclampsia) superimposed on long-standing hypertension. A survey of deaths during and following pregnancy found intracranial vascular disease to be the certain cause of death in 24 of 375 women and the probable cause in five others, totaling 7.6% of maternal deaths (Table 22-2).[8] Autopsy findings from these patients showed that some had congenital vascular abnormalities while others did not. Table 22-3 summarizes the causes of intracranial hemorrhage.[9]

Arteriovenous malformations and aneurysms can also cause intracranial hemorrhage. While these lesions occur in many different vessels, they are most common in the basilar, communicating, and middle cere-

---

TABLE 22-3

---

*Causes of intracranial hemorrhage**

1. Arterial aneurysms
   a. "Congenital" berry aneurysms
   b. Acquired arterial aneurysms
      (1) Fusiform
      (2) Mycotic

2. Arteriovenous malformations

3. Hypertensive vascular disease

4. Vascular lesions associated with primary or metastatic brain tumors

5. Systemic bleeding diatheses

6. Undetermined and miscellaneous causes

*Adapted from McDowell.[9]

---

bral arteries. Bleeding from these malformations may be preceded by significant degrees of hypertension, but often it is not.

Bleeding from aneurysms most often goes into the subarachnoid space, but an arteriovenous malformation may bleed into the subarachnoid space or the brain substance. The initial symptoms and signs of an intracranial hemorrhage often are more dramatic and severe than those of an ischemic lesion, with coma, headache, and neck pain being the usual presenting complaints.[10] When the hemorrhage is intracerebral, there may be lateralizing signs, but subarachnoid hemorrhage may produce neither reflex changes nor muscle weakness.

DIAGNOSTIC TESTS

As a rule, a spinal tap is the simplest and quickest procedure when CNS disorders are suspected (although most patients with presumed intracranial hemorrhage will benefit from angiography). A tap should be done except (1) when there is increased intracranial pressure (removal of cerebrospinal fluid in long-standing situations could lead to changes in pressure dynamics with resulting structural damage), (2) when there is displacement of the pineal gland (indicating a mass), or (3) when the skin at the puncture site is infected.[11]

The other two very useful procedures are CT scans and angiography. Often both are necessary to make a final decision concerning management of the individual patient.[11, 12] Air studies, ultrasound, and radionuclide imaging are seldom useful in emergency circumstances.

TREATMENT

The availability of better diagnostic and localizing tests, plus improved medical and surgical techniques, means that treatment possibilities now exist for more and more patients. To take full advantage of available therapy, however, it's imperative that every patient with acute CNS symptoms—no matter how atypical, mild, or confusing—be thoroughly and promptly evaluated.

REFERENCES

1. Pritchard JA, MacDonald PC: *Williams Obstetrics*. ed 16. New York, Appleton-Century-Crofts, 1980
2. Rutherford WH, Nelson PG, Weston PA, et al (eds): *Accident and Emergency Medicine*. Philadelphia, JB Lippincott, 1980
3. Barnett HJ, Jones MW, Boughner DR, et al: Cerebral ischemic events associated with prolapsing mitral valve. Arch Neurol 33:777, 1976
4. Bunsal BC, Jones MW, Boughner DR, et al: Stroke during pregnancy and puerperium in young females below the age of 40 years as a result of cerebral venous/sinus thrombosis. Jpn Heart J 21:171, 1980
5. Chopra JS, Prabhakar S: Clinical features and risk factors in stroke in young. Acta Neurol Scand 60:289, 1979
6. Aminoff MJ: Neurological disorders and pregnancy. Am J Obstet Gynecol 132:325, 1978

7. Estanol B, Rodriguez A, Conte G, et al: Intracranial venous thrombosis in young women. Stroke 10:680, 1979

8. Gibbs CE: Maternal death due to stroke. Am J Obstet Gynecol 119:69, 1974

9. McDowell FH: In Beeson PB, McDermott W, Wyngaarden JB (eds): *Cecil Textbook of Medicine*, ed 15. Philadelphia, WB Saunders, 1979

10. Amias AG: Cerebral vascular disease in pregnancy. I. Haemorrhage. J Obstet Gynaecol Br Commonw 77:100, 1970

11. Smith RR: *Essentials of Neurosurgery*. Philadelphia, JB Lippincott, 1980

12. Fayle RW, Van Horn G, Grotta JC: Cerebrovascular disease: Differential features and diagnostic test. Tex Med 77:59, Sept 1981

PART II
Gynecology

23

Vasovagal Syncope

J. STEPHEN NAULTY, MD, and
GERARD W. OSTHEIMER, MD

CLINICAL SIGNIFICANCE: Though its incidence is unknown, this syndrome is fairly common, particularly in those with a history of fainting. Although potentially life-threatening, vasovagal syncope has no sequelae if promptly recognized and managed.

Vasovagal syncope arrives without warning. Its duration is brief, and its effects unpredictable. Attempts to reproduce it in susceptible individuals have not succeeded.

Two conditions appear necessary. First, there must be actual or threatened physical injury. The threat or injury is most likely to produce vasovagal syncope if it involves a new experience or one the patient has been unable to manage in the past. Second, the injury must be one the patient is expected to face easily.[1] For example, most people would not faint at venipuncture, injection of a local anesthetic, or even the sight of a needle (Figure 23-1). However, these seemingly trivial procedures may overwhelm certain susceptible individuals. For this reason, the syndrome of vasovagal syncope is more common in men than in women. In our society, men are expected to withstand such insults more readily.

PATHOPHYSIOLOGY

The attack appears to involve a biphasic response.[2, 3] First, there must be a massive discharge from the sympathetic nervous system in response to the threat of physical injury. The pulse rate, blood pressure (systolic greater than diastolic), and cardiac output all increase. And there is a massive increase in systemic vascular resistance. The patient appears apprehensive and pale, but usually denies any stress. Then, the physical changes suddenly reverse—as though the organism gives up in the face of an overwhelming threat.

As Figure 23-2 shows, pulse, blood pressure, cardiac output, and systemic vascular resistance suddenly drop. At the same time, the capacitance of the venous system suddenly increases, which leads to circulatory failure. The patient feels weak and diaphoretic, has a sudden decrease in muscle strength, becomes lightheaded, complains of vertigo, and quickly loses consciousness as the systolic pressure declines below 80 torr. The syncopal episode may be accompanied by vomiting, seizures, and a bowel movement (Table 23-1). If the response is sufficiently severe, "sudden death" may occur. This sequence has been described in patients who suddenly die in the coronary care unit.[4]

This biphasic response has been related to the sudden activation of the fight-or-flight mechanism of the sympathetic nervous system, abruptly followed by the activation of the vagal conservation-withdrawal system. Under normal circumstances, activation of the sympathetic nervous system inhibits the parasympathetic nervous system and vice versa.[1] Under conditions of conflicting stimulation, when the organism is faced with overwhelming terror at an apparently trivial stimulus, this reciprocal inhibition may begin to break down.[5]

If both systems are activated concurrently, a syncopal episode results. For instance, a terrified dog may bark and exhibit aggressive tendencies and simultaneously urinate, defecate, pant, salivate, move aimlessly, and even momentarily doze. The analogous human response, vasovagal syncope, may represent the organism's extreme reaction to overwhelming uncertainty about whether fighting or giving up is the best response to overwhelming stress.

FIGURE 23-1

A classic case

A 17-year-old high-school senior comes to her gynecologist's office for a therapeutic abortion. She tells the nurse she always faints at the sight of needles or when blood has been drawn from her. On the examining table, she appears agitated and tremulous. The procedure is started under paracervical block anesthesia. As the first dose of local anesthetic is given, the patient appears diaphoretic and pale. During the injection, she loses consciousness and has a grand mal seizure. Following the seizure, the patient is apneic, with no pulses palpable and pupils widely dilated. An ECG reveals asystole. Cardiopulmonary resuscitation is quickly instituted and within 35 minutes the patient regains consciousness. Fifteen minutes later, her recovery appears complete with no neurologic sequelae and she insists on going home. A week later, she undergoes an uneventful therapeutic abortion, under general anesthesia, in the hospital.

THE ABCs OF MANAGING A VASOVAGAL ATTACK

Despite uncertainty about its pathophysiology, the management of vasovagal syncope is fairly straightforward. The chief ingredients are the skills and equipment needed for cardiopulmonary resuscitation (CPR) (Table 23-2). The familiar ABCs of CPR provide an excellent framework for the management of vasovagal syncope.

Assessment. Place the patient supine, preferably with the head down. Check quickly for pulse, respiration, and level of consciousness. In basic CPR this means asking patients if they are all right, listening for respiration, and palpating a carotid pulse. If you've already attached an ECG monitor, consult the tracings, but don't take the time to attach one. In vasovagal syncope, you can expect an unconscious, apneic patient with a slow or nonpalpable or absent pulse.

FIGURE 23-2

Pathophysiology of vasovagal syncope

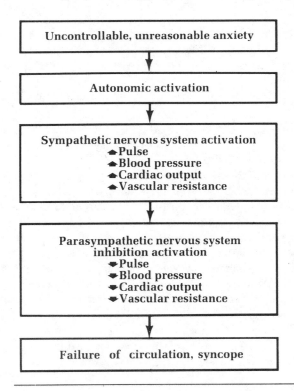

Airway. After quick assessment, establish an airway. The American Heart Association (AHA) recommends the victim's head "be tilted backward as far as possible."[6] If this doesn't clear the airway, use the jaw thrust maneuver. If she has vomited, remove the vomitus from the upper airway. Once these maneuvers are accomplished, quickly do a reassessment.

Breathing. If the patient does not rapidly begin to breathe spontaneously after you've established an airway, you must take the second step in CPR: Initiate breathing. How this is accomplished depends on the equipment available, but don't delay artificial respiration merely to obtain equipment.

The AHA recommends delivering four rapid breaths (mouth-to-mouth or by bag and mask) immediately following establishment of an airway. Follow this cycle by one breath every 5 seconds until spontaneous respirations resume. Palpate the carotid pulse again. If a pulse is present but slow, administer atropine 0.5 to 1 mg IV. If it's absent, go to the third step in CPR: Initiate circulation.[4]

Circulation. If the carotid pulse is absent, or even if there is a questionable pulse, you should use external cardiac compression to produce an artificial circulation. The AHA defines external cardiac compression as "the rhythmic application of pressure over the lower one half of the sternum, but not over the xyphoid process."[6] This maneuver should be performed 60 times/minute when two people are available, or 80 times/minute when only one is available. Always give external cardiac compression concomitantly with artificial ventilation. The techniques are well detailed in the AMA's *Standards for Cardiopulmonary Resuscitation.*[6] If after a few minutes of external compression there still is no cardiac activity, go to the fourth step in CPR: drug therapy.

TABLE 23-1

Symptoms of vasovagal syncope

SYMPATHETIC ACTIVATION	PARASYMPATHETIC ACTIVATION
Trembling	Diminished muscle tone, weakness
Diaphoresis	Urination
Pallor	Loss of bowel control
Hyperventilation	Loss of consciousness
Piloerection	Bradycardia

Drugs. The usual cardiovascular event in vasovagal syncope is cardiac asystole or a profound bradycardia. Once you establish adequate circulation and ventilation, administer atropine 0.5 to 1.0 mg IV. Repeat at 5-minute intervals until a pulse rate greater than 60 is established. The total dose of atropine should not exceed 2 mg. If atropine does not restore cardiac rhythm, further interventions will be necessary.

The interventions presuppose knowledge of the ECG and the ability to defibrillate the heart. Therefore, procedures likely to produce vasovagal syncope, such as the injection of a local anesthetic or painful procedures, should be performed only when an ECG machine and a defibrillator are available. If the ECG reveals asystole and it is unresponsive to atropine, then inject epinephrine 0.5 mg IV to convert the asystole to ventricular fibrillation.

Electrical defibrillation. If a patient is found in ventricular fibrillation, or if epinephrine has converted asystole to fibrillation, then perform direct current defibrillation using a delivered dose of 200 to 400 joules (watts/second). If an ECG is unavailable and the patient has been unresponsive to atropine, then give a dose of epinephrine and make one unmonitored defibrillation attempt.

DIFFERENTIAL DIAGNOSIS

Many conditions may mimic vasovagal syncope. The common ones include local anesthetic toxicity, profound hyperventilation, and myocardial infarction.

TABLE 23-2

ABCs of managing vasovagal syncope

Assess
Respiration, pulse, level of consciousness, and ECG (if possible)

Airway
Extend head or use jaw thrust maneuver

Breathing
Begin mouth-to-mouth resuscitation, or artificial intermittent positive pressure breathing with oxygen

Circulation
Perform external cardiac compression, 60 to 80 times/minute

Drugs
Administer atropine (0.5 to 1.0 mg IV) or epinephrine (0.5 mg IV)

Electricity
Apply direct current defibrillation (200 to 400 joules)

Local anesthetic toxicity. The accidental injection of a local anesthetic drug IV may produce symptoms like vasovagal syncope: agitation, tremulousness, and cardiorespiratory collapse with a seizure. What distinguishes the anesthetic reaction is that it occurs in the absence of a history of fainting and without the signs of anxiety and terror that usually precede a vasovagal attack. The management of the two conditions, however, is similar: Apply the basic steps of CPR. The anesthetic problem is usually brief and self-limited. If she breathes sufficient oxygen and the pulse is maintained, the patient will quickly awaken.

Hyperventilation. An extremely anxious patient may hyperventilate and lose consciousness as a result of intense cerebral vasoconstriction. This is usually a self-limited event. After this type of fainting, arterial CO_2 accumulates, vasoconstriction decreases, and the patient regains consciousness. Again, the management of hyperventilation syncope is the same as that of vasovagal syncope. Establish an airway and the patient will quickly begin breathing.

Myocardial infarction. A patient undergoing a stressful procedure, who has coronary artery disease, may develop a myocardial infarction during the procedure. Many of the same symptoms as vasovagal syncope may be produced, and, in fact, the myocardial infarction may result from the same mechanism that produces the vasovagal episode. The intense vasoconstriction and increased cardiac output stress initiates may increase the heart's oxygen requirements above what a compromised coronary circulation can provide. Myocardial ischemia and infarction may ensue, followed by vasomotor collapse, bradycardia, and profound hypotension. The patient's age, sex, and history may help you diagnose myocardial infarction.

CPR must be instituted and continued in either case, but recovery may take longer with a myocardial infarction. The patient who has had a heart attack will probably regain consciousness complaining of chest pain. If there is any doubt about whether the episode was vasovagal or myocardial, you should transfer the patient to a hospital for further evaluation and observation.

GUIDELINES TO PREVENTION

A patient who gives a history of fainting under stressful circumstances, or who appears more anxious than the nature of the procedure would warrant, may be considered susceptible to a vasovagal attack. Reviewing the entire procedure, giving reassurance, and encouraging questions may be helpful. An informative interview has been found most effective in reducing anxiety.[7] Tranquilizers or sedative drugs, given prophylactically in combination with atropine, may also help reduce the incidence or severity of attacks in susceptible individuals. Finally, when you prepare to do a potentially stressful procedure on a patient with a history of syncope, set up ECG monitoring and start an IV infusion before you begin.

REFERENCES

1. Engel GL: Psychologic stress, vasodepressor (vasovagal) syncope and sudden death. Ann Intern Med 89:403, 1978
2. Graham DT, Kabler JD, Lunsford L: Vasovagal fainting: A biphasic response. Psychosom Med 23:493, 1961
3. Tizes R: Cardiac arrest following routine venipuncture. JAMA 236:1846, 1976
4. Wolf S: Central autonomic influences on cardiac rate and rhythm. Mod Concepts Cardiovasc Dis 38:29, 1969
5. Gellhorn E: *Principles of Autonomic-Somatic Integrations.* Minneapolis, University of Minnesota Press, 1967
6. *Standards for Cardiopulmonary Resuscitation (CPR) and Emergency Cardiac Care (ECC).* JAMA 227:833, 1974
7. Egbert LD, Battit GE, Turndoff H, et al: The value of the pre-operative visit. JAMA 185:553, 1963

24

Responding to Cardiorespiratory Complications

ROBERT H. HAYASHI, MD

CLINICAL SIGNIFICANCE: Physiologic changes of pregnancy, as well as certain gynecologic conditions, can predispose patients to heart-lung problems. During pregnancy, accurate diagnosis and appropriate therapy will improve outcome for both mothers and babies.

Cardiorespiratory complications are rare in ob/gyn patients. All the more reason to stress the signs and symptoms, so the clinician can be ready to treat the occasional emergency. I'll begin by reviewing how pregnancy and various gynecologic situations alter the cardiorespiratory system. Then I will move on to management of several common clinical entities (Table 24-1).

CARDIORESPIRATORY CHANGES

Normal pregnant women often complain of excessive fatigue, shortness of breath, and peripheral edema. These complaints should not be ignored, because they are also those of patients in early congestive heart failure. The placenta provides a large arteriovenous shunt that results in a hyperdynamic cardiovascular state. Total peripheral vascular resistance decreases and midtrimester blood pressures often go below prepregnancy levels. Blood volume (proportionately more plasma volume than RBC volume) increases by 20% to 100% in midtrimester. Cardiac output increases by 30% to 50%, mainly as a result of increased stroke volume (20% to 40%); heart rate increases only 10% to 15%. Early postpartum, extravascular fluid volume rapidly shifts into the vascular compartment, requiring cardiac output that is increased 60% above prepregnancy levels.

Decreased muscular tone of the chest wall during pregnancy increases the anterior-posterior and lateral diameters of the chest, with elevation and flattening of the diaphragm. The pregnant woman's heart rotates laterally, so that the point of maximal impulse shifts to the left and the electrical axis of the ECG also shifts to the left by about 15°. The ECG can also show T-wave inversion and a Q wave in lead III. The changes in the chest cavity contribute decreased functional residual capacity and increased tidal volume. Vital capacity is unchanged. The respiratory system is not stressed in pregnancy; it becomes superefficient.

In gynecologic patients, acute cardiorespiratory complications are likely to occur during the intra- and postoperative periods. For exam-

---

TABLE 24-1

Management of ob/gyn cardiorespiratory complications

Pulmonary edema
Have patient sitting
Administer morphine 10 to 15 mg IM
Give IPPB with O_2
Infuse furosemide 40 mg IV slowly (may repeat in 15 to 20 minutes)
Prescribe digoxin 0.5 mg IV, then 0.25 mg IV q2h for total of six doses, but not if patient is hypokalemic
Treat underlying conditions

Reversal of intracardiac shunt
Identify patient at risk
Have IVs in both arms and blood ready at delivery
Replace any blood or volume loss quickly
Infuse dopamine 10 μg/kg/minute; increase by 1 to 4 μg/kg/minute q15m

Ventricular ectopic beats
Give lidocaine IV bolus of 50 to 100 mg, approximately 1 mg/kg (may repeat)
Follow with continuous infusion, 4 mg/minute, and taper over 24 hours
Or give procainamide 0.2-1.0 gm IV very slowly
Treat ventricular fibrillation with dc defibrillator (300 to 400 watts/second)

Adult respiratory distress syndrome
Give PEEP ventilation
Maintain strict intake-output fluid balance
Use diuretics cautiously
Treat underlying conditions aggressively

ple, older patients may have acute myocardial ischemia or heart damage. Hemorrhagic shock resulting in adult respiratory distress syndrome, aspiration pneumonitis, and pulmonary emboli are potential complications of gynecologic surgery.

HEART PROBLEMS

Acute pulmonary edema. Obstetric patients develop pulmonary edema in several ways. The cardiac patient with rheumatic mitral valve disease may have acute left ventricular failure. Patients are likely to go into heart failure when the changes of pregnancy demand increased cardiac output, that is, in midpregnancy, late in the second stage of labor, and immediately postpartum. As left atrial pressure increases, myocardial failure raises pulmonary venous and capillary pressures. When pulmonary intravascular pressure rises above colloid osmotic pressure (COP), free fluid leaves the vascular tree and enters the alveoli and terminal bronchioles—producing pulmonary edema.[1]

Patients with severe preeclampsia or eclampsia may develop pulmonary edema. Their total peripheral vascular resistance may rise and increase cardiac workload; their COP may fall because of hypoalbuminemia; and those with decreased intravascular volume may be easily overloaded when IV fluids are administered. Those being treated for premature labor with sympathomimetic agents, with and without corticosteroids, are also at risk for pulmonary edema.[2, 3] The cause in this case is unclear, but the edema usually follows prolonged therapy and substantial volumes of IV fluids. Pulmonary edema has been reported when large volumes of fluid are infused, when there is no heart failure.[4]

Patients with acute pulmonary edema may have suffocating dyspnea, tachypnea, anxiety, and labored breathing. Physical examination shows diffuse rales and frothy, possibly blood-tinged, sputum. Chest x-rays usually show diffuse or perihilar infiltrates in both lung fields.

Treat acute pulmonary edema by having the patient sit up, give morphine 10 to 15 mg IM to relieve anxiety, and administer oxygen by mask. Oxygen by positive pressure raises intrapulmonary pressure and decreases pulmonary venous return to the heart—this could be an added benefit. Give 40 mg furosemide as a slow IV injection, and repeat in 15 to 20 minutes, if necessary. This rapidly acting diuretic also decreases venomotor tone to promote peripheral venous pooling.[5]

Consider rapid digitalization of the cardiac patient to enhance myocardial function. But use digitalis with caution, if at all, for patients who have recently been given sympathomimetic drugs for premature labor. Such patients tend to be hypokalemic. For rapid digitalization, give digoxin 0.5 mg IV followed by 0.25 mg every 2 to 4 hours as needed, but do not exceed a total dose of 2 mg in 12 hours. A steady-state therapeutic level is 1.5 ng/mL and the half-life is 36 hours.

If left heart failure is associated with acute hypertension, lower the blood pressure to lessen the cardiac afterload. You can inject hydralazine intermittently, 5 to 10 mg IV, or in a constant infusion (50 mg in 500 mL D_5W), to lower the diastolic pressure to 90 to 110 mm Hg. Obtain hourly readings of urine output, frequent serum electrolyte levels, and periodic arterial blood gases and ECGs. Correct any hypokalemia, particularly in patients treated for premature labor.

If flow-directed catheters (Swan-Ganz) are available for monitoring pulmonary capillary wedge pressure (PCWP), use them. This type of monitoring can provide a clue to the pathophysiology of the edema. COP measurements may indicate whether an albumin infusion along with furosemide might be beneficial.

Once the edema subsides, the specific obstetric and medical problems will dictate care. Serial measurements of total pulmonary vital capacity are useful for following patients who are at risk of congestive heart failure.[6]

Reversal of intracardiac shunt. Certain congenital heart defects are associated with intracardiac left-to-right shunts: atrial and ventricular septal defects, Eisenmenger's syndrome, and tetralogy of Fallot. About two-thirds of maternal deaths associated with these conditions occur around delivery.[7] Excessive blood loss or decreased peripheral vascular resistance may reverse the left-to-right shunt, causing a bypass of the lungs. Hypoxemia will quickly ensue. The best management of these patients is preventive. Have large-bore IV catheters in both arms, and blood in the delivery suite, to correct excessive blood loss quickly. Avoid conduction anesthesia and the supine hypotension syndrome.

If a shunt reversal occurs, expand the circulating volume as quickly as possible and consider using a peripheral vasoconstrictor to increase left heart afterload pressure. If you try a dopamine infusion (800 μg/mL concentration), begin at 10 μg/kg/minute and increase gradually by 1 to 4 μg/kg/minute every 15 minutes until the patient is normotensive. At this dosage, the drug will produce an increase in cardiac output and peripheral resistance. Once the shunt reversal has occurred, the prognosis for survival is poor.

Acute myocardial infarction. One in 10,000 deliveries is complicated by acute myocardial infarction. The disorder is more frequent when older women have gynecologic procedures. Anterior chest pain and .ECG changes will clinch the diagnosis. Because myocardial ischemia is manifested by exaggerated inverted T waves, the ECG changes may include some of the following (Figure 24-1): tall T waves that indicate subendocardial ischemia (A); inverted T waves that indicate epicardial ischemia (B); RST-segment depression that indicates subendocardial injury (C); and RST-segment elevation that indicates epicardial injury

(D). ECG death is usually the equivalent of biologic death and results in QS waves in the lead facing the area of transmural infarction (E).[8]

Management of pregnant patients with an infarction would include oxygen, analgesics, intensive care, monitoring for arrhythmias, but no anticoagulants. The gynecologic patient might be given anticoagulants, depending on whether or not she is postoperative. These decisions should be made with the attending cardiologist.

Cardiac arrhythmia. Pregnant patients are more prone than nonpregnant women to episodes of paroxysmal tachycardia. A healthy woman can tolerate these episodes, but carotid sinus stimulation, the Valsalva maneuver, or digitalis or quinidine may help. If the patient has any hemodynamic embarrassment from the supraventricular tachycardia, and the vagal stimulation maneuvers fail, use direct current (dc) cardioversion. This is effective and safe during pregnancy.[9] Use the synchronizer circuit on the dc defibrillator at the low-energy level (20 to 50 watts/second). The patient should be sedated with diazepam before starting this procedure.

FIGURE 24-1

*Characteristic ECG forms of ischemic events**

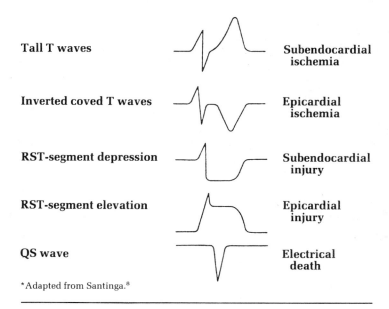

Tall T waves	**Subendocardial ischemia**
Inverted coved T waves	**Epicardial ischemia**
RST-segment depression	**Subendocardial injury**
RST-segment elevation	**Epicardial injury**
QS wave	**Electrical death**

*Adapted from Santinga.[8]

During early labor, consider using antiarrhythmic agents if warning arrhythmias appear on the ECG (frequent premature ventricular contractions, R-on-T phenomenon, multifocality, bigeminy, or short bursts of ventricular tachycardia).[10] The risk of hypoxemia or hypotension is substantial in peripartum.

Lidocaine effectively controls ventricular ectopic activity if prompt treatment is necessary.[11] Give an IV bolus of lidocaine, 10 to 100 mg (approximately 1 mg/kg), rapidly. This dose may be repeated every 3 to 5 minutes until the dysrhythmia is suppressed (doses in excess of 300 mg approach toxic levels). Follow bolus doses of lidocaine immediately with continuous infusion of 20 to 50 μg/kg/minute (or 1 to 4 mg/minute in the 70-kg patient). For example, begin a 4-mg/minute infusion immediately (1 gm lidocaine in 500 mL D_5W) after the bolus, and gradually taper during the next 24 hours.[12] Some patients will respond to depressants such as procainamide, quinidine, or disopyramide when lidocaine has failed.[10] The usual IV dose of procainamide hydrochloride is 0.2 to 1.0 gm and should be given very slowly at a rate not in excess of 25 to 50 mg/minute. For ventricular fibrillation, use the dc defibrillator at 300 to 400 watts/second.

Atrial fibrillation in a pregnant woman with rheumatic heart disease places her at risk for pulmonary embolus (23%) and heart failure.[13] Try to restore normal sinus rhythm, administer digitalis to slow the ventricular response, and then give a maintenance dose of quinidine (0.2 to 0.3 gm orally every 6 to 8 hours). If atrial fibrillation persists or recurs, seriously consider long-term anticoagulation.

WHEN THE LUNG IS INVOLVED

Adult respiratory distress syndrome (ARDS). This serious and potentially fatal pulmonary disease may complicate a variety of obstetric and

---

TABLE 24-2

Aspiration pneumonitis

Perform endotracheal suction if aspiration is noted

Infuse with hydrocortisone 1 gm IV at once and q4h

Give IPPB with O_2

Monitor arterial blood gases (patient may need intubation or tracheostomy)

Administer aminophylline 250 to 500 mg in 50 mL of D_5W over 20 minutes to counteract bronchospasm

Consider antibiotics to prevent secondary infections

gynecologic conditions: amniotic fluid embolism, aspiration, severe preeclampsia, eclampsia, massive fluid infusions, sepsis, and intra-abdominal or pelvic abscesses.[14] ARDS has been well recognized in association with massive trauma and shock.

Progressive respiratory distress and severe hypoxemia, relatively refractory to high inspired oxygen tension, characterize the syndrome. Chest x-rays show diffuse infiltrates.

The clinical picture is similar to that seen in pulmonary edema, except that the patchy or fluffy infiltrates involve the patient's entire lung field. The alveolar-capillary membrane becomes increasingly permeable, and progressive interstitial and alveolar edema results. You can differentiate cardiac from noncardiac pulmonary edema by determining the PCWP with a flow-directed catheter. In ARDS, the pulmonary artery pressures and pulmonary vascular resistance may be elevated, but the PCWP remains low or normal; in cardiogenic pulmonary edema, the PCWP is elevated.[15]

To manage ARDS, support cardiovascular and respiratory function and treat underlying or associated conditions. Positive end expiratory pressure (PEEP) ventilation has become the key in therapy. PEEP increases arterial oxygenation by increasing lung volumes and decreasing intrapulmonary shunting. The goal is to maintain arterial oxygenation of at least 60 torr. This generally requires a tidal volume of 10 to 20 cc/kg and a PEEP level of 5 to 35 cm H_2O.[15] Balance the intake and output of fluids. Use diuretics with caution, and give antibiotics and packed red blood cell transfusions as needed. The use of steroids has been controversial. Again, aggressive management is critical to recovery.

TABLE 24-3

Pulmonary embolus

Give 5,000 to 10,000 units of heparin IV initially and then repeat every 4 to 6 hours. Maintain whole blood clotting time at two to three times normal, or the activated PTT at one and a half to two times normal

Prescribe constant infusion of approximately 1,000 units of heparin per hour as acceptable alternative. Monitor the same way

Watch for hemorrhagic complications

Order O_2 and mild sedation

If repeated embolization occurs while patient is on anticoagulant therapy, surgically interrupt inferior vena cava and possibly left ovarian vein

---

TABLE 24-4

Amniotic fluid embolus

Have patient sitting

Inject morphine 10 to 15 mg IM

Give IPPB with O_2

Give aminophylline 250 to 500 mg in 50 mL D_5W over 20 minutes

Prescribe digoxin 0.5 mg IV, then 0.25 mg IV q2h for six doses

Order hydrocortisone 1 gm IV; follow with 250 mg q4h

Compress uterus to control atony

Make judicious use of blood transfusion therapy

Combat coagulopathy with fresh frozen plasma or cryoprecipitate

---

Postevacuation of molar pregnancy syndrome. Acute respiratory insufficiency in the early postevacuation period among patients with a uterus of 16 weeks' size or greater has a reported incidence of 27%.[16] The syndrome is characterized by tachycardia, tachypnea, and hypoxemia.[17] Chest x-rays demonstrate patchy or fluffy bilateral pulmonary infiltrates, and sometimes a concomitant pleural effusion. Contributing factors include deportation of trophoblastic tissue, hyperthyroidism, fluid overload, dilutional anemia, preeclampsia, and general anesthesia.[16, 17] Before evacuating a mole, document blood gases for baseline study. Watch fluids in the pre-, intra-, and postoperative periods and carefully monitor CVP. Treat aggressively any underlying condition such as hyperthyroidism, preeclampsia, or anemia. Use oxygen, sedation, and diuretics as needed. The syndrome is uniformly transient, with good outcome, but patients have been reported at risk of later having invasive mole or choriocarcinoma.[7]

Tables 24-2 to 24-4 give management protocols for treating aspiration pneumonitis, pulmonary embolus, and amniotic fluid embolus. These entities have been discussed in detail by Huff and Hayashi.[18]

REFERENCES

1. Rackow EC, Fein IA, Leppo A: Colloid osmotic pressure as a prognostic indicator of pulmonary edema and mortality in the critically ill. Chest 72:709, 1979
2. Jacobs MM, Knight AB, Arias F: Maternal pulmonary edema resulting from betamimetic and glucocorticoid therapy. Obstet Gynecol 56:56, 1980
3. Katz M, Robertson PA, Creasy RK: Cardiovascular complications associated with terbutaline treatment for preterm labor. Am J Obstet Gynecol 139:605, 1981

4. Stein L, Beraud J, Cavanilles J, et al: Pulmonary edema during fluid infusion in the absence of heart failure. JAMA 229:65, 1974

5. Dikshit K, Vyden JK, Forrester JS, et al: Renal and extrarenal hemodynamic effects of furosemide in congestive heart failure after acute myocardial infarction. N Engl J Med 288:1087, 1973

6. Kannel WB, Seidman JM, Fercho W, et al: Vital capacity and congestive heart failure: The Framingham study. Circulation 49:1160, 1974

7. Conradsson TB, Werko L: Management of heart disease in pregnancy. Prog Cardiovasc Dis 16:407, 1974

8. Santinga JT: Electrocardiographic diagnosis of anterior myocardial infarction. Univ Mich Med Ctr J 40:20, 1974

9. Schroeder JS, Harrison DC: Repeated cardioversion during pregnancy. Am J Cardiol 27:445, 1971

10. Myerburg RJ, Besozzi MC: Decisions in the treatment of ventricular ectopic activity. JAMA 240:476, 1978

11. Lie KI, Wellens JH, van Capelle FJ, et al: Lidocaine in the prevention of primary ventricular fibrillation: A double blind, randomized study of 212 consecutive patients. N Engl J Med 291:1324, 1974

12. Collinsworth KA, Kalman SM, Harrison DC: The clinical pharmacology of lidocaine as an antiarrhythmic drug. Circulation 50:1217, 1974

13. Mendelson CL: Disorders of the heart during pregnancy. Am J Obstet Gynecol 72:1268, 1956

14. Andersen HF, Lynch JP, Johnson TRB Jr: Adult respiratory distress syndrome in obstetrics and gynecology. Obstet Gynecol 55:291, 1980

15. Zapol WM, Snider MT: Pulmonary hypertension in severe acute respiratory failure. N Engl J Med 296:476, 1977

16. Cotton DB, Bernstein SG, Read JA, et al: Hemodynamic observations in evacuation of molar pregnancy. Am J Obstet Gynecol 138:6, 1980

17. Twiggs LB, Morrow CP, Schlaerth JB: Acute pulmonary complications of molar pregnancy. Am J Obstet Gynecol 135:189, 1979

18. Huff RW, Hayashi RH: Emergencies in obstetric patients: Difficulties in breathing. Contemp Ob/Gyn 11:54, Jan 1978

25

Anovulatory Bleeding

LEON SPEROFF, MD

CLINICAL SIGNIFICANCE: This type of uterine bleeding can almost always be treated medically; very few patients need surgery. Define the problem, then administer appropriate hormone therapy.

Categorizing endometrial bleeding by descriptive terms, such as hypomenorrhea, hypermenorrhea, polymenorrhea, menorrhagia, and metrorrhagia, only complicates clinical management. These are terms designed to tax one's memory. It is more straightforward and helpful to have a general understanding of normal and abnormal bleeding.

The most reproducible indication of menstrual function, in terms of quantity and duration, is the postovulatory estrogen-progesterone withdrawal bleeding response. This response is so dependable that many women, over the years, come to expect a certain characteristic flow pattern. Any slight deviation may be a cause for concern on the patient's part and may require strong reassurance from the physician. Significant deviation requires evaluation for a local or systemic problem. A thorough history and physical examination are usually sufficient for evaluating teen-agers. However, adult patients often require appropriate biopsies, including one of the current vacuum techniques for endometrial sampling.

DEFINING THE PROBLEM

Dysfunctional uterine bleeding can be defined as the bleeding manifestations of anovulatory cycles. This type of bleeding can result from systemic problems, such as hypothyroidism, obesity, and liver disease, or from psychogenic problems, such as mild anorexia nervosa. Regardless of the cause, anovulatory cycles may produce abnormal bleeding patterns and often can be managed without surgical intervention. Indeed, failure to control vaginal bleeding with medical therapy strongly suggests a pathologic condition within the reproductive tract.

Abnormal patterns include:

- Excessive or prolonged cyclic bleeding
- Delayed menses followed by heavy or prolonged flow
- Premenstrual and postmenstrual spotting
- Intermenstrual bleeding.

There are two common major categories of dysfunctional endometrial bleeding. The first, *estrogen breakthrough bleeding*, is characteristic of anovulation. The amount of circulating estrogen and fluctuations in the blood level determine the type of bleeding. Relatively low amounts of estrogen yield intermittent spotting, which may be prolonged, but the flow is generally light. High levels of estrogen and sustained availability lead to prolonged periods of amenorrhea, followed by acute and often profuse bleeds with excessive loss of blood. High levels of estrogen are most often associated with polycystic ovary syndrome, immaturity of the hypothalamic-pituitary-ovarian axis in teen-agers, and late anovulation in perimenopausal women. Without growth-limiting progesterone and periods of desquamation, the endometrium attains an abnormal height but no competent structural support. This tissue is fragile and suffers spontaneous breakage and bleeding.

The second type, *progestational breakthrough bleeding*, is encountered in patients who are anovulatory as the result of taking progestin medication, such as birth control pills, progestin therapy for endometriosis, or treatment with depot forms of progestin. Without sufficient estrogen, continuous progestational impact on the endometrium yields intermittent bleeding of variable duration, which can be heavy at times.

Estrogen and progestational breakthrough bleeding lack self-limitation, the single most important property of the estrogen-progesterone withdrawal bleed that follows the ovulatory cycle. There are three reasons for the self-limiting character of ovulatory bleeding:

- It is a universal endometrial event. The onset and conclusion of menses are related to a precise sequence of hormonal events, and menstrual changes begin almost simultaneously throughout every segment of the endometrium.
- The endometrial tissue that has responded to a sequence of estrogen and progesterone is structurally stable and the events leading to ischemic disintegration of the endometrium are orderly and progressive in character.
- The vasomotor response involved in stopping menstrual flow is a consequence of the events that start menstrual bleeding following estrogen-progesterone stimulation. Waves of vasoconstriction initiate the ischemic event to provoke menses; prolonged vasoconstriction, abetted by the stasis associated with endometrial collapse, enables clotting factors to seal off exposed bleeding sites. In the subsequent cycle, the resumed stimulation of rising estrogen levels adds to the healing effect.

CHOOSING THE THERAPY

After evaluation and examination, including biopsies if appropriate, the immediate objective of medical therapy for anovulatory bleeding is to restore the natural controlling influences—universal, synchronous endometrial events, structural stability, and vasomotor rhythmicity. Table 25-1 summarizes the principal points of treatment. Therapy involves an initial choice between high-dose progestin-estrogen combination medication and high doses of estrogen.

Any brand of progestin-estrogen oral contraceptives can control bleeding rapidly and easily. Administer one pill four times daily for 5 to 7 days. Continue this therapy even though flow usually ceases within 12 to 24 hours. If flow does not clearly diminish, re-evaluate other diagnostic possibilities, such as polyps, incomplete abortion, and neoplasia, by examination under anesthesia and D&C. If flow does diminish rapidly, the remainder of the week of treatment can be devoted to evaluating causes of anovulation, hemorrhagic tendencies, and iron or blood replacement.

TABLE 25-1

Principal points of medical therapy for anovulatory bleeding

Evaluate by history and physical examination

Begin intense progestin-estrogen therapy and maintain it for 7 days

Continue cyclic low-dose oral contraceptives for at least 3 months

For premenopausal, sexually active women, continue oral contraception

If contraception is unnecessary, induce progestational withdrawal bleeding on a monthly basis with medroxyprogesterone acetate, 10 mg for the first 10 days of each month

Give high-dose estrogen therapy—25 mg conjugated estrogen IV every 4 hours—under the following conditions:
  If bleeding has been prolonged
  If the biopsy yields minimal tissue
  If the patient is on progestin medication

If this medical therapy produces no response in 12 to 24 hours, proceed with D&C

The four-pills-a-day therapy induces structural rigidity intrinsic to the compact pseudodecidual reaction. Continued random breakdown of formerly fragile tissue is avoided and blood loss is stopped. However, a relatively large amount of tissue remains to react to withdrawal of the medication. The patient must be warned to anticipate a heavy, perhaps severely cramping flow 2 to 4 days after stopping therapy.

Continued control of bleeding requires maintaining cyclic combination birth control medication. Each successive cycle serves to prevent any regrowth that might be caused by unopposed estrogen and allows orderly regression of excessive endometrial height to normal, controllable levels.

For the patient who does not require contraception and whose endometrial tissue has been reduced to normal height, discontinue the pill and start monthly progestin therapy. Recent studies in England found that postmenopausal women needed 10 days of progestational therapy to prevent hyperplasia and endometrial adenocarcinoma.[1] Therefore, it seems wise to apply this duration of therapy to the younger anovulatory woman. Accordingly, medroxyprogesterone acetate, 10 mg orally, is given the first 10 days of every month. This induces a reasonable flow 2 to 7 days after the last pill and prevents excessive endometrial buildup. Regular shedding and the need to form new tissue each month prevent prolonged stimulation and development of hyperplasia. If bleeding occurs at an unexpected time, the occurrence of spontaneous ovulation must be suspected.

Spontaneous ovulation in the anovulatory patient is possible and unpredictable. Since there is no evidence that birth control pills increase the risk of secondary amenorrhea, the need for contraception takes precedence. For a patient who requires contraception, it is prudent to maintain pill medication.

Bleeding manifestations are frequently associated with low estrogen stimulation. There is usually intermittent vaginal spotting, and endometrial biopsy yields little tissue. Progestin treatment has no beneficial effect, because a tissue base is lacking on which the progestin may exert its organizational and strengthening action. This is also true of anovulatory patients in whom prolonged hemorrhage leaves little residual tissue. Give such patients high-dose estrogen therapy—conjugated estrogens 25 mg IV every 4 hours until bleeding diminishes. Usually treatment is maintained for 24 hours. If this high-dose estrogen therapy does not significantly diminish flow within 12 to 24 hours, D&C is necessary. If blood flow does diminish, initiate therapy with combination oral contraceptives. When bleeding is not excessive and IV therapy is not practical, a program of oral high-dose estrogen medication may be used: 10 mg conjugated estrogens for 7 days, followed by combination birth control pills.

Two problems clinicians frequently encounter are associated with progestin breakthrough bleeding: the bleeding encountered with birth control pills and that related to treatment regimens using oral or depot forms of progestin. When there is insufficient endogenous and exogenous estrogen, the endometrium becomes shallow. It is composed almost exclusively of pseudodecidual stroma and blood vessels with minimal glands. This type of endometrium is also fragile and may break down. Breakthrough bleeding in the first few months of treatment is best managed by encouragement and reassurance. If necessary, even this early pattern can be treated with exogenous estrogen.

It is helpful to explain to the patient that this bleeding represents tissue breakdown as the endometrium readjusts from its usual thick state to the relatively thin state promoted by the progestin therapy. If bleeding occurs just before the end of a pill cycle, it can be managed by having the patient stop the pills, wait seven days, and start a new cycle. If breakthrough bleeding is prolonged or distressing, it can be controlled by a short course of exogenous estrogen. Give conjugated estrogens 2.5 mg or ethinylestradiol 20 μg daily for 7 days, no matter where the patient is in her pill or treatment cycle. Have her adhere to the pill-taking schedule. Usually one course of estrogen solves the problem. Recurrence of breakthrough bleeding is unusual, but if it does recur, another 7-day course of estrogen is effective.

Increasing the dose of the progestational agent does not correct irregular bleeding. The progestin component of the pill will always dominate; doubling the number of pills doubles the progestational impact, with its decidualizing, atrophic effect on the endometrium. Adding extra estrogen while keeping the progestin dose unchanged is both logical and effective.

If a patient has recurrent bleeding despite repeated medical therapy, you must suspect submucous myomas or endometrial polyps. Even thorough curettage can miss such pathology and further diagnostic study may be helpful. Either hysterosalpingography, with slow instillations of dye and careful fluoroscopic examination, or hysteroscopy may reveal a myoma or polyp. These conditions are particularly likely in the puzzling case of a patient with abnormal bleeding and ovulatory cycles.

REFERENCE
1. Paterson MEL, Wade-Evans T, Sturdee OW, et al: Endometrial disease after treatment with oestrogens and progestogens in the climacteric. Br Med J 1:822, 1980

26
Vaginal Hemorrhage

WALTER B. JONES, MD

CLINICAL SIGNIFICANCE: First be alert to the risk, then apply correct procedures promptly, and you may prevent or control life-threatening bleeds. Definitive treatment of the underlying disease process is the ultimate goal.

The problem of vaginal hemorrhage is one that may confront the clinician at any time. Copious vaginal bleeding is a challenge not only to the oncologist but to the general gynecologist as well. In addition, the gynecologist is expected to manage the uterine hemorrhage that sometimes occurs with an underlying bleeding diathesis. Correct procedures can usually stop the bleeding. Some hemorrhage can be prevented.

PATIENTS LIKELY TO HAVE PROBLEMS

Hemorrhage can be defined as any bleeding that requires active treatment. It is often the first indication of a tumor in the vagina or cervix. It is seen most often in patients who have not consulted a physician since their last pregnancy, perhaps as long as 25 or 30 years ago. Vaginal bleeding is likely to be the first sign that a tumor exists.

Bleeding may also be the first sign of vaginal cancer in a young woman exposed in utero to diethylstilbestrol. But this has come to be the exception, because of the publicity given to the DES problem in recent years. Vaginal bleeding may be the first sign of sarcoma botryoides in very young children. Other patients at risk for severe vaginal hemorrhage are women with metastatic vaginal choriocarcinoma or metastases from primary ovarian, endometrial, or colonic tumors.

Hemorrhage from the uterus is often the hallmark of endometrial carcinoma, as every gynecologist knows only too well. It is also a characteristic sign of molar pregnancy. Occasionally uterine hemorrhage may be a complication of acute leukemia, either as the initial sign of the disease or as a side effect in patients undergoing chemotherapy. Such bleeding may also occur with aplastic anemia and von Willebrand's disease.

Under certain circumstances, postoperative hemorrhage may be anticipated. Occasionally a patient who has had cone biopsy of the cervix will have bleeding approximately 10 days to 2 weeks after the operation—the time when the catgut stitches dissolve. This type of bleeding is likely to result from faulty technique.

When hemorrhage complicates radical hysterectomy, it is usually because of incomplete hemostasis at surgery. Patients who have undergone exenteration may also hemorrhage immediately following the operation. Most of these patients have cervical cancer unsuccessfully treated with radiation. They also risk delayed hemorrhage months to years later. The source may simply be granulation tissue at the apex of the vaginal remnant, which begins to bleed spontaneously, or it may be the life-threatening rupture of hypogastric vessels.

CONTROLLING THE HEMORRHAGE

Cervical and vaginal hemorrhage. You may choose among several methods to stop cervical and vaginal bleeding. The first step is, of course, to determine the cause. Modest bleeding from a vaginal tumor may be controlled by applying a silver nitrate stick to the area. Almost as simple, and perhaps more effective, is application of Monsel's solution (ferric subsulfate), using a cotton swab or a soaked cotton ball, with direct pressure.

If the bleeding is copious, do suture ligation of the bleeding vessel with No. 0 chromic suture. If the vessel cannot be seen, suture the bleeding bed.

When this method is also unsuccessful, packing with a head-and-neck roll (gauze pack) saturated with acetone can be effective. When even this method fails, three alternatives are available—selective arterial embolization, emergency irradiation, or, as a last resort, ligation of the hypogastric vessels.

When skilled radiologists are available, percutaneous selective embolization with autologous clot, gelatin foam, or detachable silicone balloons may obviate the need for hypogastric ligation.[1, 2] Ligating the hypogastric arteries interferes with the vascularization of the tumor-bearing area, and this may jeopardize future treatment of patients who will receive radiation as definitive therapy.

Use an external high-energy beam for bleeding tumors of the cervix or vagina. Give high-dose fractions of 600 rad daily for three days through small, 10 × 10-cm portals encompassing the tumor. Alternatively, intracavitary irradiation can be employed from either a radium or a cesium source, at 1,500 to 2,000 mg/hour. Be ready to give blood transfusions as needed.

The correct treatment of a molar pregnancy is to evacuate the uterus with suction during infusion of an oxytocic agent. Then give a uterotropic agent such as ergonovine maleate. At one time, hysterotomy was the procedure of choice when the uterus was enlarged, but today evacuation can be accomplished safely from below, regardless of the size of the uterus. In metastatic trophoblastic disease, we sometimes see a mass in the vagina. Such lesions should never be biopsied or excised, because of the bleeding danger.

One patient with a vaginal metastasis, correctly treated with chemotherapy, responded with disappearance of the mass and a drop in hCG titer, though not to normal values. She failed to return for follow-up and, 6 months later, staff at another hospital informed us that she had been admitted and was hemorrhaging. She was transferred to our hospital, still bleeding profusely from a recurrence of the vaginal metastasis. We started transfusions in both arms, and attempted to stop the flow with cautery and packing. Both methods were unsuccessful, as was suturing. The tumor had a soft, spongy consistency; it was like trying to suture a pudding. We ligated the hypogastric arteries and, immediately after the operation, irradiated the vaginal tumor.

We then treated this patient with the combination chemotherapy that had been successful the first time. Within 2 months her titer returned to normal and the vaginal tumor completely disappeared. Unfortunately, the patient again failed to return for follow-up appointments.

Endometrial hemorrhage. Diagnostic D&C can also be therapeutic for an endometrial hemorrhage. If the D&C fails to stop the bleeding, the uterus can be packed. Begin by packing both cornua, then pack the central cavity. Packing should be left in place for 24 to 48 hours, then removed slowly and carefully. When this technique fails, try external radiation therapy. Should the hemorrhage continue, add intracavitary irradiation with radium or cesium.

One patient with severe uterine hemorrhage caused by aplastic anemia responded atypically. When the original packing was removed, she again began to hemorrhage; the uterus had to be repacked. Then, 2 weeks later, she started to bleed again. Remember that this patient's basic problem was a hemorrhagic diathesis, not a gynecologic condition. She was also bleeding from other orifices—bladder, rectum, mouth. Once again, the uterus was packed and a transfusion with platelets and other coagulation factors given. About a week later, the patient became febrile. Because we thought infection might be developing, we removed the packing. A pack left in place too long in a granulocytopenic patient makes infection always a possibility.

Postexenteration hemorrhage. Hemorrhage after exenteration may be the result of previous intensive radiation therapy that produced tissue necrosis, or recurrent tumor. It is sometimes possible to visualize the source of the bleeding, when a perineal opening remains. Often, the bleeding can be controlled from below by applying a clamp or a hemo-clip to the vessel. The clamp can be left in place for 24 to 48 hours, if hemostasis cannot be achieved otherwise, or until adequate replace-ment transfusion has been carried out, if exploratory surgery is planned. However, clamping the vessel from below may be unsuccess-ful, particularly in older women whose vessels may have become frag-ile. The only certain method of controlling such bleeding is to perform a laparotomy and stop the bleeding from within.

Bleeding from the distal stump of the hypogastric artery or pelvic floor vein may be severe. You can usually identify the source of the bleeding by suctioning to remove fresh blood and following the suction catheter down to the source. If you have found the source, put a large

---

FIGURE 26-1

*Relationship between hemorrhage and platelet count**

Curve shows percentage of days with hemorrhage in a 92-patient group, correlated with platelet readings. Low—and falling—counts indicate need for intervention.

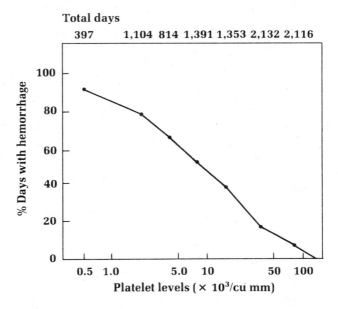

*Modified from Gaydos, Freireich, and Mantel.[4]

hemoclip on it. If not, ligate the vascular bed with silk sutures. As a last resort, apply a pelvic pack, using a head-and-neck roll.

While there is no way to prevent bleeding after exenteration, there are warning signs. A history of even minimal bleeding from the perineum may portend severe bleeding episodes. Watch for evidence of any bleeding at all. Seek the source immediately; don't wait for active bleeding to begin.

Hemorrhage in acute leukemia. For patients with acute leukemia following chemotherapy, or for those who have other hemorrhagic diatheses, D&C is not recommended. Vaginal bleeding can often be controlled by means of therapeutic amenorrhea. First, give medroxyprogesterone acetate 10 mg every 4 hours for rapid cessation of bleeding. Once active bleeding diminishes, give a combination pill containing a potent progestin, such as Ovral. In leukemic patients, continue this therapy until the bone marrow recovers sufficiently from the effects of the cytotoxic drugs so that the threat of blood loss from normal menstrual flow no longer need be feared. There is no objection to continuing therapeutic amenorrhea throughout the treatment period.

PREVENTING HEMORRHAGE

Many bleeding episodes occur because patients did not consult a physician in time. Early treatment of cervical and vaginal cancers usually makes such episodes unlikely.

Avoid biopsy of a metastatic focus of choriocarcinoma in the vagina. This can cause uncontrollable, often fatal, hemorrhage.

In solid tumors,[3] as well as acute leukemia,[4] low platelet levels may predict bleeding episodes (see Figure 26-1). If the platelet count is in the low-normal range and falling fast, give platelets immediately and be prepared to intervene surgically, if necessary.

REFERENCES

1. Smith DC, Wyatt JF: Embolization of the hypogastric arteries in the control of massive vaginal hemorrhage. Obstet Gynecol 49:317, 1977
2. White RI, Kaufman SL, Barth KH, et al: Therapeutic embolization with detachable silicone balloons. JAMA 23:1257, 1979
3. Belt RJ, Leite C, Haas CD, et al: Incidence of hemorrhage complications in patients with cancer. JAMA 239:2571, 1978
4. Gaydos LA, Freireich EJ, Mantel N: The quantitative relationship between platelet count and hemorrhage in patients with acute leukemia. N Engl J Med 266:905, 1962

27

Ruptured Pelvic Abscess

DAVID L. HEMSELL, MD, and
F. GARY CUNNINGHAM, MD

CLINICAL SIGNIFICANCE: Only about 0.3% of patients admitted to ob/gyn services require immediate surgery for ruptured pelvic abscesses. Most are in the third or fourth decade of life and may show little clinical evidence of peritonitis; all the more important that diagnosis be accurate and management appropriate. A large amount of purulent material in the peritoneal cavity can be lethal.

Patients with ruptured tubo-ovarian or pelvic abscesses have a wide spectrum of signs and symptoms. The common denominator is that they all require immediate and aggressive therapy. A large volume of purulent material in the peritoneal cavity mandates prompt surgery; leakage may respond to intensive medical management alone or to surgery after an interval of antimicrobial therapy.

Before the 1950s, when operative treatment was not the rule, 75% to 100% of patients with ruptured adnexal abscesses died. These devastating statistics prompted Collins and Mickal and their colleagues at Charity Hospital, New Orleans, and Vemeeren and TeLinde at Johns Hopkins Hospital to advocate drainage and adnexal extirpation.[1-3] This approach—coupled with new techniques for administering anesthesia, fluid replacement, and antimicrobials—has reversed the mortality/survival ratio (Table 27-1).

WHO IS AT RISK?

Patients with ruptured tubo-ovarian or pelvic abscesses make up only 0.2% to 0.3% of admissions in teaching hospitals. Gynecologists in private practice probably encounter these problems even less frequently. The incidence of leaking abscesses is undoubtedly higher, but is unknown. Women with abscesses tend to be older and of lower parity than those with uncomplicated pelvic infections. A larger number are infertile and have had previous documented pelvic infections. Most ruptured abscesses occur in the third and fourth decades, but the reported age range is from preteens to the 70s.

Women who have had pelvic inflammatory disease are more likely to develop abscesses, but occasionally abscesses complicate an initial episode of salpingitis. There is increasing evidence that IUD wearers are at higher risk. As many as 20% to 40% of adnexal abscesses may be unilateral even without an IUD. An infected ectopic pregnancy may present in this manner. Women who have recently had hysterectomies may develop abscesses, usually following pelvic and cuff cellulitis. Table 27-2 gives the common physical findings associated with pelvic abscesses.

SIGNS AND SYMPTOMS

A woman with a leaking or ruptured abscess appears ill and almost invariably complains of abdominal pain and, often, nausea, vomiting, and fever. Usually she has had nonspecific lower abdominal or pelvic pain for several days, with a recent and sudden increase in intensity. Physical findings resemble peritonitis, the severity paralleling the severity of the illness. For example, overt rupture is accompanied by generalized peritonitis and dramatic clinical symptoms. But women in their mid-40s, and especially diabetics, may have little clinical evidence of peritonitis, despite unrelenting sepsis from large amounts of purulent material free in the peritoneal cavity. When only a small amount of material has leaked, symptoms and physical findings are generally less severe and are often confined to the pelvis or lower abdomen.

TABLE 27-1

History of surgical treatment for ruptured adnexal abscess

AUTHOR	YEARS	NO.	MORTALITY (%)	SURGERY*
Vemeeren and	1925-1944	22	90	1
TeLinde[3] (Johns Hopkins)	1945-1953	25	12	13
Pedowitz and	<1947	16	100	1
Bloomfield[4] (Brooklyn)	1947-1959	127	3.1	90
Mickal and	1951-1959	54	11 ⎱	94
Sellman[2] (Charity Hospital, New Orleans)	1959-1966	55	3.7 ⎰	

*Hysterectomy, bilateral salpingo-oophorectomy.

Sometimes a pelvic mass may be palpable, but frequently peritonitis precludes adequate examination. If the abscess is well confined, with leakage but little peritonitis, then it is more likely a mass will be felt. The patient may also be hypotensive, usually because the peritonitis depletes the intravascular volume. Suspect endotoxemia if the patient shows signs of hypothermia or significant pyrexia, as well as tachypnea and mental obtundation. Any of these findings should tell you that the patient is seriously ill.

DIFFERENTIAL DIAGNOSIS

The following conditions in a young woman can mimic a leaking or ruptured abscess:
- Other adnexal pathology
- A perforated appendix or one that is gangrenous, with either localized or generalized peritonitis
- Purulent peritonitis with uncomplicated salpingitis
- Inflammatory bowel conditions such as Crohn's disease
- Complications of elective termination of pregnancy, usually following infection after perforation during suction curettage
- Uterine perforation during attempts to retrieve a lost IUD.
  In the older woman, be suspicious when there is:
- Bowel pathology
- Appendicitis and any of its attendant complications
- Perforation of a colonic diverticulum or of carcinoma
- A gastric or duodenal ulcer
- Acute pancreatitis.

AIDS IN DIAGNOSIS AND MANAGEMENT

Ruptured pelvic abscesses are usually diagnosed clinically; however, some lab tests can help pinpoint associated conditions.

Hemogram. Leukocytosis with a shift to the left usually occurs with peritonitis; but leukopenia may suggest septicemia. The platelet count is usually normal, but thrombocytopenia may also accompany septicemia. The hematocrit will reflect dehydration and chronic infection, but if it is less than 30, there is probably concomitant blood loss. Request 6 to 8 units of cross-matched whole blood when you expect to operate.

Urinalysis. Acetonuria reflects dehydration and metabolic acidosis. Glucosuria should prompt you to check for diabetes, which may be precipitated by peritonitis or may actually mimic its signs and symptoms. Pyuria unaccompanied by bacilluria frequently indicates bacterial peritonitis. Although bacteriuria suggests urinary tract infection, this is almost never confused with intraperitoneal infection.

Serum chemistries and enzymes. At a minimum, determine serum sodium and potassium, to guide electrolyte replacement, and creatinine clearance, to assess renal function. With septicemia and peritonitis, invariably there is prerenal azotemia, and endotoxin is nephrotoxic. Hyperamylasemia suggests pancreatitis, usually a nonsurgical condition. Temporary abnormalities of liver function are frequent and suggest the presence of toxic hepatitis from septicemia.

Sonography. When you can't do an adequate pelvic examination, try sonography. Ultrasound can also help you measure palpated masses. Frequently, the sonolucent cavity will be smaller than the conglomerate tumor, because of edema and inflammation in the bowel wall and omentum adjacent to, or part of, a pelvic abscess.

X-rays. Plain and upright films of the abdomen usually are consistent with paralytic ileus. Free air may indicate a perforated, hollow viscus, but may also be due to gas-forming organisms. Chest films are generally normal. A sympathetic pleural effusion may coexist with peritonitis, but when accompanied by an infiltrate, it suggests primary pulmonary damage from sepsis.

Culdocentesis. Culdocentesis will confirm hemoperitoneum, which can produce abdominal pain, fever, leukocytosis, and mild to moderate anemia. This procedure is a must in the older or diabetic woman whose history is consistent with any of these conditions, but whose examination results may not reflect the severity of the process. The procedure is not as helpful in the differential diagnosis when there is a palpable cul-de-sac abscess or when there is generalized peritonitis.

TABLE 27-2

Common presenting symptoms with pelvic abscesses

SYMPTOM	RUPTURED	LEAKING
Peritonitis	Generalized, appears toxic	Lower quadrants
Fever	Hyperthermia or hypothermia	Hyperthermia or normal
Volume status	Hypervolemia, hypotension	Usually isovolemic
Pelvic mass	Usually nonpalpable	Palpable
Ileus	Generalized	Segmental

MEDICAL MANAGEMENT

Immediate resuscitation is necessary to correct any systemic derangements resulting from severe infections. Replace fluids with balanced isotonic salt solution and continue until urine output is at least 30 mL/hour, more optimally 60 mL/hour. It is not unusual for a woman to require 4 to 6 liters of saline or Ringer's solution to prompt such a diuresis. After the woman is isovolemic, determine the hematocrit again and, if it's less than 30, give whole blood or packed red blood cells. Before general anesthesia, add potassium as needed to correct hypokalemia. Rapid fluid replacement will correct metabolic acidosis.

Antimicrobial therapy. Begin broad-spectrum antimicrobial coverage and IV fluid replacement after taking blood and cul-de-sac samples for anaerobic and aerobic cultures. In our experience, any one of several regimens is suitable. Base your selection on your own experience and the patient's history of allergies (Table 27-3).

We have had good results using newer cephalosporins as single-agent therapy for pelvic abscesses that did not require surgery. We have treated 41 women with cefotaxime (Claforan) 2 gm every 8 hours; 95% responded favorably. Only one (5%) required the addition of chloramphenicol, and none required surgery. Eighty-five per cent of these abscesses measured at least 6 cm clinically, with sonographic confirmation of the size. Moxalactam (Moxam) has also been used.

TABLE 27-3

Antimicrobial regimens used for intra-abdominal sepsis

Drugs
1. Penicillin G—5 million units q6h
2. Cefamandole—2 gm q4h
3. Cefoxitin—2 gm q4h
4. Clindamycin—1,200 mg q6h
5. Chloramphenicol—50-100 mg/kg in four divided doses
6. Gentamicin—1.5 mg/kg q8h
7. Cefotaxime—2 gm q8h
8. Moxalactam—2 gm q8h

Regimens
1 + 4 + 6
1 + 5 + 6
2 + 5
3 + 5

Adjunctive measures. The following procedures may also be necessary: central venous pressure determinations, nasogastric suction, supplemental oxygen, assisted ventilation for respiratory failure, or IV adrenal corticosteroids in pharmacologic doses. Methylprednisolone succinate 15 to 30 mg/kg as an initial dose, repeated every 4 to 6 hours for four doses, should be considered if there is clinical evidence of septicemic shock.

TIMING SURGERY

You may postpone surgery if there is a prompt response to medical management. For generalized peritonitis, however, plan celiotomy as soon as you have restored fluids and electrolytes and corrected metabolic acidosis.

Immediate laparotomy. When you must operate, make a lower midline incision with adequate preparation to allow for extension to the xiphoid. Upon entry, take samples of peritoneal fluid for anaerobic and aerobic cultures. After identifying the site of the abscess, carefully dissect away the involved omentum and bowel in order to prevent perforation. Make sure that all pelvic structures are completely free of contiguous structures before extirpating the adnexa or uterus. Because the tissue planes are distorted and dissection is bloody, surgery will be safer and less blood will be lost if you isolate the pelvic structures before beginning a hysterectomy.

Bring multiple Penrose or Jackson-Pratt drains out through the vaginal cuff or through a posterior colpotomy incision if you don't remove the cervix or uterus. You may want to place indwelling abdominal catheters for postoperative irrigation, but we seldom use them. Before closing the abdomen, copiously irrigate the peritoneal cavity with warm saline, and remove all purulent material from the upper abdomen. Frequently, you may have to lyse adhesions and remove loculations of pus. Close the fascia with monofilament sutures using the Smead-Jones technique. Leave the skin and subcutaneous layers open and pack with fine-mesh gauze soaked in povidone-iodine solution. Remove this 3 to 4 days later, and close the incision secondarily. Retention sutures may be beneficial.

Delayed operative intervention. In some cases, you can delay surgery safely for several days while you assess response to antimicrobial therapy. If peritonitis improves with 3 to 5 days of aggressive medical management, but no further, then operate. If fever and signs of peritonitis, albeit less severe, persist, then it is unlikely medical management alone will succeed. Obviously, surgical exploration is indicated if the patient's condition worsens.

Interval surgery. Some leaks respond to aggressive medical and antimicrobial therapy, but usually you have to operate. We discharge patients who have been afebrile and asymptomatic for several days, place them on a regimen of oral antimicrobials, follow them closely, and schedule elective surgery in 6 to 12 weeks. If symptoms of infection occur before surgery is scheduled, we promptly readmit them, treat with IV antimicrobials, and perform surgery on the same admission—its urgency dictated by the patient's condition.

Most patients are best served by hysterectomy and bilateral adnexectomy. Conservative surgery, when possible, is more appropriate for women who desire fertility. Ginsburg and colleagues at the Johns Hopkins Hospital found that after even conservative surgery for unruptured abscess, fertility was poor.[5] Rivlin and Hunt, however, reported fertility *potential* in 42.5% and retained hormonal and menstrual function in 73.5% of 113 women after conservative surgery for generalized peritonitis due to ruptured abscesses.[6] Obviously, the extent of disease and the patient's overall medical condition and desire for future childbearing will influence the type of operation performed.

REFERENCES

1. Collins CG, Nix FG, Cerrha HT: Ruptured tuboovarian abscess. Am J Obstet Gynecol 72:820, 1956
2. Mickal A, Sellman AH: Management of tubo-ovarian abscess. Clin Obstet Gynecol 12:252, 1969
3. Vemeeren J, TeLinde RW: Intra-abdominal rupture of pelvic abscesses. Am J Obstet Gynecol 68:402, 1954
4. Pedowitz P, Bloomfield RD: Ruptured adnexal abscess (tubo-ovarian) with generalized peritonitis. Am J Obstet Gynecol 88:721, 1964
5. Ginsburg DS, Stern JL, Hamod KA, et al: Tubo-ovarian abscess: A retrospective review. Am J Obstet Gynecol 138:1055, 1980
6. Rivlin ME, Hunt JA: Ruptured tuboovarian abscess—is hysterectomy necessary? Obstet Gynecol 50:518, 1977

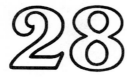

Laparoscopy

RICHARD M. SODERSTROM, MD, and
STEPHEN L. CORSON, MD

CLINICAL SIGNIFICANCE: Bleeding, penetrated viscus, and bowel burn are complications of laparoscopy that require immediate attention—with no time for observation or procrastination. Treat all injuries as emergencies. Laparoscopy is also useful in situations such as ectopic pregnancy, abdominal injury, or uterine rupture, where it can often replace emergency laparotomy.

EMERGENCIES DURING LAPAROSCOPY

The possible complications of laparoscopy include acute bleeding, penetrating injuries, thermal injury to the bowel, instrument failure, problems with anesthesia, postoperative pain, sepsis, and urinary tract damage. Late complications are symptoms due to unrecognized bowel burns and ectopic pregnancy. Laparoscopy can, however, be most useful in diagnosing and treating extrauterine gestation, exploring the abdomen following blunt trauma, uterine perforation, or postoperative bleeding, relieving adnexal torsion, and removing foreign objects from the abdomen. It also has value as an adjunct to laparotomy—and can sometimes replace it.

Acute bleeding. Acute bleeding is always serious, whether it results from poor placement of the insufflating needle or sharp trocar before the laparoscope is inserted, or from operative maneuvers. The unexpected may also take the form of a penetrated viscus, a burn, or an anesthesia problem.

Mesosalpingeal tears can accompany either electrical or nonelectrical methods of sterilization. Usually unipolar electrocoagulation will stop even brisk arterial bleeding. An insulated 3- or 5-mm suction cannula-coagulator attached to a unipolar, low-voltage generator allows discrete coagulation and an accurate view of the bleeding site. The experienced laparoscopist can apply clips and bands directly to aid hemostasis.

Fortunately, the most dreaded vascular accident during laparoscopy—penetrating the great vessels of the abdomen and pelvis—rarely happens anymore. Education, experience, and the increasing use of open laparoscopy for difficult cases should make this sobering event practically nonexistent. When it occurs, it usually means there has been a departure from standard precautions during trocar insertion, frequently in a teaching session. Exploratory laparotomy and vessel repair are mandatory, whether the vessel is penetrated during the insertion of the smaller Veress needle, large trocar, or secondary trocar. However, don't panic. Make an incision large enough to maintain digital pressure on the laceration. This will control the bleeding until a vascular surgeon can assess the damage.

Occasionally, despite transillumination of the abdominal wall, the right or left deep epigastric vessels in the wall will be lacerated when the secondary trocar is inserted. If electrocoagulation fails to halt the bleeding, ligature may become necessary. You need not extend the incision for the secondary trocar if you use a through-and-through ligature. Under laparoscopic direction, place the suture with a large curved needle through the incision into the abdominal cavity (Figure 28-1).

Penetrating injuries. The needle used to create a pneumoperitoneum may accidently enter a hollow viscus such as the bowel, stomach, or bladder. Usually the entry is innocuous and the defect seals itself. However, it is important to recognize when the wrong space is being distended. If you attach a 20-mL syringe barrel filled with saline, you will be aware of a problem when blood, urine, or bowel contents appear in the syringe. Don't discontinue the procedure. Place another sterile needle and continue—for no other reason than to assess possible damage created by the initial needle insertion. Place an indwelling catheter if hematuria from a bladder puncture persists. Copious lavage with a suction cannula should cleanse the peritoneal cavity when there is minimal leakage of bowel contents.

Most serious injuries accompany trocar entry. Often, they result from excessive force, either because the trocar is dull or because the incision is inadequate. Open laparoscopy (technique of Harrith M. Hasson, MD, Grant Hospital of Chicago) may be the best choice when patients have had surgery or radiation therapy that may have produced bowel adhesions to the anterior abdominal wall.[1] The very thin or obese may also pose problems.

General anesthesia increases the risk of stomach injury. When a ventilation mask is used alone to administer anesthetic agents, the stomach may become distended. Most procedures are performed with an endotracheal cuff, but occasionally a false entry into the esophagus can distend the stomach. To prevent such problems, pass a nasogastric tube before any surgical manipulation.

Even with good technique and attention to details, accidents happen. Should the telescope enter the lumen of the stomach, intestine, or bladder, prepare for laparotomy but don't remove the laparoscope. Otherwise the defect may partially close and become difficult to find.

Make an incision parallel to the trocar sheath tract and use the laparoscope to elevate the damaged organ. After identifying and exposing the site, place and tie a simple pursestring suture as the laparoscope is withdrawn. This minimizes peritoneal contamination. Copious irrigation is the next step.

The consulting surgeon may decide suction drains are necessary. Whenever possible, place the incision so the surgeon can carry out the original procedure—for example, a sterilization. For severe injuries, wall off the area with packs before removing the laparoscope.

Thermal injury. Both unipolar and bipolar coagulating devices can produce bowel burns. Because the extent of tissue damage cannot be as-

---

FIGURE 28-1

Through-and-through ligature

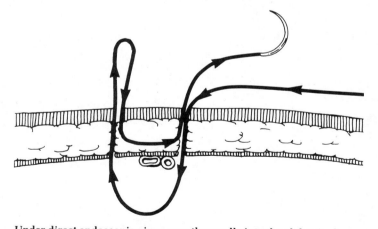

Under direct endoscopic view, pass the needle into the abdominal cavity, under the epigastric vessels, and take it out through the abdominal skin medial to the incision. Then reverse the needle and direct it back through the exit site, bringing it out through the trocar incision. Confirm placement and security endoscopically, once the ligation has been completed.

sessed immediately, it is best to be prudent and do a wide resection in the small bowel—usually 5 cm on either side of the burn.[2]

The large bowel seems more resistant than the small bowel to breakdown by thermal injury, and colon burns are rare. In most cases, debridement is appropriate and complete resection probably unnecessary.

Instrument failure. Equipment problems during surgery are usually a nuisance rather than an emergency—for example, when a faulty bulb in the light source needs replacement. Electrical problems, however, are more vexing and potentially dangerous. Never increase the rheostat setting if there is inadequate or intermittent current flow. Serious injury can result if there is a break in the circuit. To identify the source of an electrical problem, proceed as follows:
● Withdraw the instrument gently from the abdomen.
● Check the return (dispersive) electrode on unipolar instruments. Some generators have a safety feature that prohibits current flow if the return electrode is not properly applied and connected.
● Have someone check the plugs connecting the generator to the foot switch and to the wall source of electricity.
● Use the foot switch to close the circuit. Usually a light on the generator will show the integrity of that part of the circuit.
● If the problem seems to be in the forceps itself or in the cord connecting it to the generator, try a different cord and then a different forceps. A minute break within the cord or an insulation defect in the forceps may not be readily visible.

Should a plastic trocar sleeve break within the abdomen, remove the fragments with accessory grasping instruments. If an instrument locks in the jaws-open position, you may have to enlarge the incision to remove it. A 30° cystoscope or hysteroscope can be substituted for a broken laparoscope. In fact, the angle of view is usually greater, similar to that of a culdoscope.

Rarely, a Silastic band applicator may misfire during a sterilization procedure and trap the grasping tongs on the tube. Don't apply traction, which could cause avulsion of the tubal segment and produce major bleeding. Instead, cut the band by inserting laparoscope scissors through a separate trocar sleeve.

Anesthesia emergencies. Certain problems are unique to laparoscopy. Cardiac arrhythmias, with severe bradycardia, may result from increased pressure from abdominal insufflation. Proper assisted ventilation will usually correct this problem.

Though rare, gas embolism can occur during abdominal insufflation or during the actual operation. The classical "mill-wheel murmur" can be heard over the precordium, and is associated with profound hypotension. Anyone administering an anesthetic for laparoscopy should be skilled in managing this serious emergency.

Susceptible patients receiving succinylcholine for intraoperative relaxation may develop a pseudocholinesterase deficiency syndrome. Continued ventilatory support is necessary until the agent has been metabolized.

Table 28-1 summarizes the intra- and postoperative complications of laparoscopy.

POSTOPERATIVE EMERGENCIES

Increasing pain. Pain, particularly in healthy women, should diminish steadily after the procedure. Most laparoscopies are performed on an outpatient or short-stay basis; therefore, increasing pain may be the only clue to a problem. If a patient telephones and asks for more analgesics, question her closely. Examine *all* patients who report increasing pain. If hospitalization is necessary, consider repeat laparoscopy shortly after admission.

Fortunately, delayed postoperative bleeding is rare. Repeat laparoscopy is not contraindicated if the patient's vital signs are stable and fluid replacement is adequate. Bleeding often occurs at the site of intraabdominal surgery (that is, lysis of adhesions), but don't overlook unexpected bleeding at a trocar site.

Sepsis. Intraperitoneal infection or systemic sepsis is uncommon following laparoscopy. Hemostasis during laparoscopy helps prevent infections. But, as with any procedure that mobilizes pelvic structures, laparoscopy can exacerbate pre-existing infectious disease, especially salpingitis. If you encounter salpingitis at laparoscopy, take intraperitoneal samples for aerobic and anaerobic cultures to guide your selection of antibiotics. Whenever a fever develops after laparoscopy, rule out concurrent respiratory or urinary tract infection.

TABLE 28-1

Laparoscopic emergencies

During the procedure	**Following the procedure**
Acute bleeding	Delayed bleeding
Anesthetic problems	Delayed thermal injury
Instrument failure	Ectopic pregnancy
Thermal injury	Increasing pain
Penetration of viscus	Sepsis
	Urinary tract injury

Urinary tract damage. Uroperitoneum may follow laparoscopy-related injury to the urinary tract. Frequently the bladder is involved. Ureteral damage has been reported with adnexal surgery such as ovarian biopsy. The XO streak ovary seems to pose a special threat, because it is located in the broad ligament and lacks mobility.

Take special care when removing endometriotic implants by electro-surgery. Be sure you specifically locate the ureter when implants are found near its course. The peritoneum is not pulled taut with a retractor, as in laparotomy. Thus, it is easy to follow the paths of the great vessels and ureter in the pelvic side wall during laparoscopy.

Unrecognized burns. Bowel burns characteristically produce symptoms late in the postoperative period. Several days to more than a week may pass before the symptoms of perforation develop in what appeared to be a surface burn of the intestine at the time of injury. Exploratory laparotomy that includes a thorough evaluation of the entire GI tract is mandatory, and copious intra-abdominal lavage, with appropriate drainage, is recommended. Though the extent of electrical injury may seem obvious, prudence dictates a wide resection or extensive debridement of the injured area. Figure 28-2 illustrates the proper management of a bowel burn.[2]

Ectopic pregnancy. All methods of tubal sterilization produce some failures. Women who conceive after a sterilization attempt are at increased risk for ectopic gestation because their tubes are damaged.

Pregnancy may occur if a fistula forms at the proximal stump of the tube. The failure may be a result of loss of blood supply following elec-

---

FIGURE 28-2

The proper management of a bowel burn (by Wheeless)

Place no sutures within 4 cm of burned area.

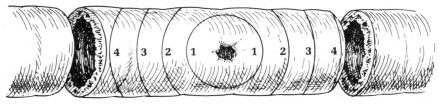

Resect intestinal burned area.

---

trosurgical procedures or, conversely, from regeneration, healing, and re-establishment of luminal patency. Motile sperm may exit from the defect in the proximal tube and find their way to the fimbriated end. Fertilization then occurs as usual, but the blastocyst becomes trapped in the distal segment.

Therefore, even years after a woman has been sterilized, treat symptoms or signs of pregnancy with great respect and expediency. It's mandatory to use a sensitive pregnancy test. If the result is positive, use ultrasound or laparoscopy to locate the gestational sac.

At the time of exploratory surgery, part of the problem is deciding how to prevent a recurrent ectopic pregnancy. A small fistula may be invisible. Distal salpingectomy will not eliminate continued leakage of sperm into the abdominal cavity and the continued risk of ovarian implantation. A cornual resection with imbrication of the intramural portion of the tube may be difficult, because of postelectrosurgical fibrosis. In such cases, it may be necessary to consider hysterectomy for permanent sterilization.

NO TIME FOR WAITING

Any surgical procedure has inherent problems and some that are unique to it. This form of remote control surgery demands a thorough knowledge of risks and their proper management. Patients subjected to laparoscopic operations should expect to recover rapidly and progressively. Immediately evaluate any patient whose postoperative course takes a turn for the worse. There is little place for observation and procrastination in early or late laparoscopic complications—each should be treated as an emergency.

EMERGENCY USES OF LAPAROSCOPY

Extrauterine gestation. Women who have had tubal surgery, salpingitis, endometriosis, or a tubal pregnancy are considered at risk for extrauterine gestation. Most ectopic pregnancies, however, occur without any such history. Spotting and vague, moderate pelvic pain may appear late in the evening, 6 to 9 weeks after the last menstrual period. The tubal mass can rarely be palpated, and unless rupture has occurred the hemoglobin level may be unremarkable. Sensitive pregnancy tests and, in particular, quantitative serial β-hCG serum sampling can diagnose early pregnancy. Coupled with an intrauterine gestational sac visible on real-time ultrasound, pregnancy tests will differentiate impending or incomplete abortion from ectopic pregnancy.

The patient may benefit from emergency laparoscopy if the result of a sensitive urinary test (250 mIU/mL or less), which reflects functioning trophoblastic tissue at any location, is positive. Death rates from ectopic pregnancy usually correlate with delay in diagnosis.[3] With early diagnosis, there is less need for transfusion and morbidity in general is reduced. Chances of salvaging the affected tube are better, too.

Before performing an emergency laparoscopy, make sure that banked blood is available and the operating suite is ready for immediate laparotomy. Of course, laparoscopy is contraindicated in obvious hypovolemic shock. Culdocentesis, while helpful, is associated with both false-positive and false-negative results.

There are a number of advantages to using laparoscopy when you suspect an ectopic pregnancy. The differential diagnosis of ectopic gestation versus ruptured hemorrhagic corpus luteum can be made by inspection, after you aspirate blood with a 5-mm suction cannula. Often, bleeding from an ovarian source may cease spontaneously, requiring no further treatment. However, if necessary, a bleeding point can be coagulated under laparoscopic view. In the event that abortion of the tubal pregnancy is complete, laparotomy is not needed.

FIGURE 28-3

Removing an early ectopic pregnancy with the Soderstrom snare

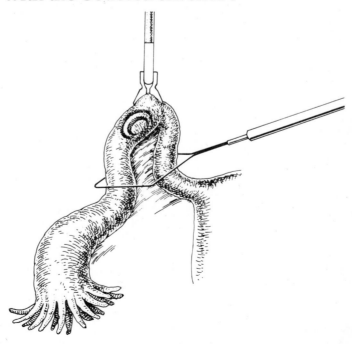

If the laparoscope discloses a tubal gestation, you might perform a minilaparotomy while the patient remains in stirrups. A uterine elevator can bring the uterus and adnexa up to the anterior abdominal wall. A few technically gifted laparoscopists have performed partial salpingectomy via the laparoscope, using a multitrocar approach or specialized laparoscopic equipment such as a snare (Figure 28-3).

Abdominal injury. In the mid 1970s, Gazzaniga and Bartlett assessed the value of laparoscopy for patients with blunt injuries.[4] Following the usual tests for postural hypertension and needle abdominal lavage, laparoscopy was performed before planned exploratory laparotomy. In general, 20% of patients who were made ready for laparotomy required no exploration after laparoscopy. Conversely, 20% of those who did not meet the criteria for immediate laparotomy did require such exploration after laparoscopy disclosed unsuspected intraperitoneal damage. Laparoscopy also furnishes a quick, expedient answer when there is a question of a stab wound of the abdominal wall having entered the abdominal cavity.

Uterine perforation. During D&C or D&E, the abdominal cavity may be entered accidentally. If the mishap is recognized during dilation, postpone the rest of the procedure and observe the patient to see whether problems develop. However, if the perforation is noticed during evacuation or after, use laparoscopy to evaluate the integrity of the abdominal cavity. Should the D&E be incomplete, as with abortion procedures, a second surgeon can complete the evacuation while the laparoscopist observes the perforated site. It is rare to need electrocoagulation or sutures to repair the uterine wall.

Uterine perforation occurs at a rate of 1 to 3:1,000 during IUD insertions. As soon as it is clear that a perforation has occurred, remove the IUD if it contains copper, because an intense tissue reaction will occur around the device. If you delay laparoscopic exploration, adhesions may form and removal via this route will be difficult or impossible. Hysteroscopy may help rule out partial perforation, but an ultrasonic search for the true intra-abdominal IUD is seldom of value. Therefore, preoperative posterior-anterior and lateral x-rays of the *entire* abdomen are helpful. Repeat x-ray during the laparoscopic procedure may be necessary if the IUD disappears from view. An operating laparoscope usually makes it easier to retrieve the IUD through the laparoscope trocar sleeve, but experienced laparoscopists do equally well using the multitrocar approach.

Postoperative bleeding. Occasionally, unexpected bleeding follows major or minor surgery. Laparoscopy may be of value for locating and assessing the source if the patient is stable and has had adequate fluid and blood replacement. Liver biopsy sites that continue to bleed can be dealt with by tamponade under laparoscopic vision. Small bits of gelatin foam can be inserted into the puncture site. Electrocoagulating the surface doesn't help, because the bleeding comes from a deeper source.

Laparoscopy can help pinpoint the source of intra-abdominal bleeding that follows vaginal hysterectomy, when there is no active bleeding from the extraperitoneal stumps, and helps make the "decision about the size of the incision." Occasionally the bleeding may have stopped by the time exploration is under way. Laparoscopy can confirm this finding and direct the placement of one or more intra-abdominal drains to evacuate the blood.

Acute adnexal torsion. Adnexal torsion seems a likely diagnosis when a patient develops unilateral adnexal pain that is abrupt and intense, with rupture of a cystic structure as a strong alternative. Laparoscopy can help identify which cystic structure is twisted. Usually it is an ovarian cyst, but a particularly long-pedicled cyst of Morgagni or a paraovarian cyst can behave similarly. Simple cysts can be aspirated and a biopsy taken from the wall, for diagnosis and to prevent re-formation. If a cystic lesion has spontaneously ruptured, use a suction cannula to aspirate the contents from the cul-de-sac and to irrigate with saline. You can place a drain using accessory trocar sleeves and bring it out to suction without resorting to laparotomy. If there is no accompanying pathology, and the incident is only a few hours old, the structure can be untwisted and observed to see whether normal color and circulation are restored. If this simple maneuver does not suffice, follow the patient's white cell count, temperature, and level of pain as indicators for removal.

Removing a foreign body. On rare occasions, at the completion of vaginal hysterectomy with concomitant colpoperineal repair, a sponge may be missing. After radiologic confirmation, laparoscopic exploration can often locate the sponge, which may then be extracted through the subumbilical incision.[5]

Indwelling intra-abdominal drainage shunts used in hydrocephalic patients have occasionally become lost or clogged after placement. Laparoscopy can aid in locating, retrieving, and properly placing them.

Unexpected malignant disease. Many gynecologic procedures are performed through a lower transverse incision. If an unexpected—usually ovarian—cancer is encountered, it's difficult to explore the upper reaches of the abdominal cavity, especially the liver and diaphragm. Under these circumstances, insert the laparoscope through the wound. By using broad retractors, you can inspect the liver, lymphatics, and the upper surface of the diaphragm. Under the directed lighting and magnification of the laparoscope you can identify small surface lesions and take samples for histologic confirmation.

PRELUDE TO LAPAROTOMY

Laparoscopy can be valuable when laparotomy is contemplated, yet it is rarely performed in the acutely ill patient. Using it can improve the ability to make an accurate diagnosis, for example, when a young woman has lower abdominal pain, an elevated white blood cell count, and fever. Diagnosing pelvic inflammatory disease solely on the basis of these symptoms has an error rate of approximately 35%.[5]

Unnecessary laparotomy in women of reproductive age is to be discouraged. Laparoscopy can help pinpoint the exact cause when diagnoses to be considered include appendicitis, mesenteric adenitis, regional enteritis, ovarian cysts, and endometriosis, and when findings are negative.

When atraumatic forceps are used, it's usually possible to visualize the appendix. It may aid in placing the incision if the appendix is fixed and retrocecal, with pus and inflammation along the cecal edge.

SUMMARY

Numerous emergencies can arise when a complication of laparoscopy occurs. The operator must be prepared to manage these complications promptly and effectively in order to minimize morbidity.

Laparoscopy can aid the surgeon in acute emergencies and can guide the plan of management so that an expedient diagnosis can be made and excessive exploration prevented. A command of the multiple trocar approach to operative laparoscopy can, in experienced hands, correct a number of emergent problems without resorting to laparotomy.

REFERENCES

1. Hasson HM: Open laparoscopy: a report of 150 cases. J Reprod Med 12:234, 1974
2. Wheeless CR Jr: Gastrointestinal injuries associated with laparoscopy. In *Endoscopy in Gynecology*. Downey, Calif, American Association of Gynecological Laparoscopists, 1978, p 317
3. Schneider J, Berger CJ, Catell C: Maternal mortality due to ectopic pregnancy. Obstet Gynecol 45:557, 1977
4. Gazzaniga AB, Bartlett RH: Blunt and penetrating injuries to the abdomen. In Phillips JM (ed): *Laparoscopy*. Baltimore, Williams & Wilkins, 1977, p 113
5. Jacobson L, Weström L: Objectivized diagnosis of acute pelvic inflammatory disease. Diagnostic and prognostic value of routine laparoscopy. Am J Obstet Gynecol 105:1088, 1969

29

Evisceration and Dehiscence

JOHN T. QUEENAN, MD

CLINICAL SIGNIFICANCE: A rare complication, evisceration is preventable in most instances. Since it is associated with substantial morbidity and even mortality, proper management of surgical patients is mandatory. Wound dehiscence, a more common occurrence, is also preventable.

From 0.2% to 2% of ob/gyn patients have wound dehiscence.[1-5] The incidence of evisceration is considerably less. "Dehiscence" and "evisceration" are often used interchangeably, but they are distinct entities. Dehiscence entails the separation of one or more layers of the abdominal wall; the peritoneum may or may not be involved. If only the skin and subcutaneous layers separate, the problem may be upsetting to the patient but should be manageable nonsurgically. Evisceration means that the intestines are externalized and therefore all five abdominal layers are disrupted. This represents an acute emergency associated with serious morbidity and mortality of 10% to 20%.

Wound dehiscence can follow any type of incision, but a midline incision is more likely to dehisce than a transverse. The likelihood of dehiscence increases if the incision extends above the umbilicus.

SIGNS AND SYMPTOMS

Such conditions as a chronic cough or severe distention should alert the clinician to the possibility that the wound may separate. Certain signs and symptoms are suggestive of impending wound separation and possible evisceration. Bulging at the incision site suggests hematoma or separation of deeper abdominal wall layers; local pain often precedes separation. Serosanguinous drainage is a classic sign; wound infection is another. The most likely time for a wound to dehisce is 5 to 10 days after the operation, but the time can range from 2 to 17 days.

CAUSES

Fortunately, failure to heal is an uncommon problem. Certain factors contribute to dehiscence. These may be grouped in four categories:

Poor tissue. Patients who are malnourished have tissue that does not heal well. Obesity, alcoholism, vitamin deficiency, poor diet, and old age also are associated with failure to heal on the basis of poor tissue.[3-6] Patients who are on steroids or who have had radiotherapy also heal poorly. The same is true of those with extensive cancer. Physicians should anticipate the possibility of wound dehiscence in malnourished patients and choose the type of closure accordingly.

Infection. A common cause of dehiscence,[3, 4] wound infection may start with a cellulitis that progresses to an abscess or an infected hematoma and, finally, to breakdown of the wound. Infection causes a particularly difficult clinical situation, because of the large amount of infected and necrotic tissue at the site of dehiscence.

Mechanical causes. Certain stresses such as coughing, retching, and vomiting tend to cause wound separation. So can severe abdominal distention due to paralytic ileus, mechanical obstruction, or ascites. Occasionally a hematoma can separate tissues to the degree that they fail to heal. This may happen even without infection. Pfannenstiel incisions rarely dehisce; when they do, a hematoma is often the cause.

Improper closure. If the abdominal wall is not closed with the proper surgical technique, failure to heal and wound dehiscence may result. When the abdominal wall is closed with a continuous suture, the risk of separation is greater than when interrupted sutures are used. Catgut sutures also increase the risk of wound separation.[7-9] Nonabsorbable sutures, such as stainless steel wire, nylon, or polypropylene, or the syn-

---

TABLE 29-1

Causes of wound dehiscence

Poor tissue	Mechanical
Obesity	Vomiting
Poor diet	Coughing
Old age	Hematoma
Disseminated cancer	Abdominal distention
Steroid therapy	Ascites
Irradiation therapy	Improper closure
Infection	

FIGURE 29-1

Smead-Jones abdominal incision closure

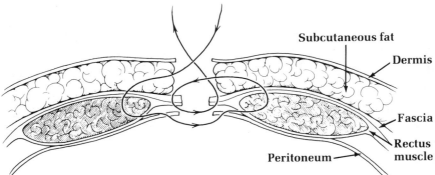

Subcutaneous fat

Dermis

Fascia

Rectus muscle

Peritoneum

A. Suture takes small bites of peritoneum and passes twice through rectus muscle on each side of incision

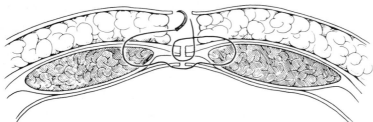

B. Technique minimizes amount of suture material left inside abdominal cavity

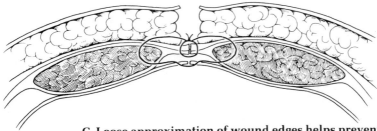

C. Loose approximation of wound edges helps prevent ischemia and necrosis

Reprinted, witn permission, from Sanz L: Choosing the right wound-closure technique. Contemp Ob/Gyn 21 (special issue):142, 1983

thetic absorbable sutures like Dexon and Vicryl have distinct advantages over catgut in this respect.[1-3, 7-11]

The causes of wound dehiscence may be multiple or not well defined. The patient may have several interacting factors—for example, hematoma that becomes infected plus abdominal distention due to paralytic ileus. Table 29-1 summarizes the problems the physician should be on the alert for.

MANAGEMENT

1. Evaluate the severity of the separation. If the separation does not involve the fascia, the problem can be managed without surgical closure. Unless you are certain that the separation is superficial, explore the wound in the operating room with the patient under general anesthesia. If the fascia is separated, chances are the peritoneum is involved. Inspect the wound thoroughly, remove any foreign bodies, and debride if necessary.
2. If the wound is clean and there is no obvious infection, close it secondarily with the Smead-Jones technique (Figure 29-1). Close the subcutaneous layer and skin with interrupted sutures. Some surgeons prefer a through-and-through closure.

If there is infection, it is better to debride, irrigate, and then close the fascia with the Smead-Jones technique. Leave the subcutaneous layer and skin open. The wound can then be cleaned daily to allow the subcutaneous and skin layers to granulate.
3. If the peritoneum is disrupted, use this protocol for evisceration:
- Replace bowel as aseptically as possible.
- Move the patient to the operating room for secondary closure.
- Apply a warm saline pack while taking the patient to the OR.
- Treat such additional complications as shock, intestinal or other hemorrhage, and infection.
- Remove any foreign bodies.
- Explore the area for damaged or necrotic bowel.
- Culture for aerobes and anaerobes.
- Debride wound edges.
- Close with the Smead-Jones technique (Figure 29-1). Close the skin separately. If the wound is infected, leave the skin open. Or close the wound with through-and-through sutures.
- Use silver wire, stainless steel, heavy polypropylene, or No. 2 nylon. To avoid infection, use only monofilament sutures.
- Place Smead-Jones sutures at 2-cm intervals, approximately 2 cm from wound edges.

Postoperatively, allow the patient nothing by mouth and institute a regimen of IV feeding, gastroduodenal suction, and parenteral antibiotics. The patient should be considered seriously ill and her vital signs, intake and output, and clinical progress monitored meticulously.

If Smead-Jones sutures are used, they are not removed. Through-and-through sutures are generally removed after 2 to 3 weeks. If the patient makes good progress and recovers before the sutures can be removed, she may be discharged, followed at home, and return as an outpatient for suture removal.

COMPLICATIONS

Usually an incision closed secondarily by Smead-Jones or through-and-through sutures heals well and recovery is uneventful. Occasionally a patient may have a complication involving the incision, usually an incisional hernia. If she is well and her tissues are of good quality, this can be repaired easily at a later date.

PREVENTION

When operating on a patient who has a chronic cough, the surgeon may choose to use a Smead-Jones suture technique to prevent dehiscence. If the patient is obese, meticulous attention to hemostasis is necessary to prevent a hematoma in the subfascial and subcutaneous layers. In some patients drains may be helpful. If there is gross infection, it may be best to close with a Smead-Jones technique, leaving the skin open for irrigation and drainage. If the patient has disseminated carcinoma, poor healing can be anticipated and a Smead-Jones closure should be elected.

Retention sutures have the advantage of strength by incorporating the entire abdominal wall. Their disadvantage is that they remain 2 to 3 weeks and can produce discomfort and local infection. The Smead-Jones closure has almost completely replaced through-and-through closure. The surgeon can choose among several options in the way the skin is managed. It can be left open, irrigated, and closed secondarily. Or it can be closed in a separate layer, without cumbersome through-and-through sutures. If wound separation is a risk, the Smead-Jones closure is ideal.[10-12]

According to Lacey and co-workers, Smead-Jones closure is the method of choice in patients at risk for abdominal wound disruption, and is superior to through-and-through retention sutures.[13] This technique is also recommended by Malt, who states that the sutures should be placed at least 1.5 cm from the fascial edges and not more than 1 cm apart.[14] No dehiscences were noted in 747 cancer patients who had Smead-Jones closures for midline abdominal wounds. This result was compared with the results in 545 lower-risk patients on a gynecologic service, who had layered wound closures. There were five wound dehiscences (0.9%) in the latter group. All had had midline vertical incisions, and separations occurred on postoperative day 5 or 6.[9]

Goligher and colleagues compared three methods of closing vertical incisions: catgut without retention sutures, catgut with retention sutures, and steel wire closure with the Smead-Jones technique. The last was best for preventing wound separation and evisceration.[11]

REFERENCES

1. Baggish MS, Lee WK: Letters to the editor. Obstet Gynecol 48:730, 1976

2. Baggish MS, Wing KL: Abdominal wound disruption. Obstet Gynecol 46:530, 1975

3. Braun TE Jr: Wound dehiscence. In Schaefer G, Graber EA, eds: *Complications in Obstetrics and Gynecology Surgery*. Hagerstown, Md, Harper & Row, 1971, Ch 12

4. Helmkamp BF: Abdominal wound dehiscence. Am J Obstet Gynecol 128:803, 1977

5. Mattingly RF: Opening and closing the abdomen. In *TeLinde's Operative Gynecology*, ed 5. Philadelphia, JB Lippincott, 1977, Ch 9

6. Pitkin RM: Abdominal hysterectomy in obese women. Surg Gynecol Obstet 142:532, 1976

7. Laufman H: Is catgut obsolete? Surg Gynecol Obstet 145:587, 1977

8. Laufman H, Rubel T: Synthetic absorbable sutures. Surg Gynecol Obstet 145:597, 1977

9. Wallace D, Hernandez W, Schlaerth JB, et al: Prevention of abdominal wall disruption utilizing the Smead-Jones closure technique. Obstet Gynecol 56:226, 1980

10. Galitano AL, Hondi ES: Closure of abdominal wounds in cancer patients. J Surg Oncol 8:413, 1976

11. Goligher JC, Irwin TT, Johnston D, et al: A controlled clinical trial of three methods of closures of laparotomy wounds. Br J Surg 62:823, 1975

12. Jones TE, Newell ET, Brubaker RE: Alloy steel wire in abdominal wound closure. Surg Gynecol Obstet 72:1059, 1941

13. Lacey CG, Morrow CP, Disaia PJ, et al: Letters to the editor. Obstet Gynecol 48:730, 1976

14. Malt RA: Abdominal incisions, sutures, and sacrilege. N Engl J Med 297:722, 1977

30

Acute Adrenal Insufficiency

WILLIAM R. GOLD JR., MD

CLINICAL SIGNIFICANCE: A serious, sometimes fatal condition, acute adrenal insufficiency affects about 1:25,000 persons. But many more are at risk of developing Addison's disease because they are receiving corticosteroids for nonendocrine disorders. Since the stress of delivery or surgery can precipitate adrenal crisis, it is important to identify patients at risk and take preventive measures.

Glucocorticoids are being prescribed for a growing number of nonendocrine disorders. As a result, the obstetrician-gynecologist will see an increasing number of patients who may be at risk for relative adrenocortical insufficiency. When exposed to the stress of infection or surgery, these patients may develop adrenal crisis.

Primary adrenocortical insufficiency (Addison's disease), characterized by progressive destruction of the adrenal cortex, is relatively rare. Addison's disease is usually idiopathic, but granulomatous infections and hemorrhage are possible causes. The disease, which affects both sexes with equal frequency and may occur at any age, is slowly progressive. The manifestations range from mild fatigue to overwhelming shock. Tiredness, weakness, nausea and vomiting, anorexia, and weight loss are the most common symptoms; pigmentation of the skin and mucosa is the most characteristic sign.

Secondary adrenocortical insufficiency, much more common, results from a deficiency of pituitary ACTH. This deficiency may be due either to exogenous glucocorticoids or to a pituitary disorder that affects ACTH production. Patients with secondary adrenocortical insufficiency have symptoms similar to those of Addison's disease. But since their ACTH and melanocyte-stimulating hormone levels are low, they do not have the hyperpigmentation that characterizes the primary disorder.

Long-term steroid therapy, the most common cause of secondary adrenocortical insufficiency, produces hypothalamic-pituitary-adrenal suppression and eventual atrophy of the adrenals as ACTH stimulation falls. Recovery from long-term adrenal suppression may take a few days to months. Until the hypothalamic-pituitary-adrenal response returns to normal, patients may be vulnerable to acute adrenocortical insufficiency, or adrenal crisis, when exposed to stress.

Normally, stressful stimuli are followed by increased secretion of corticotropin-releasing hormone from the hypothalamus. This in turn causes ACTH to be released by the pituitary, which increases circulating levels of cortisol. Depending on the nature and duration of the stimulus, circulating cortisol levels may increase from 10 μg/dL to 35 μg/dL.[1] In adrenocortical insufficiency, the response is impaired and patients risk a crisis when exposed to surgery, infection, fasting, exercise, dental extractions, or other forms of stress.

When the adrenals have atrophied during long-term steroid therapy, rapid withdrawal of exogenous steroids may precipitate such a crisis in a stressful situation. Certain patients may respond to stress with overwhelming intensification of the symptoms of chronic adrenal insufficiency. Other patients may demonstrate acute insufficiency as a result of hemorrhagic destruction of the adrenals due to infection or anticoagulant therapy. The manifestations of acute adrenal insufficiency may be marked nausea, vomiting, and severe abdominal pain. The lethargic patient may become somnolent. Fever may be high. Hypovolemic vascular shock may lead to cardiovascular collapse. While recognition and treatment of the crisis may be simple under certain clinical circumstances, it may be difficult to recognize adrenal crisis as the cause of overwhelming shock in the operating room.

PATIENTS AT RISK

Patients at risk for acute adrenocortical insufficiency fall into three groups (Table 30-1). First are those with undiagnosed Addison's disease. This is a rare cause of the acute stage, but a high index of suspicion should be maintained in the preoperative evaluation of patients who have nausea, lethargy, weight loss, and hyperpigmentation.

TABLE 30-1

Patients at risk

Undiagnosed Addison's disease
Current steroid therapy
Previous long-term steroid therapy (within past 12 months)

Patients currently receiving corticosteroids are definitely at risk, with the duration of therapy and the dose level determining the degree of risk. Patients who receive steroids for longer than a week, in doses greater than the equivalent of 7.5 mg prednisone a day, are considered at risk when exposed to a stressful stimulus. Commonly used glucocorticoids and their relative potencies are listed in Table 30-2. Patients on physiologic doses (7.5 mg prednisone daily) are not at risk; but if in doubt about the status of a patient, manage her as if she were at risk.

Patients who have previously been treated with corticosteroids may still have an impaired responsiveness to stress. Preoperative evaluation should always include questions about past steroid therapy. Those who have been managed with pharmacologic doses of a corticosteroid within the past year should be considered at risk.[2] Again, if there is a question as to whether a patient is at risk, err on the side of safety.

Patients who are at risk for adrenal crisis will need special preparation for obstetric and gynecologic procedures. Serious pelvic infection, vaginal or cesarean delivery, and all operative gynecologic procedures may induce enough stress to precipitate a crisis. Identifying patients at risk and providing adequate care will prevent adrenal crisis in most instances, but it may occur with little warning. Emergency care then is necessary.

MANAGEMENT OF ADRENAL CRISIS

Early recognition and adequate therapy for the patient in adrenal crisis may be lifesaving. Profound hypotension during surgery that does not respond to fluid replacement may be due to acute adrenocortical insufficiency. It may turn out that the patient was, in fact, at risk for an adrenal crisis. Rarely, this may be the first indicator of a new case of Addi-

---

TABLE 30-2

Commonly used glucocorticoids

DRUG	EQUIVALENT GLUCOCORTICOID DOSE (mg)
Short-acting	
Cortisol (hydrocortisone)	20
Cortisone	25
Prednisolone	5
Prednisone	5
Long-acting	
Betamethasone	0.60
Dexamethasone	0.75

son's disease. Rapid elevation of circulating glucocorticoids and adequate replacement of sodium and water are necessary. Start an IV infusion with 1 liter of normal saline containing 100 mg hydrocortisone immediately (see Table 30-3). The infusion should be given over 30 to 60 minutes. Then give additional normal saline with 50 mg hydrocortisone per liter. In severe emergencies, give 100 mg hydrocortisone IV as a bolus. Whenever managing an adrenal crisis, give glucocorticoids IM as well as IV, in case the infusion infiltrates or is stopped inadvertently. Careful attention to salt and water replacement is necessary to reverse the hypotension. Do not treat hyperkalemia, hypercalcemia, and acidosis separately; these abnormalities will respond to steroid replacement.[3] Continue steroids parenterally until adequate GI absorption is assured. Then start giving an oral preparation and taper the dose gradually until the previous steroid dose is reached.

PREVENTION

Preventing adrenal crises should be the goal of all physicians who care for patients with relative adrenocortical insufficiency from whatever cause. Identifying those at risk and developing a plan for prophylaxis is

---

TABLE 30-3

Management of adrenal crisis

Administer 100 mg hydrocortisone IV as bolus

Start IV infusion of 1,000 mL normal saline with 100 mg hydrocortisone. Give first liter over 30 to 60 minutes

Monitor BP, ECG, serum electrolytes, urine output

Give normal saline with 50 mg hydrocortisone/liter to control BP

Do not treat electrolyte imbalance. It will respond to steroid treatment

---

TABLE 30-4

Situations that can provoke a crisis

Obstetric	**Gynecologic**
Vaginal delivery	Pelvic infection
Cesarean section	Operative procedure

crucial. Table 30-4 outlines the clinical situations in obstetrics and gynecology where stress may provoke a crisis.

When normal persons with intact adrenals respond to major stress, they may produce more than 100 mg of cortisol daily, but probably not more than 300 mg/day.[4] Therefore, those at risk for adrenal crisis should receive the equivalent of 300 mg of cortisol in preparation for major stress. It may not always be possible to anticipate stress so that the patient may be prepared adequately.

Surgical emergencies or nonelective surgical procedures may produce an immediate problem in steroid management, but it is possible to achieve adequate plasma levels of cortisol under all conditions. The following are two management plans: one for patients undergoing elective surgical procedures and one for those in emergency situations requiring surgery.

Elective surgery. When planning to do an elective procedure such as hysterectomy or repeat cesarean section on a patient with adrenal insufficiency, increase the level of cortisol the night before surgery (Table 30-5). Since most of the stress occurs on the day of surgery, provide 300 mg of cortisol (hydrocortisone) or its equivalent. When the major stress of surgery is over, decrease the dosage of steroid by 50% each day until you reach either the starting dose or the physiologic dose.[4] If the patient was not on long-term steroid therapy in the immediate preoperative period, slowly taper the dose to avoid the steroid withdrawal syndrome (nausea and vomiting, anorexia, muscle weakness, and lethargy). Complications of surgery may require that additional glucocorticoids be given. It is far better to err on the side of overtreatment in situations of acute stress than to precipitate a crisis. Short-term overtreatment produces few symptoms, though prolonged overtreatment will produce symptoms and signs of Cushing's syndrome.

TABLE 30-5

Elective procedures

Day before surgery	Usual steroid dose in AM 50 mg hydrocortisone IM hs
Day of surgery	100 mg hydrocortisone IM before surgery 100 mg hydrocortisone IV infusion during surgery 100 mg hydrocortisone IV infusion in recovery room
Postoperative day 1	150 mg hydrocortisone IV infusion
Postoperative day 2	75 mg hydrocortisone IV infusion

TABLE 30-6

Nonelective or emergency procedure

Before surgery	100 mg hydrocortisone IV bolus or infusion
During surgery	100 mg hydrocortisone IV infusion
Recovery room	100 mg hydrocortisone IV infusion
Postoperative day 1	150 mg hydrocortisone IV infusion
Postoperative day 2	75 mg hydrocortisone IV infusion

Emergency surgery. When a patient at risk requires emergency surgery or is in a situation that necessitates rapid elevation of cortisol levels—a patient who presents in spontaneous labor at term would be a typical example—start a hydrocortisone infusion immediately. Give 100 mg before delivery or the surgical procedure. Give another 100 mg during the procedure and another in the immediate postoperative or postpartum period (Table 30-6). Reduce the dosage postoperatively as previously outlined.

OTHER CONSIDERATIONS

Patients who have been on long-term steroid therapy may be at risk for two postoperative complications: Wound healing may be impaired, and the patient may be predisposed to wound separation or evisceration. Smead-Jones closure or retention sutures should be considered.

Another effect of steroid therapy is weakening of the gastric mucosal barrier and susceptibility to gastric ulcers. Watch for early signs and symptoms of ulcers. Cimetidine has been used effectively to reduce the incidence of ulcer formation in these patients. Also warn these patients against taking aspirin.

REFERENCES

1. Oyama T: Influence of general anesthesia and surgical stress on endocrine function. In Brown BR (ed): *Anesthesia and the Patient With Endocrine Disease.* Philadelphia, FA Davis, 1980, p 177
2. Axelrod L: Glucocorticoid therapy. Medicine 55:39, 1976
3. Valenta LJ, Afrasiabi MA: Adrenocortical insufficiency. In *Handbook of Endocrine and Metabolic Emergencies.* Flushing, NY, Medical Examination Publishing Co, 1981, p 246
4. Liddle GW: The adrenals. In Williams RH (ed): *Textbook of Endocrinology.* Philadelphia, WB Saunders, 1981, p 284

SUGGESTED READING

• Azarnoff DL (ed): *Steroid Therapy.* Philadelphia, WB Saunders, 1975
• Condon RE, Nyhus LM (eds): *Manual of Surgical Therapeutics.* Boston, Little, Brown, 1981

PART III
Anesthesia

31

Anesthetic Emergencies

RAYMOND R. SCHULTETUS, MD, PhD

CLINICAL SIGNIFICANCE: The incidence of anesthetic emergencies may be as high as 1%. If improperly managed, loss of airway control, pulmonary aspiration, and total spinal or local anesthetic toxicity can cause serious morbidity and death. Be aware of the potential for complications, know treatment modalities, and make sure appropriate equipment is available.

Careful adherence to good standards of practice usually results in safe anesthesia, but occasionally, in spite of reasonable precautions and good intentions, emergencies arise. These emergencies are encountered by obstetricians as well as by anesthesiologists.

AIRWAY CONTROL

Loss of airway control, the most acute emergency, may follow failure to intubate the trachea after induction of general anesthesia. It also may be secondary to local anesthetic toxicity, total spinal anesthesia, or pre-eclampsia-eclampsia.

Preoperative assessment of the airway is the first step in preventing a potentially fatal problem.[1] Inspect the face and neck for obvious maxillofacial deformities such as a hypoplastic mandible. Palpate the neck to determine that the trachea is in the midline. Note neck and jaw mobility and the size of the tongue. Inspect the mouth for dentures and loose teeth. Ascertain any history of goiter, neck surgery, previous intubation, or tracheostomy. Every patient should be evaluated as though she were to be intubated.

Obesity poses special airway problems.[2] About 20% of patients near 175% of their ideal weight will have such problems once they are unconscious. Roughly 80% of those who exceed 300% of their ideal weight will have a tenuous airway. While upright, the obese patient may appear to have an adequate airway, yet when she is supine and unconscious, her head and neck may become trapped in folds of adipose tissue. Pendulous breasts and chest fat may make it virtually impossible to open the mouth and insert a laryngoscope blade. The extra chest and abdominal mass compresses the thorax and increases the amount of airway pressure required to inflate the lungs. For these patients and others with tenuous airways, consider oral or nasal endotracheal intubation while they are still awake, before the initiation of general anesthesia.[3]

If tracheal intubation is necessary for an unconscious patient, it is mandatory to do it smoothly and rapidly. Therefore, all necessary intubation equipment should be available and ready to use (Figure 31-1). This includes:
• Sterile cuffed endotracheal tubes with stylets. If there is time, check the cuff of the appropriate endotracheal tube (7-mm ID for most adult females) for leaks before insertion.
• Two laryngoscope handles with blades of appropriate size (No. 3 MacIntosh and No. 3 Miller), batteries, and bulbs. During an emergency, you will not have the time to look for spares.

FIGURE 31-1

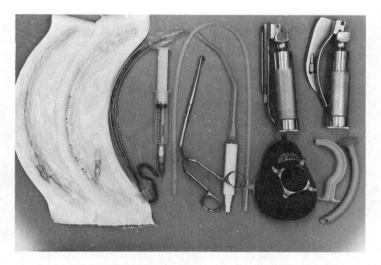

Intubation equipment includes (left to right) endotracheal tubes with stylets and syringe; Magill forceps; Yankauer suction instrument; suction catheter; laryngoscope handles with Miller (left) and MacIntosh (right) blades; and (bottom right) mask with oral and nasal airways

- An oxygen supply and a means for delivery such as an Ambu bag and mask and a Yankauer suction instrument with an adequate vacuum source.
- An oral and a nasal airway of appropriate size.

Laryngoscopy and endotracheal intubation are not difficult. All physicians should be able to perform them rapidly. Although training mannequins are available, intubation skills are best developed in the operating room under the supervision of a trained laryngoscopist, using anesthetized, paralyzed patients. To facilitate laryngoscopy, place a 3- to 4-inch-thick pad under the patient's head. This thrusts the head forward into the "sniffing position," aligns the axes of the trachea, pharynx, and mouth, and makes the larynx easier to visualize. Hold the laryngoscope in the left hand and open the patient's mouth with the right (Figure 31-2, left). Insert the laryngoscope along the right side of the mouth, sweeping the tongue to the left (Figure 31-2, right). The tip of a curved blade (MacIntosh) should rest between the epiglottis and the base of the tongue. Place the tip of a straight blade (Miller) on the epiglottis, to lift it. To visualize the larynx, lift the laryngoscope at a 45° angle away from you; don't use the patient's teeth to provide leverage. Insert the endotracheal tube from the right side of the mouth—not down the center of the laryngoscope blade—between the vocal cords and advance it until the

FIGURE 31-2

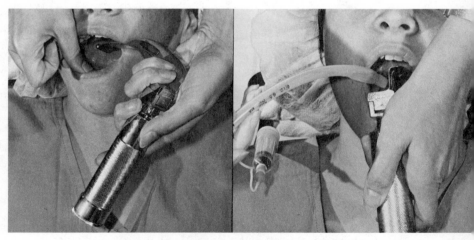

How to perform laryngoscopy and tracheal intubation. Left: Hold the laryngoscope in the left hand and open the patient's mouth with the right. Right: Insert the laryngoscope along the right side of the mouth, sweeping the tongue to the left

cuff has passed 1 to 2 cm beyond them. Inflate the cuff and auscultate the chest for bilaterally equal breath sounds.

If intubation proves impossible, use a mask to ventilate the patient. Quickly check the airway for vomitus and clear it if necessary. Apply a mask to the face with the head extended and the jaw thrust forward, and provide positive pressure ventilation (PPV) with 100% oxygen. Although regurgitation during PPV will force gastric contents into the trachea, the risk of hypoxic death outweighs the risk of aspiration.

Because the lower esophageal sphincter has an opening pressure of approximately 18 to 20 cm H_2O, high-pressure ventilation by mask introduces gas into the stomach. The resulting gastric distention further increases the likelihood of regurgitation and aspiration. Therefore, use the lowest airway pressure that will ventilate the patient adequately. Adequacy of ventilation is best judged by chest auscultation but can be inferred from the movement of the chest during PPV.

Application of firm, posteriorly directed pressure to the cricoid cartilage by a second person affords some protection from aspiration (Figure 31-3). This occludes the esophagus and prevents passive regurgitation. Because of the high pressures developed, cricoid pressure will not prevent regurgitation during active vomiting. Under these conditions, continued pressure on the cricoid could result in esophageal rupture.

FIGURE 31-3

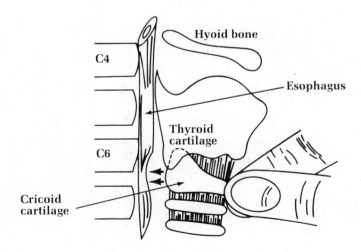

Firm, posteriorly directed pressure applied by a second person to the cricoid cartilage affords some protection from aspiration

---

If intubation cannot be accomplished and ventilation by mask is inadequate, a cricothyrotomy can sustain the patient until she can breathe or until a tracheostomy can be performed (Figure 31-4). Introduce the 12-gauge cannula into the trachea through the cricothyroid membrane and withdraw the needle. Use a 3-mm endotracheal tube adapter to connect the plastic catheter to an Ambu bag or an anesthesia machine and ventilate the patient with 100% oxygen.

Frequently, regional or local anesthesia is proposed for patients with potentially difficult airways. Remember, however, that the treatment for local anesthetic toxicity or high spinal anesthesia includes securing the airway and providing adequate ventilation, which may prove impossible. A well-planned general anesthetic with oral or nasal intubation while the patient is still awake may be a wiser choice.

PULMONARY ASPIRATION

All unconscious patients are at risk from regurgitation and pulmonary aspiration, even those who have been fasting for 8 hours. Pregnancy

---

FIGURE 31-4

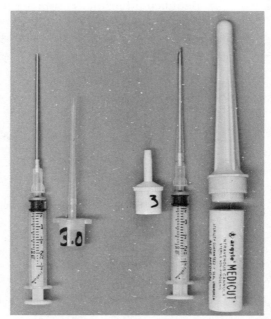

A cricothyrotomy can sustain the patient either until she can breathe or until a tracheostomy can be done. Cannula package (right) consists of needle (left), plastic catheter, and adapter

imposes additional risks. Esophageal sphincter tone decreases during pregnancy—perhaps because of hormonal changes—allowing the esophageal reflux that results in the common complaint of heartburn.[4] Concurrently, intragastric pressure increases, possibly in association with increased abdominal girth.

Decreased sphincter tone and increased intragastric pressure predispose the patient to regurgitation. The onset of labor increases the risk, particularly when narcotics are administered.[5] Narcotics prolong gastric emptying time, and intragastric volume may quadruple as a result. When the woman in labor is obese, intragastric contents are further enlarged. As if all this weren't bad enough, patients in labor frequently have eaten recently and so are at extremely high risk of substantial regurgitation and severe aspiration.

To be safe, all laboring patients should be treated as though they had just eaten. To protect their lungs from reflux of gastric contents, they should never have general anesthesia without an endotracheal tube in place. If you administer inhalation or intravenous analgesia, the patient must remain alert, to protect her airway should regurgitation occur.

Acid aspiration causes chemical burns of pulmonary tissue.[6] As the pH of the aspirate nears 1.5, the severity of the damage increases. Below pH 1.5 little additional damage is produced. Within minutes after aspiration, severe reflex bronchospasm and marked intrapulmonic shunting of blood occur. Pao_2 falls to 50 to 60 torr. During the next few hours, epithelial and alveolar cells degenerate and septal necrosis begins. Hemorrhagic pulmonary edema develops and destruction of surfactant causes alveolar collapse.

The pathophysiology of the damage produced by the aspirated food depends in part upon particle size. Large particles can obstruct the large airways and cause suffocation and cardiovascular collapse. Aspiration of small particles produces hemorrhagic pneumonia, with peribronchiolar reactions centering on the particles. The pulmonary edema that results is less severe than the edema caused by acid aspiration, but hypoxemia occurs just as rapidly and may be equally profound. The aspiration of acidic food combines the effects of both types of aspiration and produces the severest lung damage.

Clinically, pulmonary aspiration of food produces tachycardia, cyanosis, dyspnea, and bronchoconstriction. Arterial oxygen tension, which falls within minutes of pulmonary aspiration, is the earliest and most reliable sign that clinically significant aspiration has occurred. A chest x-ray typically reveals scattered, soft, mottled, confluent densities, but these changes may lag behind clinical signs by several hours.

Because physiologic changes occur rapidly, begin therapy as soon as you suspect aspiration. Intubate the trachea to prevent further aspiration of food particles and remove any remaining material by suction.

Because aspirated material rapidly disperses, prolonged or vigorous suctioning is not useful. Obtain an arterial blood sample for blood gas analysis and give supplemental oxygen.

Liquid aspirate disperses so quickly that little, if any, can be removed through the bronchoscope.[7] Do bronchoscopy only if you see large particles in the aspirate or suspect they are present. Lavage with large volumes of saline or bicarbonate is not recommended. Most studies show it produces no improvement and may actually increase the damage.[8] Solid material obstructing large airways can be removed by judicious lavage under direct vision.

Oxygen therapy and PPV improve arterial oxygenation and survival.[9] Positive end expiratory pressure reduces atelectasis and allows the use of lower concentrations of inspired oxygen. The clinical course and blood gas analyses dictate what ventilatory support to use. Therapy should be aimed at keeping arterial oxygen tension above 60 torr.

Significant amounts of intravascular fluid may be lost into the lung tissue, so fluid monitoring is necessary—perhaps with a central venous or pulmonary artery catheter. Fluid therapy should be directed at maintaining normal intravascular volume and cardiac output.

There is no conclusive evidence that steroids are beneficial in aspiration therapy, although some authors continue to recommend them.[10]

Although pulmonary aspiration may introduce a wide variety of infectious organisms, prophylactic antibiotics are not indicated. Indeed, retrospective analyses of clinical courses of patients given prophylactic antibiotics showed no advantage.[11] Instead, watch for clinical signs of infection and choose antibiotics according to culture results.

TOTAL SPINAL ANESTHESIA

Injection of a large volume of local anesthetic into the subarachnoid space—which might occur with accidental puncture of the dura during an epidural anesthetic or cephalad migration of a smaller dose during spinal anesthesia—results in progressive and widespread neuroblockade. As anesthesia rises to the T_4 level, the intercostal muscles cease to contribute to ventilation. Although the diaphragm can maintain normal minute ventilation, the ability to cough and clear the airway is lost. A lack of sensation in the chest wall frequently gives patients a feeling that they can't breathe; however, they usually respond positively to reassurance that they are breathing adequately. As anesthesia progresses to C_4, phrenic nerves will be blocked and the diaphragm paralyzed. In addition to chest wall paralysis, total spinal anesthesia can markedly alter cardiovascular tone.

As the local anesthetic diffuses cephalad, it is diluted by CSF. Eventually, the agent is too dilute to penetrate large motor or sensory fibers effectively. Sympathetic fibers arising from preganglionic cells located in spinal cord segments T_1 through L_4 are smaller and may still be affected. This results in a sympathetic blockade usually at least two segments higher than the sensory. Thus, spinal anesthesia to a sensory level of T_4 could occur concurrently with a sympathetic blockade to T_1. Since the sympathetic nervous system maintains vascular tone, a total sympathetic blockade allows venous pooling of blood.

Sympathetic cardiac accelerator fibers, which maintain heart rate, are found at spinal cord levels T_1 through T_4. High spinal anesthesia blocks these fibers and produces bradycardia. The marked decrease in cardiac output caused by the reduced venous return and slowed heart rate produces severe hypotension, which can result in medullary ischemia and respiratory arrest.

Total spinal anesthesia requires adequate ventilation with oxygen and cardiovascular support. Usually the patient needs to be intubated to ensure adequate ventilation and to secure the airway against aspiration. Circulatory support involves displacing the uterus to the left to relieve aortocaval compression, raising the legs to improve venous return, and administering fluid therapy and drugs to restore peripheral vascular tone. Ephedrine is best as the first-line vasopressor. It produces both vasoconstriction and cardiac stimulation and restores cardiac output and blood pressure without decreasing uterine blood flow. Use normal saline, Ringer's lactate, or albumin to expand intravascular volume. Because several liters of fluid may be required, don't give fluids containing dextrose for resuscitation. The infusion of even very small amounts of dextrose can produce neonatal hypoglycemia.[12]

The incidence of total spinal anesthesia is low (less than 0.1%), yet it remains a serious potential complication of epidural, spinal, and caudal anesthesia.[13]

TOXIC REACTIONS TO LOCAL ANESTHETICS

Allergic reactions to local anesthetics are rare; toxic reactions to a high plasma concentration of local anesthetic occur more frequently. The incidence of seizures induced by anesthetics during epidural blockade is estimated at 0.2%.[14] High blood concentrations result from intravascular injection, rapid uptake from highly vascular tissues, or, simply, too high a dosage. Early signs of toxicity include nervousness, dizziness, tinnitus, and tremors. The patient may be confused and have blurred vision and nystagmus. As drug levels increase, tonic-clonic seizures occur. Drug-induced CNS depression may closely follow an initial period of excitation. At high blood levels, you may see respiratory arrest and cardiovascular depression with hypotension, bradycardia, and cardiac arrest. Some early signs of toxicity (nervousness, tremor, and headache) may be difficult to distinguish from the effects of epinephrine, often used in conjunction with local anesthetic agents.

Seizures induced by local anesthetics are generally brief (usually less than 1 minute), because of the rapidity with which these drugs are redistributed. To treat, maintain the airway and give oxygen. In animal studies, this therapy alone markedly reduced the morbidity and mortality from such seizures.[15] Cardiovascular depression requires treatment with fluids and vasopressors. The use of benzodiazepines (2.5 to 5 mg IV) and short-acting barbiturates (50 to 100 mg IV) to terminate seizure activity is controversial because such drugs may depress the cardiovascular system further and delay return to consciousness. Terminating a seizure with these agents, however, may permit effective ventilation, restore cardiovascular stability, and improve cerebral oxygenation. Giving the muscle relaxant succinylcholine (20 to 40 mg IV) to produce paralysis allows ventilation during a seizure. Succinylcholine neither depresses the myocardium, alters consciousness, nor blocks cortical seizures. However, muscle relaxants should never be used unless adequate ventilation can be assured after paralysis has been induced.

Preventing toxicity is preferable to treating it. Inject local anesthetic agents slowly and check frequently for blood return to avoid intravascular injection. Follow recommended dosage limits (see Table 31-1; the limits refer to the maximum for a single injection). With repeated injections, the maximum is lower, because of the long half-lives of most local anesthetics and the resultant cumulative effect. Additional dosage corrections are required to allow for a patient's physical condition and any special problems, such as renal or hepatic disease, that alter metabolism and excretion. Finally, local anesthesia should never be used unless resuscitation equipment is available.

To respond appropriately to emergencies, you must be alert to potentially serious complications of anesthesia. This chapter is designed to stimulate the practice of old skills and the pursuit of new ones.

TABLE 31-1

Recommended maximum dosage of commonly used local anesthetic agents

AGENT	DOSAGE LIMIT (mg/kg)
Lidocaine (plain)	4
Lidocaine (epinephrine)	7
Bupivacaine (plain)	3
2-Chloroprocaine	10-15

Note: A 1% solution contains 10 mg/mL.

REFERENCES

1. Ament R: A systematic approach to the difficult intubation. Anesthesiol Rev 5(7):12, 1978

2. Lee JJ, Larson RH, Buckley JJ, et al: Airway maintenance in the morbidly obese. Anesthesiol Rev 7(1):33, 1980

3. Donlon JV Jr: Anesthetic management of patients with compromised airways. Anesthesiol Rev 7(2):22, 1980

4. Brock-Utne JG, Dow TBG, Dimopoulos GE, et al: Gastric and lower oesophageal sphincter (LOS) pressures in early pregnancy. Br J Anaesth 53:381, 1981

5. Roberts RB, Shirley MA: Reducing the risk of acid aspiration during cesarean section. Anesth Analg 53:859, 1974

6. Wynne JW, Modell JH: Respiratory aspiration of stomach contents. Ann Intern Med 87:466, 1977

7. Hamelberg W, Bosomworth PP: Aspiration pneumonitis: Experimental studies and clinical observations. Anesth Analg 43:669, 1964

8. Taylor G, Pryse-Davies J: Evaluation of endotracheal steroid therapy in acid pulmonary aspiration syndrome (Mendelson's syndrome). Anesthesiology 29:17, 1968

9. Cameron JL, Sebor J, Anderson RP, et al: Aspiration pneumonia. Results of treatment by positive-pressure ventilation in dogs. J Surg Res 8:447, 1968

10. Chapman RL Jr, Downs JB, Modell JH, et al: The ineffectiveness of steroid therapy in treating aspiration of hydrochloric acid. Arch Surg 108:858, 1974

11. Cameron JL, Mitchell WH, Zuidema GD: Aspiration pneumonia. Clinical outcome following documented aspiration. Arch Surg 106:49, 1973

12. Knepp NB, Shelley WC, Kumer S, et al: Effects on newborn of hydration with glucose in patients undergoing cesarean section with regional anesthesia. Lancet 1:645, 1980

13. Dawkins CJM: An analysis of the complications of epidural and caudal block. Anaesthesia 24:554, 1969

14. Kandel PF, Spoerel WE, Kinch RAH: Continuous epidural analgesia for labour and delivery. Review of 1000 cases. Can Med Assoc J 95:947, 1966

15. Feinstein MB, Lenard W, Mathios J: The antagonism of local anesthetic induced convulsions by the benzodiazepine derivative diazepam. Arch Int Pharmacodyn Ther 187:144, 1970

32

Complications of Paracervical Block

THOMAS M. WARREN, MD, and
GERARD W. OSTHEIMER, MD

CLINICAL SIGNIFICANCE: Paracervical block produces complications in about 0.5% of obstetric patients, and bradycardia in about 20% of fetuses. In the mother, vasovagal syncope and intravascular injection, though rare, can cause serious morbidity and mortality. Fetal bradycardia is associated with hypoxia and acidosis and can produce neonatal depression and death.

The popularity of paracervical block (PCB) for relieving pain during cervical dilation has been in decline. For outpatient gynecologic procedures, however, its use has increased. The technique can cause complications for the surgical patient, the parturient, and the fetus; so when you use it, be prepared. Surgical or maternal complications are vasovagal syncope and intravascular injection. Fetal complications include bradycardia and direct fetal injection.

ANATOMY, PHYSIOLOGY, AND TECHNIQUE

Visceral afferent fibers from the uterus, cervix, and upper vagina travel with the sympathetic nerves close to the blood vessels that supply these areas and converge bilaterally to form the left and right pelvic or inferior hypogastric plexus. This plexus is located in the parametrium at the base of the broad ligaments, very near the uterine artery and vein. From the plexus the left and right hypogastric nerves sweep posteriorly and cephalad over the pelvic brim. These connect to the lumbar and lower thoracic segments of the sympathetic chain and then enter the spinal cord at the level of T_{11} and T_{12}, with occasional branches to T_{10} and L_1.

To block sensation in the uterus, cervix, and upper vagina, you can interrupt this pathway at any point. PCB achieves its effect by blocking the pelvic plexus as it passes through the base of the broad ligament.

Blockade is best performed with the patient in the lithotomy position. After preparing the perineum and vagina, use the index and middle fingers to direct a Kobak needle or a 20-gauge needle, within an Iowa trumpet, into the vagina. The needle should meet the cervicovaginal junction at 3 o'clock or 9 o'clock. Then direct it cephalad and dorsolaterally through the guide, so that the mucosa is penetrated no more than 0.5 cm (Figure 32-1). Advancing the needle any farther increases the chance of a poor or failed block. In the obstetric patient, exercise extreme care to avoid injecting the fetal presenting part. After careful aspiration, inject 5 to 10 mL of local anesthetic; repeat the procedure on the opposite side. Table 32-1 summarizes the dosage per injection site, and the onset and duration of action in minutes for the local anesthetics most commonly used for PCB.

VASOVAGAL SYNCOPE

This syndrome is characterized by intense activity of the sympathetic nervous system, followed abruptly by the onset of intense parasympathetic activity.[1] Activation of the sympathetic system represents a re-

---

FIGURE 32-1

Site for administering paracervical block

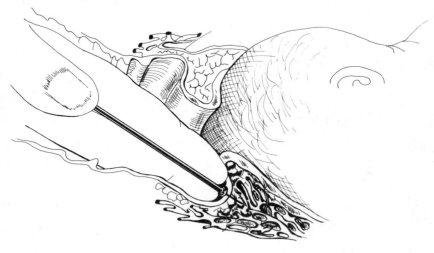

Two reasons for extra caution: (1) the rich vascular supply of the paracervical tissue; and (2) the proximity of the needle site to the fetal head.

sponse to the threat of physical injury. The sudden onset of parasympathetic activity indicates that the organism has "given up" in the face of an overwhelming threat. The patient is initially tremulous, diaphoretic, pale, and tachycardic. This stage is followed by weakness, bradycardia, hypotension, and loss of consciousness. Loss of bowel and bladder function is not unusual, and occasionally a seizure occurs. Resuscitation failure is rare, but has been reported.[2]

Use the same series of steps for vasovagal syncope that you would use for cardiopulmonary resuscitation (Table 32-2). Place the patient supine, with her head down, if possible. Assess her vital signs and consult the ECG if it is already attached. The typical patient is unconscious, apneic, and has a slow or nonpalpable pulse. An airway should be established and cleared. Initiate artificial respiration immediately, if spontaneous breathing fails to begin once the airway is established. If the pulse is absent or questionable, begin external cardiac compression. Give atropine 0.5 to 1.0 mg or epinephrine 0.5 mg IV if the patient is still bradycardic or in asystole. In ventricular fibrillation, direct current defibrillation will be necessary.[2]

INTRAVASCULAR INJECTION

Injection of local anesthetic directly into the artery or vein is a complication of PCB that must always be kept in mind. The paracervical tissue is extremely vascular, especially in late pregnancy, when the gravid uterus causes pelvic venous engorgement. In addition, the uterine artery and vein course through the parametrium in close proximity to the injection site. Frequent aspiration, both before and during injection of the local anesthetic, helps prevent this complication. Continually mov-

---

TABLE 32-1

Local anesthetics in current use for PCB

DRUG	DOSE PER INJECTION SITE* (mL)	(mg)	ONSET OF ACTION (minutes)	DURATION OF ACTION (minutes)
2-Chloroprocaine 1% to 2% (Nesacaine)	5-10	50-200	3-5	45-60
Lidocaine 1% (Xylocaine)	5-10	50-100	5-10	60-90
Mepivacaine 1% (Carbocaine)	5-10	50-100	5-10	60-90

*Usually there are two injection sites; multiply by two for total dose.

ing the needle back and forth during the injection is an alternative technique. Intravascular injection of a local anesthetic results in a major toxic reaction in the central nervous and cardiovascular systems.

CNS toxicity. Local anesthetics initially block inhibitory cortical neurons, allowing facilitory neurons to operate unopposed. As the blood level of the anesthetic increases, the facilitory neurons also become blocked. The syndrome of CNS toxicity includes initial excitatory signs and symptoms that lead to a generalized convulsion, followed by a generalized state of CNS depression. The patient first complains of lightheadedness, dizziness, a metallic taste, visual and auditory disturbances, disorientation, and a sense of twitching. Other signs of toxicity include euphoria, dysarthria, vomiting, shivering, and fasciculation. Either clonic or tonic-clonic convulsions ultimately occur. The generalized CNS depression that follows the convulsions is a serious consequence and can cause death from respiratory arrest.[3]

Cardiovascular toxicity. Cardiovascular effects following an intravascular injection are produced by direct cardiac and peripheral vascular action. Toxic blood levels of lidocaine increase atrioventricular and intraventricular conduction times, with a prolonged P-R interval and QRS period the result. Decreased automaticity causes sinus bradycardia, which can progress to asystole. Direct hemodynamic effects of toxicity include decreased myocardial contractility, increased diastolic volume, decreased intraventricular pressure, and decreased cardiac output.

TABLE 32-2

ABCs of managing vasovagal syncope

Assess
Respiration, pulse, level of consciousness, and ECG (if possible)

Airway
Extend head or use jaw thrust maneuver

Breathing
Begin mouth-to-mouth resuscitation, or artificial intermittent
    positive pressure breathing with oxygen

Circulation
Perform external cardiac compression, 60 to 80 times/minute

Drugs
Administer atropine (0.5 to 1.0 mg IV) or epinephrine (0.5 mg IV)

Electricity
Apply direct current defibrillation (200 to 400 joules)

In the peripheral vasculature, local anesthetics exert a direct relaxant effect on the smooth muscle of the arterioles. Thus, the clinical picture is one of a bradycardic patient with profound hypotension and circulatory collapse. Usually the toxic cardiovascular effects that follow an intravascular injection do not develop until after the patient has convulsed and suffered respiratory arrest.[3]

Treatment. If you notice prodromal signs or symptoms of CNS excitement while injecting local anesthetic, stop the injection immediately. Administer oxygen by mask and prepare to treat a seizure. If the patient convulses, give 100% oxygen by mask and bag. Maintaining an oral or nasal airway may be necessary. Give diazepam in incremental doses of 2.5 mg or thiopental in incremental doses of 50 mg to stop the convulsion. If the seizure still does not stop and the patency of the airway is in question, administer succinylcholine 1.0 to 1.5 mg/kg; then intubate and institute controlled ventilation with 100% oxygen.

If the seizure stops after you administer diazepam or thiopental, assess the patient's respiratory status. If she resumes spontaneous ventilation, continue 100% oxygen and assisted ventilation. If spontaneous ventilation does not resume, intubation and controlled ventilation are indicated. Perform intubation in the significantly obtunded obstetric patient, whether or not spontaneous ventilation has resumed, to protect her airway from the risk of regurgitation and aspiration.

Once the respiratory system is stable, direct attention to the cardiovascular system. Use atropine and epinephrine to treat bradycardia and asystole. Perform external cardiac compression if there is a decreasing or nonpalpable pulse. Electrical defibrillation may be indicated. Treat hypotension with crystalloid solution and vasopressors. Ephedrine is the vasopressor of choice in the obstetric patient. In the nonpregnant patient, use a vasoconstrictor such as Neo-Synephrine or norepinephrine to counteract decreased systemic vascular resistance induced by the local anesthetic. Remember that during cardiopulmonary resuscitation of the undelivered parturient, the gravid uterus should be displaced to one side or the other, to allow venous return via the inferior vena cava and adequate perfusion of the uteroplacental circulation.

After stabilizing the respiratory and cardiovascular systems, assess the fetus. If it is in jeopardy, immediate delivery is indicated. However, if you determine that the fetus is stable, delay delivery to allow the mother to dispose of the anesthetic.

Prevention. CNS and cardiovascular toxic reactions to local anesthetics are simply manifestations of elevated blood levels. Systemic toxic reactions can occur even without frank intravascular injection, if excessive amounts are injected locally and absorbed. The paracervical area is very vascular, and systemic absorption therefore occurs rapidly. Staying within the dosage guidelines outlined in Table 32-1 will help prevent toxic systemic reactions due to rapid vascular absorption.

Ester-linked local anesthetics (such as 2-chloroprocaine) are rapidly metabolized in the bloodstream by plasma pseudocholinesterase. Amide-linked local anesthetics (such as lidocaine and mepivacaine) are slowly metabolized in the liver. Following an intravascular injection, blood levels of an ester-linked agent will fall much faster than those of an amide-linked agent. The maternal plasma half-life of 2-chloroprocaine, for example, is 21 seconds, compared with that of mepivacaine, which is approximately 3 hours.[4] Thus, the incidence and severity of systemic toxic reactions will be much less when an ester-linked agent is used.[5] In fact, for 5 years, Brigham and Women's Hospital has used nothing but 1% 2-chloroprocaine for paracervical block for therapeutic abortions. Over 10,000 paracervical blocks have been performed with this agent without producing a single convulsion.

FETAL BRADYCARDIA

Associated with fetal hypoxia and acidosis, bradycardia indicates fetal distress and an increased risk of neonatal depression. Bradycardia typically develops 2 to 10 minutes after the block is performed and lasts from 3 to 30 minutes. The high frequency of fetal bradycardia following PCB has kept us from using this technique for pain relief during labor. The incidence of this complication is 20% or greater, depending on what study is quoted.

PCB probably induces bradycardia both by raising fetal blood levels of local anesthetic and by decreasing uterine blood flow (Table 32-3). The high fetal blood levels are caused by rapid systemic absorption in the highly vascular paracervical area and direct transarterial diffusion of local anesthetic into the uterine arteries. In fact, fetal blood levels can be higher than simultaneously drawn maternal levels.[6] Uterine blood

---

TABLE 32-3

Causes of fetal bradycardia

High fetal blood levels of local anesthesia
Rapid systemic absorption
Transarterial diffusion

Decreased uterine blood flow
Direct mechanical compression of uterine vasculature
Local-anesthetic-induced uterine artery vasoconstriction
Local-anesthetic-induced increase in uterine tone

flow is decreased mechanically by direct compression of the uterine arteries by the local anesthetic solution and pharmacologically by local-anesthetic-induced uterine artery vasoconstriction.[7, 8] Another recently elucidated mechanism for decreasing uterine blood flow after PCB is increased uterine activity, with subsequent reduction in uteroplacental blood flow.[9]

Continuous electronic monitoring of the fetal heart rate is considered mandatory if PCB is to be used in labor. If evidence of fetal distress (persistent bradycardia, late decelerations, or variable decelerations) develops after PCB, obtain serial fetal scalp capillary blood samples for pH determinations. If the bradycardia is persistent and the scalp pH progressively deteriorates (to 7.20 or less), immediate delivery is indicated. If the bradycardia resolves and the fetal scalp pH is not persistently abnormal, delay delivery to permit transplacental transfer of local anesthetic to the mother, to decrease the fetal blood level. In either case, have neonatal resuscitative drugs and equipment ready, in case the newborn should be depressed.

The best way to prevent fetal bradycardia is not to exceed the dosages listed in Table 32-1 and to avoid maternal intravascular injection. Paracervical block is contraindicated in cases of uteroplacental insufficiency, prematurity, or pre-existing fetal distress.[10]

DIRECT FETAL INJECTION

Injecting local anesthetic directly into the fetus produces severe CNS and cardiovascular depression manifested by convulsions, bradycardia, cyanosis, apnea, unresponsiveness to positive pressure ventilation—and frequently death. Dodson believes that forced neonatal diuresis is the safest and most effective way to enhance excretion of local anesthetic.[11] Some success in treating these neonates has been reported with gastric lavage and exchange transfusions.[10]

Obviously, the best way to prevent this complication is to pay strict attention to detail. Exercise extreme care in directing the needle and avoid advancing it too deeply. This is especially important during the later stages of labor, when the cervix is dilated beyond 7 cm. PCB should not be given when the cervix is fully dilated and completely effaced or if the fetal presenting part is at a low station.

REFERENCES

1. Engel GL: Psychologic stress, vasodepressor (vasovagal) syncope and sudden death. Ann Intern Med 89:403, 1978
2. Naulty JS, Ostheimer GW: CPR for vasovagal syncope. Contemp Ob/Gyn 18:20, July 1981
3. Covino BG: Pharmacology and physiology of local anesthetics. ASA Refresher Courses in Anesthesiology, vol 5. Philadelphia, JB Lippincott, 1977, p 33

4. Bromage PR: Choice of local anesthetics in obstetrics. In Shnider SM, Levinson G (eds): *Anesthesia for Obstetrics*. Baltimore, Williams & Wilkins, 1979, pp 109-120

5. Grimes DA, Cates W Jr: Death from paracervical anesthesia used for first-trimester abortion, 1972-1975. N Engl J Med 295:1397, 1976

6. Asling JH, Shnider SM, Margolis AJ, et al: Paracervical block anesthesia in obstetrics. II: Etiology of fetal bradycardia following paracervical block anesthesia. Am J Obstet Gynecol 107:626, 1970

7. Greiss FC, Still JG, Anderson SG: Effects of local anesthetic agents on the uterine vasculatures and myometrium. Am J Obstet Gynecol 127:889, 1976

8. Cibils LA: Response of human uterine arteries to local anesthetics. Am J Obstet Gynecol 126:202, 1976

9. Morishima HO, Covino BG, Yeh MN, et al: Bradycardia in the fetal baboon following paracervical block anesthesia. Am J Obstet Gynecol 140:775, 1981

10. Ralston DH, Shnider SM: The fetal and neonatal effects of regional anesthesia in obstetrics. Anesthesiology 48:34, 1978

11. Dodson WE: Neonatal drug intoxication: Local anesthetics. Pediatr Clin North Am 23:399, 1976

INDEX

A

Abdomen, 3, 5*
  acute, 8-16
  bleeding, 240
  distention, 133, 243, 245
  exploration, 231, 239
  foreign objects, 231, 240
  insufflation, 234
  lavage, 236
  mass, 175
  muscle rigidity, 10, 15
  pain, 12, 14, 96, 97, 175, 227, 241, 249
  tenderness, 96
  trauma, 20, 231, 239
Abortion, 26, 100
  ectopic pregnancy, 238
  elective, 226
  in hemolytic anemia, 137
  incomplete, 216, 237
  saline, 114
  septic, 25, 26, 179
  spontaneous, 8, 10, 59, 65
  therapeutic, 59
  threatened, 34, 237
Abruptio placentae, 34, 40, 61, 72, 73, 87-91
  blood loss, 100
  with coagulopathy, 114, 117
  concealed, 117-118
  delivery, 88-89, 105
  diagnosis, 60, 88
  eclampsia, 80
  and fetal anemia, 128, 131
  hemorrhagic shock, 105
  hypertension with, 88, 148
  management, 88-91
  mortality, 88
  and postpartum hemorrhage, 158
  renal failure and, 25, 26
  third-trimester bleeding, 84, 85
  uterine rupture and, 95
Abscess, 243
  abdominopelvic, 179, 182, 183
  intra-abdominal, 211
  intraperitoneal, 61
  pelvic, 170, 173, 174, 182, 211, 224-229
  perinephric, 182
  ruptured, 11, 224-230
  signs and symptoms, 225-226, 227
  surgery, 229
  tubo-ovarian, 10-11, 183, 224

Acidosis, 75
  in adrenal insufficiency, 251
  in diabetics, 44-52
  fetal, 53, 148, 153, 266, 271
  in hemorrhagic shock, 101, 105
  intracerebral, 53
  metabolic, 48-49, 101, 180, 226, 228
  in renal failure, 27
  respiratory, 180
  in shock, 177, 180, 186
  in sickle cell crisis, 36
ACTH, 11, 45, 188, 248, 249
Acute abdomen, 8-16
Addison's disease, 248-251
Adnexal torsion, 10, 34, 231, 240
Adnexectomy, 230
Adrenal (adrenocortical) insufficiency, 248-253
  infection and, 248-250, 251
  management, 250-251
  patients at risk, 249-250
  prevention, 251-253
  primary. See Addison's disease
  secondary, 248-249
  surgery in, 252-253
β-Adrenergic agents, 53, 61, 62
Adult respiratory distress syndrome (ARDS), 178, 181, 182, 186, 206, 207, 210-211
Airway, 151, 201, 202, 203, 256-264, 268, 269, 270
Albumin
  administered, 153, 185, 208, 263
  serum, 68, 207
  urine, 69
Alcoholism
  pancreatitis and, 15
  sickle cell crisis and, 32
  wound dehiscence and, 243
Alkalosis, 49, 180
Amenorrhea, 4, 215, 217, 223
Amniocentesis, 60, 83, 128, 131, 135
Amniotic fluid
  decreased volume, 76
  embolus/ism, 25, 26, 114, 158, 211, 212
  meconium in, 120, 149, 153
  polyhydramnios, 127, 135, 157
  in preterm cervical dilation, 60
Amniotomy, 83, 90
Analgesics, analgesia, 16, 36, 41, 209, 261

*Italic numbers indicate illustrations.

Anemia, 37, 158, 227
  aplastic, 219, 221
  dilutional, 212
  fetal/neonatal. See Fetal/neonatal
    anemia
  hemolytic, 128, 171
  infection and, 128, 138
  microangiopathic hemolytic, 25, 69, 70,
    73, 115
  and postpartum endometritis, 170, 171
Anesthesia, 106
  avoidance of, 131
  in cerclage, 62
  conduction, 41, 123, 208
  in eclampsia, 83
  general, 131, 157, 212, 228, 232, 256,
    260, 261
  general endotracheal, 62
  high spinal, 260
  in laparoscopy, 231, 234-235
  local, 260
  paracervical block. See Paracervical
    block
  pudendal block, 83
  in shoulder dystocia, 142, 147
  and sickle cell crisis, 31-32, 41
  spinal, 83
  total spinal, 256, 262-263
  and uterine atony, 157
Anesthetic emergencies, 256-264
Anesthetics, 75
  fetus and, 266, 272
  local, 83, 262, 264, 271
  maximum dosage, 264
  neonatal respiration and, 148
  paracervical block, 268
  procedure for administering, 264
  toxicity, 202, 203, 256, 260, 263-264, 270
  vasovagal syncope and, 199, 202
Aneurysm, 16, 128, 179, 193
Angiography, 75, 193, 194
Anorexia
  in Addison's disease, 248
  in cholecystitis, 14
  nervosa, 214
Anovulation, 215, 216
Antibiotics, 2, 3, 27, 36, 54, 187
  in adult respiratory distress syndrome,
    211
  in aspiration, 262
  in aspiration pneumonitis, 210
  in cholecystitis, 14
  in postpartum endometritis, 173-175
  in septicemia, 183, 184
  in shock, 105
  in urinary tract infection, 60
Anticoagulants, 133, 209, 210, 249. See
  also Heparin

Anticonvulsants, 191, 193
Antidiuretic hormone, 76
Antiemetics, 16, 54
Antifungals, 184
Antimicrobials, 173-175, 184, 224, 228,
  230
Antinuclear antibiotics (ANA), serum, 68,
  71, 72
Antishock (MAST) trousers, 104, 185, 187
Apgar scoring, 150, 151
Apnea, 199, 268, 272
Appendicitis, 8-11, 15, 34, 61, 172, 179,
  226, 241
Apt test, 130, 131, 152
ARDS. See Adult respiratory distress
  syndrome
Arrhythmia, cardiac, 178, 179, 209-210,
  234
Arteriovenous malformations, 193, 194
Ascites, 28, 67, 76, 135, 154, 243
Asphyxia
  antenatal, 127, 153
  perinatal, 88, 148-152
  pulmonary aspiration and, 261
Aspiration, 211
  acid, 261
  adnexal cysts, 240
  blood, 238
  in convulsion, 191
  gastric contents, 62
  meconium, 153
  with paracervical block, 268
  in perinatal asphyxia, 149
  pneumonitis, 207, 210
  prevention, 259, 263, 270
  pulmonary, 259-262
Aspirin, 14, 54, 110, 113, 133, 188, 253

B
Bacteria. See also individual organisms
  in amniotic fluid, 60
  in appendicitis, 8
  in blood, 177-179, 183, 188
  in gallbladder disease, 13
  in postpartum endometritis, 171-174
  in salpingitis, 11
  septic shock and, 177
  in urine, 10
Bacteroides, 11, 171, 173, 174, 184
Barbiturates, 83, 133, 264
Bilirubin, 134, 135
Biopsy
  adnexal cysts, 240
  in anovulatory bleeding, 214, 216, 217
  cone, of cervix, 59, 220
  liver, 240
  ovarian, 236
  tumor, 223

Bladder, 97, 98
  distention, 141
  function, loss of, 268
  injury, 232-233, 236
  periurethral lacerations and, 165
  rupture, 21
Bleeding. *See also* Hemorrhage
  aneurysms, 194
  anovulatory, 214-218
  arteriovenous malformations, 194
  birth trauma, 132-133
  concealed, 96, 97
  in curettage, 158
  diathesis, 29, 158, *193*, 219
  excessive, 215, 217
  fetal, 130, 131, 133
  genital tract, 106
  internal iliac vein, 106
  intra-abdominal, 240
  intracranial, 133
  intraperitoneal, 6
  intrapulmonary, 133
  irregular, 4, 214-218
  during laparoscopy, 231-232, *235*
  maternal drugs and, 133
  neonatal, 132-133
  peptic ulcer and, 14
  postoperative, 231, 239-240
  postpartum, 91
  in septic shock, *178*, 179
  third-trimester, 84-91, 130
  urinary, *71, 178*
  uterine, 117
  uterine rupture and, 96, 98, 167
  vaginal, 59, 60, 63, 85, 88, 97, 156, 157, 168
Blood, *22*
  ABO incompatibility, 134-135
  atypical antibodies, 158
  complement, 134, 186, 188
  component therapy, 116
  loss, 11, 20, 31, 84, 85, 89, 97, 98, 100, 127, *128, 136,* 138, 152, 156, 158, 180, 208, 226
  loss, fetal, 130, 137
  placental, heparinized, 153
  replacement, 2, 11, 14, 42, 87, 104, 105, 154, *206,* 216, 240
  septicemia, *73,* 183, 184, 186, 226, 227, 229
  in stool, 13
  uremia, 27, *72, 75*
  vomiting, 14
  whole, 116-117, 185, 187, 226, 228
Blood flow/circulation
  enhancing, 36
  peripheral reduced, 152
  renal, 100

in shock, 100-101
uterine, 20, 78, 123, 263, 270-272
venous return, 20, 101, 183, 207, 263, 270
Blood gases, 41, 49, 105, 149, 180, 186, *187,* 208, *210,* 212, 262
Blood pressure, *28, 66, 68,* 82, 84, 152, 159, 179, 183, 185, 205, 208, *251,* 263, 269. *See also* Pressure
  in eclampsia, *79,* 80, 82-83
  in pregnancy, 19, 20
  pulmonary, 183, 207
  in shock, 101, *102*
  in vasovagal syncope, 198, 199, *200*
  venous, 19. *See also* Central venous pressure
Blood studies, 20, *70, 71, 72, 73, 74, 75,* 192. *See also* Partial thromboplastin time; Prothrombin time; Thrombin time
  in abruptio placentae, 89
  blood urea nitrogen, 180
  coagulation, 41
  complete blood count, 60
  cultures, 172, 173, *180,* 181, 228
  diabetic ketoacidosis, 49
  eclampsia, 82
  hematocrit, 11, 19, *28, 66,* 76, 79, 82, 89, 129, *136,* 137, 138, *159,* 160, 180, 226, 228
  hemorrhagic shock, 105
  in preeclampsia, 76
  ruptured abscess, 226-228
  septic shock, 180
  serum glutamic-oxaloacetic transaminase, *67,* 73, 76
  whole blood clotting time, *211*
Blood transfusion, 85, 91, 97, 104, *212,* 221, 238
  exchange, 31, 35, 42, 136, 154, 272
  fetofetal, 127, *128,* 133, 152
  fetomaternal, 152
  incompatible, *114*
  intrauterine, 129, 135
  massive, 97, *114,* 116
  partial exchange, 37, *38,* 39-40, 41
Blood volume
  diastolic, 269
  fetal, 130
  increase, 19, 36, 65, 205, 269
  intravascular, 61, 152, 185, *187*
  maintenance, 20
  neonatal, 131, 152
  in pregnancy, 19, 205
  reduction, 20, 47, 79, 83
  replacement, 152
  restoration, *103,* 104, 185
Bradycardia
  anesthesia and, 234, 263, 270

in cardiovascular toxicity, 269
in concealed hemorrhage, 97
following myocardial infarction, 203
postpartum, 97, 151
in vasovagal syncope, 201, 202, 268
Bradycardia, fetal, 120-126
anesthesia and, 126, 271-272
assessment, 122, 124, 125
causes, 271

C

Calcium, 81, 109
administration, 27, 82
hypercalcemia, 251
hypocalcemia, 16
Cancer
adenocarcinoma, 217
carcinoma, 219, 226, 246
cervix, 84, 85, 220, 223
choriocarcinoma, 212, 219, 223
laparoscopy and, 240-241
leukemia, 72, 138, 177, 219
stomach, 15
vagina, 219, 223
wound dehiscence and, 243
Cardiac arrest, 53, 81, 158, 263
Cardiac output
assessment, 183
decreased, 177, 179, 263, 269
dialysis and, 28, 29
increased, 185, 186, 203, 205, 207, 208, 263
maintenance, 41, 101
in pregnancy, 205, 207
in vasovagal syncope, 198, 199, 200
Cardiopulmonary resuscitation, 20, 199,
    200-203, 270
Cardiopulmonary system
failure, 101
intrapulmonary shunting, 211, 261
Cardiorespiratory system
collapse, 203
complications, 205-212
complications, management, 206
illness, 192
in pregnancy, 205-207
Cardiovascular system
collapse, 249, 261, 270
depression, 263, 264, 272
evaluation, 182-185
support, 263
toxicity, 269-270
Catecholamines, 45, 46, 53, 68, 100
Central nervous system
depression, 263, 269, 272
disturbances, 190, 194
excitement, 270
failure, 101
toxicity, 269

Central venous pressure, 28, 105
monitoring, 11, 20, 90, 103, 104, 117,
    184-185, 212, 229
in pregnancy, 19
Cerclage, cervical, 58, 60, 62-63
Cerebrospinal fluid, 52, 75, 76, 262
Cerebrovascular accident, 75, 80
Cervical dilation, preterm, 56-63
Cervix
cancer, 84, 85, 220, 223
cervicitis, 84, 85
cone biopsy, 59, 220
Dührssen's incisions, 59
ectopic pregnancy and, 2, 3
effacement, 56, 59-60
hemorrhage, 220
incompetence, 56-59, 62
insufficiency, 61
laceration, 58, 59, 96, 156, 160, 163, 167
neural pathways, 266
nondilated, 90, 123
trauma, 84, 85
tumor, 219
unfavorable, 83
Cesarean section, 76, 93, 105, 167, 168, 178
in abruptio placentae, 88-90
in adrenal crisis, 250, 251, 252
and anemia, 128
anesthesia in, 41
blood loss in, 130, 156
complications, 86-87
dangers, 130-131
history of, 85, 95, 97
indications for, 83, 98, 106, 123, 146-147
in intestinal surgery, 13
in peptic ulcer perforation, 15
in placenta previa, 86
postmortem, 22
and postpartum endometritis, 170, 171
and uterine atony, 157
and uterine rupture, 95, 97
Chemotherapy, 219, 221, 223
Chlamydia, 171
Cholecystitis, 13-16, 34, 61, 179
Chorioamnionitis, 25, 26, 60, 61, 63, 157,
    160
Clostridium, 135, 171, 172, 184
Coagulation
inhibition, 112, 113
labor and, 114
laparoscopy and, 238
normal physiology, 108-113
pregnancy and, 113-114
procoagulants. See Coagulation factors
tests, 112-113
Coagulation factors (procoagulants), 27,
    104, 105, 108, 109, 111, 113, 115-
    117, 158, 215, 221

Coagulopathy, 104, 108-118
abruptio placentae, 89-91
clinical conditions with, *114*, 117-118
disseminated intravascular coagulation, 115-116
excess clotting, 116
hemorrhagic shock, 105
postpartum hemorrhage and, 158, 160
renal failure and, 25
with shock, *114*, 179, 187
therapy, 91, 116-117, 187, *212*
Colloid osmotic pressure (COP), 207, 208
Colloids, 11, *103*, 104, 151, 185
Coma, *75*, 191-194
Computed tomography (CT) scan, 75, 174, 182, 193, 194
Congestive heart failure, 37, 42, 127, 153, 154, 186, *187*, 205, 208
Constipation, 12
Convulsions, 75. *See also* Seizures
clonic, 269
in CNS toxicity, 269
eclamptic, 78, *79*, 80, 82, 190-191
epileptic, 190, 191
fetal, 272
infection and, 191
ischemic disorders, 193
in paracervical block, 270, 272
postpartum, 191
tonic-clonic, 190, 269
treatment, 191
Coombs test, *68*, 137, 138, 139
Corticotropin-releasing hormone, 249
Cortisol, 45, 249, 252, 253
Cough, *178*, 242, 243, 246, 262
Creatinine clearance, *68, 71*, 76, 82, 180, 227
Crystalloids, 11, 14, 20, 61, 89, *103*, 104, 185, 270
Culdocentesis
ectopic pregnancy, 6, 238
intraperitoneal hemorrhage, 6, 21
ruptured abscess, 11, 227
Curettage, 157, 158, *159*, 218. *See also* Dilation and curettage
suction, 59, 226
uterine perforation and, 226
uterine rupture and, 95
Cyanosis, 80, *102*, 138, *178*, 179, 261, 272

D
Defibrillation, 202, *206*, 210, 268, *269*, 270
Dehiscence, 168, 242-247
Dehydration
diabetic ketoacidosis and, 44-46, 51, 54
in ruptured pelvic abscess, 226
and sickle cell crisis, 31, 35, 36

Delivery, 117
in abruptio placentae, 88-90
and adrenal crisis, 248, 250, *251*
blood loss in, 127
cesarean. *See* Cesarean section
coagulopathy, 118
delaying, 85, 86, 270
early, 63, 76, *81*, 105, 123, 152
in eclampsia, *81*, 83
in hemorrhagic shock, *103*
hydropic infant, 154
indications for, 27, 123, 126, 131, 270, 272
postpartum endometritis and, 170-171
in preeclampsia-eclampsia, 118
second-trimester, 59
in sickle cell crisis, 41-42
symphysiotomy, 146
trauma during, 132-133, 156-157, 163-169
uterine rupture in, 96
Diabetes, *71, 132*, 147, 177, 191, 226
Diabetic ketoacidosis, 16, 44-54, 179
Dialysis, renal, 25, 27-28, *29*, 65
Diethylstilbestrol, 59, 219
Digitalization, *103*, 105, 186, *187*, 207, 210
Dilation and curettage, 6, 59, 216, 217, 221, 223, 239
Disseminated intravascular coagulation, 25, *26*, 70-72, 80, 101, 115-116, 118
diagnosis, 27, 61, 69, 180
laboratory findings, *115*
Diuresis
neonatal, 272
osmotic, 45-47
Diuretics
in adult respiratory distress syndrome, *206*, 211
in molar pregnancy, 212
in renal failure, 26
Drain, drainage
abscess, 11, 183, 224
bladder, 165
"dog-ear," 11
hematoma, 165
intra-abdominal, 240
serosanguinous, 242
suction, 233
surgical wound, 242, 246
Drug abuse, 32, *34*, 36, 191, 193
Dual pregnancy, 6
Dyspnea, 61, *178*, 179, 207, 261

E
Eclampsia, 75, 76, 78-83, 190, 211. *See also* Preeclampsia-eclampsia
delivery, 83
diagnosis, 79-80

pulmonary edema and, 207
treatment, 80-83
Ectopic pregnancy, 2-7, *34*
  causes, 3-4, 236-237
  diagnosis, 4-6, 231, 237-239
  emergency laparoscopy and, 231, 237-239
  infected, 225
  and laparoscopy complications, 231, 236-237
  recurrence, 7
  ruptured, 100, 106
  sites/frequency, 2, *3*
  surgery, 6-7, 106
Edema, 8, 14, *28*, 135, 165, *181*, 193, 205, 227. See also Hydrops fetalis
  cerebral, 50-52, 80
  in preeclampsia-eclampsia, 65, 73, 78, 190
  pulmonary, 61, 80, *178*, 179, 182, 185, 188, 190, *206*, 207-208, 211, 261
Electrocardiogram/graphy, *180*, 182, *199*, 200, 202, 204, 206, 208-209, *251*, 268,   269
Electrocoagulation, 231-233, 240
Electrolytes, 27, 49, *180*, *251*. See also Calcium; Potassium; Sodium
  bicarbonate, 46, 47, *51*, 52-53, 180
  depletion, 47
  disturbances, 191
  magnesium, 80-82
  monitoring, 82, 208
  in pancreatitis, 16
Embolus/ism
  amniotic fluid, 25, *26*, *114*, 158, 211, *212*
  gas, 234
  intracranial, 192
  pulmonary, *34*, 42, 179, 182, 207, 210, *211*
  and renal failure, 25, *26*
Embolization, 106, *159*, 160, 188, *211*, 220
Endomyometritis, 34, 41, 42, 170, 178, 179
β-Endorphin, 188
Enterobacter, 171, 177
Enterobacteriaceae, 188
Enzymes
  amylase, serum, 16, *22*, 227
  diastase, 16
  liver, 74
  proteolytic, and pancreatitis, 15
EPH gestosis. See Preeclampsia; Preeclampsia-eclampsia
Episiotomy, 41, 91, 142, 147, 163, 164
Erythroblastosis fetalis, 40, 129, 133, 139
Erythrocytes
  abnormal, 135
  hemolysis. See Erythroblastosis fetalis; Hemolysis
  in injury, *22*
  megaloblastic crises, 33
  packed, 37, *116*, 185, 211, 228
  reticulocytopenia, 33
  schistocytes, 69, *73*
  in sickle cell crisis, 33
  in sickle cell disease, *32*
  spherocytosis, 33, 135, 139
  transfer, in Rh isoimmunization, 133
  in urine, *68*
  values during gestation, *137*
Escherichia coli, 11, 34, 171, 177
Estrogen, endogenous, 215, 217, 218
Estrogens, exogenous
  in anovulatory bleeding, 216-218
  conjugated, 217, 218
  and gallstones, 13
Evisceration, 179, 242-247

F
Fallopian tube
  ectopic pregnancy and, 2, 3, 6
  occlusion, 3
  surgery, 6-7, 11
Fasting
  and adrenal crisis, 249
  and diabetic ketoacidosis, 44, 45, 54
Fetal distress, *61*, 63, *89*, 120, 123, 128, 133, 271, 272
Fetal heart block, 126
Fetal heart rate, 85
  anemia and, 127, 129, *139*
  decrease, 120, 151
  early decelerations, 120, *121*
  flat, 126
  late decelerations, 120, 121, 123, 127, 129, 272
  monitoring. See FHR monitoring
  in uterine rupture, 168
  variability, 120, 121, 123
  variable decelerations, 120, 121, 123, 272
Fetal/neonatal anemia, 127, *128*, 129-135, *136*, 137-139
Fetal scalp blood sampling, 41, 120, 121, *122*, 123, 127, 129, 133, 139, 272
Fetus
  condition, 60, 85, 130
  death, 9, 12, 25, 44, 53, 63, 69, *73*, 78, 80, 88, *114*, 118, 133, 272
  electronic monitoring, 60, 61, 123, 127, 131, 139, 171
  heart tones, 96
  ketoacidosis and, 53
  local anesthetic injection, 266, 272
Fever, 54, 60, 174, 179, 192, 193, 227, 241
  adrenal insufficiency, 249
  appendicitis, 9

hemoperitoneum and, 227
after laparoscopy, 235
ovarian vein syndrome, 175
pancreatitis, 16
postpartum endometritis, 170, 173
pyelonephritis, 9
ruptured abscess, 11, 225, 226, 229
salpingitis, 9
sickle cell crisis, 31, 36
FHR monitoring, 120, 121, *122, 124, 125,*
272
in diabetic ketoacidosis, 49
in sickle cell disease, 37, 41
Fibrillation
atrial, 210
ventricular, 202, *206,* 210, 268
Fibrin, *110,* 111, 115, 180
Fibrinogen, 61, 69, 80, 91, 109, 113, 115-
117, 180
Fibrinolytic system, *111,* 112-115
Fluid, 49, 101, 205, *206,* 211, 262
administration, 2, 16, 20, 27, 36, 42, 50-
51, 54, *79,* 89, 97, 101, 185, 207, 211,
224, 228, 240, 250, 251
assessment, 27, *28*
intestinal, 9, 12, 13, 15
overload, 65, 186, 212
peritoneal cavity, 8
water, 45, 251
Folate, 33
Fracture, pelvic, 21
Fundal height, 60, 84, 97

G
Gallbladder, 14
bile salts, 13, 15
bile stasis, 13
cholangitis, 179
disease, 15
duct obstruction, 13
gallstones, 13, 15, *34*
infection and, 13
Gastrointestinal tract. *See also* Intestines;
Stomach
hemorrhage, 76
transit time, 19, 20
Gelatin foam, 106, *159,* 160, 220, 240
Gestational age
determining, 59, 60
error in, 56, *57*
Glomerular filtration rate, 24, 45, 79
Glucagon, 45, 46
Glucose, 28, 46, 47, 51, 52
blood levels, 45, 50, 53, 54, 61
hyperglycemia, 46, 47, 49-54, 61
hypoglycemia, 50, 51, *75,* 153, 263
in urine, 46, 49, 54, 226
Gonococcus, 3, 11

H
Head compression, fetal, 120, *121*
Heart
asystole, 202, 269, 270
damage, 207
defects, congenital, 208
disease, rheumatic, 210
external compression, 201, *202,* 268,
269, 270
intracardiac shunt, reversal of, *206,* 207
mitral valve disease, 207
mitral valve prolapse, 192
problems in pregnancy, 207-210
rate, 185, 188, 205, 263
ventricular ectopic beats, *206*
Heart failure, 76, 207, 208, 210
HELLP (hemolysis, elevated liver
enzymes, low platelet count)
syndrome, 74, 115
Hematoma, 65, 72, 74, *128, 132,* 165, *167,*
168
prevention, 246
wound dehiscence and, 242-243
Hemoglobin
fetal, 130, 137, 152
hemoglobinopathies, 31-42, *128,* 129
Hemolysis, *26,* 74, 133-137, 171
Hemolytic uremic syndrome, 65, 69, *73,*
135
Hemorrhage, 34, 245. *See also* Bleeding
in abruptio placentae, 90
and Addison's disease, 248
anovulatory, 217
antepartum, 106
cerebral, 80, *192*
cervical, 220
delayed, 220
diathesis, 221, 223
in ectopic pregnancy, 2
endometrial, 221
fetal, *128,* 130, 133
gastrointestinal, 76
intracerebral, *75*
intracranial, 133, *192*
intraperitoneal, 21
intraventricular, 76
in leukemia, 223
in placenta previa, 85, 87
postexenteration, 220-223
postoperative, 220
postpartum. *See* Postpartum hemorrhage
renal failure, 25, *26*
in septic shock, *178,* 179
subarachnoid, *75*
in trauma, 19, 21
uterine, 219, 221
in uterine rupture, 98
vaginal, 219-223

Hemorrhagic shock, 100-102, *103*, 104-106, 177, 207
Heparin, 25, 27, 70, 105, 174
  coagulopathy, in, 118, 187
  endogenous, 111
  neutralization, 111
  pulmonary embolus, in, *211*
  resistance, 113
Hormones. *See* specific hormones
Hydration, 11, 36, 42, 60, 83
Hydrops fetalis, 127-129, *132*, 133, 136, *139*, 153-154
Hypertension, 65, 69, 74-76, 159, 188, 192
  abruptio placentae, 88, 148
  acute, pathophysiology of, 78-79
  differential diagnosis, 67-68
  in eclampsia-preeclampsia, 65, 67, 73, 78, 80, 148, 190
  essential, 67, *68*
  heart failure, 208
  hydropic fetus and, 127
  intracranial hemorrhage and, 193
  pregnancy-induced, 19, 36. *See also* Preeclampsia; Preeclampsia-eclampsia
  preterm labor and, 59
  renal function, 24, 27
Hyperventilation, 47, 180, *201*, 202, 203
Hypervolemia, 20, *227*
Hypotension, 61, 159, 188, 203, 208, 234-235, 270
  in abruptio placentae, 88
  with abscess, 226
  adrenal insufficiency and, 250, 251
  in anesthesia, 123, 263, 270
  in anesthetic toxicity, 263
  in asphyxia, 152, 153
  in concealed hemorrhage, 97
  in convulsion, 191
  in diabetic ketoacidosis, 51
  in hemorrhage, 84, *102*
  intestinal obstruction and, 12
  in labor, 210
  in pelvic abscess, *227*
  peptic ulcer perforation and, 15
  in septic shock, *178*
  in uterine rupture, 96
  in vasovagal syncope, 268
  volume depletion, 47
Hypovolemia, 100
  in anemia, 70
  in diabetic ketoacidosis, 51
  postpartum, 163
  in preeclampsia-eclampsia, 74, 76
  in renal failure, 27
Hypovolemic shock, 18, 20, 89, *114*, 153, 156, 157, 238, 249

Hypoxemia, 37, 208, 210-212, 261
  fetal, 120, 148, 153
Hypoxia, 12, 101
  cerebral, 192
  in convulsion, 191
  fetal, 88, 120, 136, 266, 271
  neonatal, 141
  in shock, 177, 186
Hysterectomy
  and abscesses, 225
  adrenal insufficiency and, 252
  bleeding control, 87, 91, *103*, 157, *159*, 161
  hemorrhage in, 220
  ruptured abscess, 229, 230
  ruptured uterus, 93, 97, 98, 106, 169
  sterilization, 237
  vaginal, bleeding in, 240
Hysterosalpingography, 63, 218
Hysterotomy, 95, 97

I
Idiopathic thrombocytopenic purpura, 69, 72, 158
Immunosuppressed patients, 177, 181, 184, 187
Infection, 3, 8, *73*, 74, 171, 172, 245, 262
  intra-amniotic, 179
  intraperitoneal, 235
  and hemolysis, 135
  packing and, 221
  pancreatitis, 15
  pelvic, 183, 224, 225
  TORCH, *74*
  treatment, 183-184
Injury. *See also* Trauma
  abdominal, 20, 231, 239
  accidental, 18-22
  penetrating, 231-233, *235*
  thermal, 231, 233-234, *235*
  urinary tract, 231, *235*, 236
Insulin, 44-46, 53
  administration, 49-50, 53, 54
  deficiency, 44-46, 54
  in hyperkalemia, 27
  regular, 49, 50, 54
  resistance, 45, 49, 50, 53
  treatment, 49-50, *51*, 52
Intestinal obstruction, 9, 12-14, 16, *34*, *178*, 182, 227, 243,
Intestines
  air in, 9, 12, 13
  bowel function, loss of, 268
  burn, 231, 233-234, *235*, 236
  diverticulitis, 179
  diverticulum, 226
  enterocolitis, 148
  fecalith, 8

inflammation, 227
inflammatory bowel disease, 179, 226
ischemic disease, 15
pancreatitis, 16
perforation, *178*, 179, 182, 229, 232-233, 236
tumor, 219
volvulus, 12, 13
Intracranial disorders, 192-194
Intrauterine growth retardation, 69, 76, 118, 127, 133, *139*
Intubation, 104, 154, *210*, 263, 270
endotracheal, *103*, 151-153, 191, 256-259, 261
equipment, 257-258
nasogastric, 20, 82, 233, 260
oral, 260
procedure, 258-259
IUDs
abscesses and, 225
ectopic pregnancy and, 4
uterine perforation and, 239

J
Jaundice, 13, 25, 65, *74*, *138*, 139, 171, *178*, 179

K
Kernicterus, 128, 134, 148
Ketones, 45-48, 53, 54
Kidneys, 188
abscess, 27, *178*, 182
biopsy, *70*
disease, 16, 24-26, 59, 65, 67, *68*, *70*, *71*, 80, 264
drugs and, 10, 186
dysfunction, 10, 24, 79
failure. *See* Renal failure
function, 227
hydronephrosis, 19
infection, 27
ischemic damage, 25
lesion, 24, 79
necrosis, 24, 25, 29, *70*, 89, 100
nephrotic syndrome, *68*, 69, *71*, 171
pregnancy and, 24
prerenal azotemia, 227
prerenal disease, 26, 27
septic shock, in, 180
Klebsiella, 11, 171, 177
Kleihauer-Betke test, 130, 132

L
Labor
abnormal progress, 147
acceleration, 58
blood loss in, 127, 130-131
contraindications, 168

improper management, 157
inhibition, drug, 57-58, 61, 62
neglected, 95
postpartum endometritis and, 171
precipitous, 156, *157*
premature, 9, 12, 53, 56-59, 61, 62, *74*, 86, 207, 208
prolonged, *157*, 171
regurgitation and, 261
sickle cell crisis in, 40-42
trial of, 97, *98*
uterine rupture during, 96, 97
Laparoscopy
complications, 231-237
contraindications, 238
diagnostic, 6
repeat, 235
uses, 231, 237-241
Laparotomy, 10, 16, 91, 98, 158, 222, 229, 238
diagnostic, 8, 165
emergency, 6, 168, 233
exploratory, 6, 232, 236, 239
hematomas, 165
indications for, 6
mini-, 239
Laryngoscopy, 153, 258
Lavage
abdominal, 236
gastric, neonatal, 272
isotonic saline, 14
peptic ulcer, 14
peritoneal, 21, *22*, 232
in pulmonary aspiration, 262
Leukocytes, 60, 240
aggregation, 186
in amniotic fluid, 60
in appendicitis, 8, 9
coagulation and, 115
elevated, 241
karyotyping, 63
leukocytosis, 180, 226, 227
leukopenia, 226
low, 180
in pregnancy, 9, 19
in sickle cell crisis, 35
transfusion, 187
in trauma, 19, *22*
Ligation, 87, 91, 98, 220, 232, *233*
hypogastric artery, *103*, 106, 157, *159*, 161, 220, 221
internal iliac artery, 106
ovarian artery, 106, *159*, 161
uterine artery, *159*, 161
Liver
biopsy, 240
coagulation factors in, 112, 115
congestion, 179

disease, 66, 72-74, *75*, 214, 264
dysfunction, 67, 72, 73, *74*, *178*
enzymes, elevated, 74
failure, 101, 191
fatty, 25, *26*, *74*
glycogenolysis, 53
hematoma, 65, 74
hepatitis, 65, 69, *73*, *74*, 91, 117, 227
hepatomegaly, 153, *178*
periportal necrosis, 80
in pregnancy, 19
rupture, 19, 74
Lochia, 170, 171, 175
Loss of consciousness, 203
in eclampsia, 190
in hyperventilation, 203
in vasovagal syncope, 199, *201*, 268
Lungs, 188
alveolar collapse, 261
alveolar filling pattern, *28*
consolidation, 179
edema, 61, 80, *178*, 179, 182, 185, 188,
190, *206*, 207-208, 211, 261
effusions, 16, *28*, 212, 227
hemorrhage, *178*
infiltrates, 207, 211, 212, 227
rales, *28*, 207
venous pattern, *28*
vital capacity, 208
volumes, increasing, 211

M
Magnesium sulfate, 62
convulsions, therapy for, 80-83, 191
prophylactic, 156
Mannitol, 26, 52
Mass(es)
abdominal, 175
adnexal, 4, 6
in cholecystitis, 14
ovarian cysts, 10
pelvic, 179, 226, 227
in uterine laceration, 167
vaginal, 221
Meconium, 83, 120, 121, 123, 149, 171
Membranes
evaluation, 60
postpartum endometritis and, 170, 171
premature rupture, 57
prolonged rupture, 170, 171
ruptured, *61*, 63, 106
Menstrual cycle, 11, 215
Microangiopathic hemolytic anemia. *See
under* Anemia
Molar pregnancy, 212, 219, 220
Mucus, 8, 13, 14
Muscle relaxants, 264
Mycoplasma, 34, 171

Myocardial contractility, 51, 185, 269
Myocardial infarction, 127, 202, 203, 208-
209

N
Narcotics, 14, 36, 83, 105, 261
Nausea
in Addison's disease, 248
in adrenal insufficiency, 249
in appendicitis, 9
in cholecystitis, 14
in diabetic ketoacidosis, 47
in ischemic vascular disorders, 193
in pregnancy, 190
in pyelonephritis, 9
in ruptured abscess, 225
in salpingitis, 9
in shock, 15, *178*, 179
Neonatal distress
cardiac massage, 151
cardiovascular collapse, 152-153
drugs, 151
equipment, resuscitation, 148-149
hydrops fetalis. *See* Hydrops fetalis
meconium aspiration, 153
perinatal asphyxia, 148-152
resuscitation procedures, 149-152
Neoplasms, 12, 192, 216

O
Obesity, 68
airway obstruction in, 256-257
anovulatory bleeding and, 214
dialysis and, 28, *29*
postpartum endometritis and, 171
regurgitation and, 261
shoulder dystocia and, 147
wound dehiscence and, 243, 246
Oral contraceptives, 58-59, 192, 215, 223
in anovulatory bleeding, 216-218
ectopic pregnancy and, 4
Ovarian vein syndrome, 172, 175
Ovary
biopsy, 236
cancer, 240
cysts, 10, *34*, 215, 240, 241
ectopic pregnancy and, 2, *3*
surgery, 10, 11
torsion, 10, *34*, 231, 240
tumor, 219
XO streak, 236
Ovulation, 59, 217
Oxygen. *See also* Hypoxemia; Hypoxia
in anesthetic toxicity, 203, 264
bradycardia, prolonged, 126
consumption, myocardial, 185
in convulsion, 191
depressed neonate, 150, 151

in diabetic ketoacidosis, 46, 53
in eclampsia, 82
in hemorrhagic shock, 103-104
in intubation, 258, 262
in molar pregnancy, 212
in myocardial infarction, 209
in ominous decelerations, 123
placental, 148
in pulmonary edema, 207
in pulmonary embolus, *211*
in ruptured abscess, 229
in septic shock, 186, *187*
in sickle cell crisis, 37, 41
in vasovagal syncope, *202*
in ventilation, *206, 210, 212*, 259, 260,
  263, *269*
Oxygenation, 148, 185, 211. See *also*
  Hypoxemia
Oxytocics, 41, 91, 105, 117, 159, 220
Oxytocin, 83, 90, 91, 97, 105, 123, 158-159

P
Pain
  abdominal, 12, 14, 96, 97, 175
  in abruptio placentae, 88
  adnexal, 240
  in adrenal insufficiency, 249
  in appendicitis, 8, 9
  chest, 61, 208
  in cholecystitis, 13
  convulsions, preceding, 190
  in ectopic pregnancy, 4, 5, 6, 237
  epigastric, 190
  in hemoperitoneum, 227
  in intestinal obstruction, 12
  lacerations, 165
  in myocardial infarction, 208
  neck, 194
  in ovarian vein syndrome, 175
  in pancreatitis, 16
  pelvic, 237
  in peptic ulcer, 14, 15
  postoperative, 231, 235
  in preeclampsia-eclampsia, 79
  in pyelonephritis, 9
  right upper quadrant, *67, 73, 74*
  in ruptured abscess, 225
  in salpingitis, 11
  in sickle cell crisis, 33
  in third-trimester bleeding, 84
  in tubo-ovarian abscess, 11
  in urolithiasis, 10
  in uterine rupture, 96, 168
  in wound dehiscence, 242
Pancreatitis, 15-16, *34*, 61, 179, 226, 227
Paracentesis, 21, 154, 165
Paracervical block, 126, 266-272
Parenteral hyperalimentation, 177, 181, 184

Partial thromboplastin time, 27, *112, 115*,
  180, 211
Pelvic inflammatory disease, 3, 11, 225,
  241
Peptic ulcer disease, 14-15
Perineum, lacerations of, 163-165, *166*
Peritoneal cavity, 224, 225
  ectopic pregnancy and, 2
  fluid in, 8
  lavage, 232
  peptic ulcer perforation, 14
  tubo-ovarian abscess rupture, 11
Peritoneum, 245
  abscess, 61
  irritation, 9
  hemo-, 6, 227
  pneumo-, 15, 232
  uro-, 236
Peritonitis, 8, 9, 61
  acute, 10
  with cholecystitis, 14
  ovarian cyst and, 10
  in peptic ulcer perforation, 15
  with ruptured abscess, 225-227, 229
  subacute granulomatous, 10
  septic shock, in, *178, 179*
  tubo-ovarian abscess, ruptured, 11
pH, 41, 129
  aspirate, 261
  blood, 53, 180
  cerebrospinal fluid, 53
  in diabetic ketoacidosis, 47, 53
  fetal scalp blood, *122*, 123
  membranes, 60
  in perinatal asphyxia, 148
Phosphorus depletion, 46
Physical examination, *20*, 59-60
  digital, 85
  hemorrhage, in, 106
  pelvic, 172
  speculum, 85, 106
Placenta, 134, 138, 205
  abruption. See Abruptio placentae
  accreta, 87, *114*, 157, 158
  blood samples, 129
  circumvallate, 84, *85*
  drugs crossing, 82
  enlargement, 135
  fragments, retained, 157, 158, *159*
  fundus, implanted in, 157
  hypoperfusion, 88
  increta-percreta, 95
  insufficiency, 118, 148
  premature separation, 20
  previa. See Placenta previa
  uterine atony and, *157*
Placenta previa, 25, *26*, 84-87, 157
  anemia and, *128*

blood loss and, 100
cesarean delivery, 86-87
diagnosis, 85-86
fetal bleeding in, 131
hemorrhagic shock, 105
management, 86-87
risk factors, 85
uterine atony and, 157
vaginal delivery, 87
Plasma, 11
fresh frozen, 36, 91, 104, 116, 117, 187, 212
volume, 65, 67, 70, 117, 180, 185. See also Hypervolemia; Hypovolemia
Platelets
adhesions, 69
administration, 91, 104, 187
aggregation, 71, 108-111, 188
in coagulation, 109-112
concentrate, 116
count, 27, 41, 61, 66, 112-114, 117, 118, 222, 226
decreased, 69, 74, 115, 116, 180, 223
function, 76, 112, 116
in pregnancy, 113
in sickle cell crisis, 35
transfusion, 221
Pneumococcus, 34
Pneumocystis, 184
Pneumonia, 16, 34, 153, 261
Polydipsia, 47, 53
Polyps, 216, 218
Positive pressure ventilation, 104, 150-151, 153, 207, 259, 262, 272
intermittent, 202, 206, 210, 212, 269
Postpartum endometritis, 170-175
Postpartum hemorrhage, 25, 26, 87, 91, 100, 105, 106, 142, 156-161, 163, 165
Potassium, 227
administration, 51, 52, 228
depletion, 53
hyperkalemia, 27, 46, 251
hypokalemia, 46, 50, 52, 61, 206, 207, 208, 228
Preeclampsia, 78, 79, 190, 193. See also Preeclampsia-eclampsia
EPH gestosis, 66-67, 71, 75
hypertension with, 148
molar pregnancy and, 212
pancreatitis and, 15
postpartum hemorrhage and, 156
pulmonary edema and, 207
renal failure and, 24, 25, 27
severe, 65-77, 211
type A EPH gestosis, 66, 68
type B EPH gestosis, 65, 66, 69, 73, 74, 76, 77
uterine atony and, 157

Preeclampsia-eclampsia, 74
airway and, 256
coagulopathy and, 114, 115, 118
renal failure and, 24, 26
Premature ventricular contractions, 210
Prematurity, 83, 85, 86, 88, 131, 272
Presentation, fetal, 83-85, 133
Pressure
arterial oxygen, 37, 41, 121, 148, 180, 261, 262
carbon dioxide, 180
intragastric, 261
perfusion, 185
positive end expiratory, 206, 211, 262
pulmonary artery wedge, 185
pulmonary capillary wedge, 208, 211
Progesterone, 13, 14, 19, 215
Progestin, 215-218
Prostaglandin
analogs, 91, 159, 160
endotoxin and, 188
metabolism, abnormalities, 25
in postpartum hemorrhage, 106
uterine contractions and, 91, 117-118
Protein, 70, 154
Proteinuria, 24, 76
differential diagnosis, 68-69, 70-71
in pancreatitis, 16
in preeclampsia-eclampsia, 65, 73, 75, 78-80, 190
Proteus, 11, 171, 177
Prothrombin, 109
Prothrombin time, 27, 112, 115, 180
Pseudomonas, 177, 184, 187
Pulse
in assessment, 200, 202
fluid status and, 28
in neonatal distress, 151, 152
in peptic ulcer perforation, 15
in pregnancy, 18
in third-trimester bleeding, 84
in vasovagal syncope, 198-201, 202, 268, 269
Pyelonephritis, 9-10, 25, 26, 34, 53, 59, 71, 178, 179

R
Radiation, 220, 221, 243
Red blood cells. See Erythrocytes
Reflexes, 62, 79, 81, 82
Renal failure, 16, 74, 192
acute, 24-29, 100, 171
associated conditions, 26
causes, 24-25
chronic, 24
coagulopathy and, 117
hemolysis, 171
hemorrhagic shock and, 100, 101

infection and, 25, *26*
nutrition, 28, 29
postpartum, 24, 25, *26, 73*
preeclampsia, 76
in septic shock, *178*
therapy, 26-29
Respiration, 203
artificial, 201, *202*, 268, *269*
assessment, 200, *202*
in diabetic ketoacidosis, 54
Kussmaul, 47
labored, 207
in peptic ulcer perforation, 15
shortness of breath, 205
in vasovagal syncope, *269*
Respiratory failure, 188
arrest, 263, 269, 270
in pancreatitis, 16
paralysis, 81
in septic shock, 180, 186, *187*
Respiratory system
depression, 191
infection, 37, 235
insufficiency, 212
in pregnancy, 206
Rh disease, 128, 153. *See also*
Erythroblastosis fetalis; Hemolysis;
Rh isoimmunization
problems, 129
incompatibility, 129, 133-135
Rh isoimmunization, 127, 131, 133
Ringer's lactate, 36, 39, *51*, 105, 123, 228,
263

S

Saline, 105
irrigation, 229, 240
isotonic, 14, 36, 228
lavage, 14
loading, 26
normal, 51, 53, 82, *159*, 185, 251, 263
Salmonella, 34
Salpingectomy, 6, 239
Salpingitis, 3, 9-11, 225, 226, 235, 237
Salpingostomy, 6
Secundines, *103*, 105, 106
Sedatives, 203, *211*, 212
Seizures, 67, 69, 75, 203. *See also*
Convulsions
anesthetics and, 263, 264
differential diagnosis, *75*
in eclampsia, 79, 80
mortality, 79
in neonatal distress, 152
in vasovagal syncope, 199, 268
Sensorium derangements, sudden, 190-194
Sepsis, 11, 14, 180, 188, 211
anemia and, *139*

with coagulopathy, *114*
with laparoscopy, 231, 235
puerperal, 25, *26*
shock and, 177-188
Septic shock, 177-188
clinical manifestations, *178, 179*
diagnosis, 179-183
incidence, 177
infection and, *178*, 179, 183-184, *187*
laboratory tests, *180*
pathogens, 177
risk factors, 177
surgery, 183, *187*
treatment, 183-188
Serratia, 177
Shock, *73*, 96, *139*, 154, 157, 229, 245. *See
also* Hemorrhagic shock;
Hypovolemic shock; Septic shock
in abruptio placentae, 88
acute blood loss and, 127, 130, *136*, 138,
152
in Addison's disease, 248
adrenal crisis and, 249
adult respiratory distress syndrome and,
211
asphyxial, 152
cardiogenic, 179
with coagulopathy, *114*, 179
in diabetic ketoacidosis, 51
in intestinal obstruction, 12
in intra-abdominal injury, 133
neonatal, 152, 153
in peptic ulcer perforation, 14-15
in tubo-ovarian abscess rupture, 11
in uterine rupture, 96, 98, 167, 168
Shock lung. *See* Adult respiratory distress
syndrome
Shoulder dystocia, 95, 96, 141-147
management, 142-146
"obstetric shoehorn," 143, *146*
Sickle cell anemia, 31, *71*, 129
Sickle cell crisis, 31-42
Sickle cell thalassemia, 31
Smead-Jones technique, *244-247*
Sodium, 79, 227
hyponatremia, 46, 51, 76
loss, 45, 46
replacement, 251
Sodium bicarbonate, 28, 49, 53, 105, 151
Spleen, 19, 33-35, *73*
Staphylococcus, 11, 184
Sterilization, *159*, 161, 236, 237
Steroids
in adrenal insufficiency, 248-249
in adult respiratory distress syndrome,
211
in aspiration therapy, 262
cortico-, 52, 53, 229, 248, 250

glucocorticoids, 130, 186, *187*, 248, *250*,
  251
hydrocortisone, 11, *210*, *212*, 251-253
  overtreatment, 252
  replacement, 251
  in shock, 105
  withdrawal syndrome, 252
  wound dehiscence and, 243
Stomach
  acid, 14
  distention, 232, 233, 259
  mucus, 14
  penetration, accidental, 232-233
  ulcer, 226, 253
Streptococcus, 11, 171-173, 175, 184
Stress, 203
  adrenal crisis and, 248, 249
  diabetic ketoacidosis and, 45, 49, 53
  hormones, 44-46, 54
  impaired responsiveness to, 250
  sepsis and, 188
  sickle cell crisis and, 32
  vasovagal syncope and, 198-199
Stroke, *75*, *192*
Suctioning, 82, 222
  endotracheal, 153, *210*, 261
  nasogastric, 14, 16, 82, 229
Surgery, 4, 12, 15, 28, *29*, 193, *211*, 229
  abscess, 11, 183, 224, *225*, 229, 230
  acute abdomen, 8
  adnexal, 235
  adrenal crisis and, 248-250, *251*, 252-253
  cholecystitis, 14
  closure, 243-244, *245*, *246*, *247*, 253
  complications, 207
  ectopic pregnancy, 6-7, 106
  electro-, 236
  exploratory, 222
  genital tract bleeding, 106
  infection and, 177-178
  intestinal obstruction, 13
  ovarian, 10
  postpartum hemorrhage, 106, 158, *159*,
    160-161
  septic shock and, 177-178, *187*
  sutures, 243-244, *245*, *246*, *247*, 253
  tubal, 237
  uterine, 95, 106
Systemic lupus erythematosus, 24, 67, *68*,
  71, *72*

T
Tachycardia, 60, 61
  anemia and, 127, 129, *139*
  in concealed hemorrhage, 97
  fetal, 60, 61, 120, 123
  in hemorrhage, 84, 101, 105
  in hypovolemic shock, 18

  in labor, 210
  management, 209
  in molar pregnancy syndrome, 212
  in pregnancy, 209
  pulmonary aspiration and, 261
  in septic pelvic thrombophlebitis, 174
  in septic shock, *178*, 179
  tubo-ovarian abscess, ruptured, 11
  in uterine rupture, 96, 168
  in vasovagal syncope, 268
  in volume depletion, 47
Tachypnea, *102*, *178*, 179, 207, 212, 226
Tamponade, 97, 179, 240
Temperature. See *also* Fever
  fluctuations, *178*, 179, 187
  low, 15, 42, 47, 179, 192, 226, *227*
  monitoring, 240
  restoration, *187*
  thermal homeostasis, 151
Tenderness, 5
  abdominal, 96
  in abruptio placentae, 60
  Alder's sign, 9
  in appendicitis, 9
  in cholecystitis, 13
  in chorioamnionitis, 60
  in ovarian cysts, 10
  in peptic ulcer perforation, 15
  rebound, 9
  in salpingitis, 9
  in tubo-ovarian abscess, ruptured, 11
  uterine, 60, 84, 88, 170
  in uterine rupture, 96, 168
α-Thalassemia, 128, 136
β-Thalassemia, 129, 136
Thrombi, 25, 111, *128*
Thrombin, 111, 116
Thrombin time, *180*
Thrombocytopenia, 65-67, 69-73, 76, 115,
  118, 226
Thrombophlebitis, *34*, 170, 172-174
Thromboplastin, 115
Thrombosis, *70*, *75*, 116, 192
Thrombotic thrombocytopenic purpura,
  65, 69, *73*, *75*, 158
Tracheostomy, *210*, 260
Tranquilizers, 203
Trauma
  abruptio placentae and, 87
  adult respiratory distress syndrome and,
    211
  cervical, 84, *85*
  coma and, 192
  during delivery (birth trauma), 132-133,
    141, 142, 156-157, 163-169
  genital tract, 156-158, 163-169
  intracranial, 191
  pancreatitis and, 15

postpartum endometritis and, 170
response to, 108
sickle cell crisis and, 31
soft tissue, 170
thrombocytopenia and, 71
uterine rupture and, 95, 96
vaginal, 84, *85*
vasovagal syncope and, 198
Triglycerides, blood, 46, *68*
Tumors, 13, *72*, 75, 84, *85*, *128*, 142, 177.
   See also Cancer
   brain, *193*
   cervix, 219 ·
   colon, 219
   convulsions and, 191
   endometrium, 219
   leiomyomas, *34*
   myomas, 218
   ovary, 219
   pheochromocytoma, 67, *68*
   sarcoma botryoides, 219
   vagina, 219-221
Twin-twin transfusion syndrome, 127,
   128, 133

U
Ulcer/ulceration, 8, 14, 15, 226, 253
Ultrasound, 61, *68*, *73*, 74, 85, 86, 131, 133,
   158, *183*
   abruptio placentae, 88
   abscess, 174, 182, 227
   anemia, diagnosing, 127, 129, 139
   ectopic pregnancy and, 5-6, 237
   hemorrhage and, 129, 133
   routine, 59, 60
Umbilical cord
   abnormalities, *128*, 130, 142
   blood gases, 149
   clamping, 131, 149
   compression, 120, *121*
   entanglement, 130
   hematoma, *128*
   rupture, *128*, 130
Ureter, 19, *180*, 182, 236
Uric acid, *68*, 76
Urinary tract
   damage, 231, *235*, 236
   infections, 9-10, *34*, 42, 60, *71*, 172,
      235
Urination, 9, 59, *201*
Urine, 171
   anuria, *102*, 179, 190
   bacilluria, 226
   bacteriuria, 10, 226
   dysuria, 9
   hematuria, 21, 98, 232
   oliguria, 65, 80, 82, 90, 138, 179, 180,
      190

output, 11, 12, 21, 45, 81, 89, *102*, 105,
   116, 117, 185, 208, 228, *251*
polyuria, 47, 53
pyuria, 10, 226
sugar, 46, 49, 54, 226
urolithiasis, 10
Urine tests, 60, *70*, *71*, *73*, 82, 237
cultures, *180*, 181
electrolytes, *180*
pregnancy, 59
specific gravity, 11, *180*
urinalysis, 60, *70*, 82, 192, 226
urogram, *180*
urography, 182
Uterine contractions, 56, 57, 59, 60, 84, 85,
   87, 91, 163, 168
Braxton-Hicks, 57, 61
cessation of, 96, 168
fetal heart rate and, 120
frequent, 123
lack of, 158
suppression of, 53
Uterine rupture, *34*, 58, 89, 93-98, 158, 163,
   167-169
antepartum, 168
blood loss and, 100
categories, 93, *94*, 95, 168
causes, 95
coagulopathy, with, *114*
diagnosis, 90, 96-97
during delivery, 96
incidence, 93, *94*, 157
management, 97-98
postpartum, 168
signs, 167, 168
surgery, 106
suspected, 97-98
Uteroplacental insufficiency, 120, *121*, 272
Uterus, 9, 12, 13, 20, 59, 170
abnormalities, 59
activity, 82, 90, 272
atony, 89, 91, 105, 142, 156-160, *212*
bleeding, 117
blood flow, reduced, 20, 78
carcinoma, 219
compression, *212*
Couvelaire, 89, 117
decompression, 87
evacuation, 220
hemorrhage, 219, 221
hypertonic, 89
infection, 226. *See also* Endometritis
inversion, 157, 160
manual exploration, 157-158, *159*
massage, 91, *159*, 160, 163
neural pathways, 266
overdistended, *157*
packing, *159*, 160, 221

perforation, 95, 226, 231, 239
rupture. *See* Uterine rupture
scars, 93, *94*, 95-97
surgery, 11, 95
tenderness, 60, 84, 88, 170
tone, 160

V
Vagina, 5
    bleeding, 59, 60, 63, 85, 88, 97, 156, 157, 168
    cancer, 219, 223
    discharge, 11, 59, 170, 171, 175
    hemorrhage. *See* Hemorrhage, vaginal
    lacerations, 96, 105, 156, 160, 163-167
    neural pathways, 266
    packing, 220, 221
    trauma, 84, *85*
    tumor, 219-221, 223
Vasa previa, 84, *85*, 130, 152
Vascular system, 82, 191, 192, 199, 203, 205, 232
    capillary filling time, 152
    circulatory failure, 180, 199, *200*
    collapse, 11, 16, 152-153, 188
    ischemic coronary artery disease, 15
    lesions, *193*
    perfusion, peripheral, 152, 153
    resistance, peripheral, 205, 207, 208
    resistance, systemic, 198, 199, *200*
Vasoconstriction, 69, 100, 108, 110, *178*, 179, 185, 188, 203, 215, 263, 270, 272
Vasodilation, 157, 179, 185, 186
Vasopressors, 185, 263, 264, 270
Vasospasm, 78, *79*
Vasovagal syncope, 198-204
    conditions, 198
    differential diagnosis, 202-203
    drug therapy, 202, 268
    management, 200-202, 268, *269*
    paracervical block and, 266-268
    pathophysiology, 198-199, *200*
    prevention, 203-204
    symptoms, *201*
Veins, 8, *28*, 70, *178*, 179, 263
Ventilation, 154, 191, 229, 234, 260, 263, 264, 270. *See also* Positive pressure ventilation; Pressure
    mechanical, 151, 152, 186, *187*

Version, external cephalic, 131-132
Viruses, 8, 31, *73*, 135
Visual/eye disturbances, 76, 79-80, 190, 263, 269
Vitamin E, 33, 136
Vomiting
    in Addison's disease, 248, 249
    in appendicitis, 9
    in cholecystitis, 14
    in CNS toxicity, 269
    in diabetic ketoacidosis, 47, 49
    in intestinal obstruction, 12
    magnesium sulfate and, 62
    with ovarian cysts, 10
    in peptic ulcer, 14, 15
    in pregnancy, 25, *26*, 190
    in pyelonephritis, 9
    regurgitation, 259-261, 270
    in ruptured abscess, 225
    in salpingitis, 9
    in shock, 15, *178*, 179
    in vasovagal syncope, 199
    water loss and, 45
    wound dehiscence and, 243
Von Willebrand's disease, 158, 219

W
White blood cells. *See* Leukocytes

X
X-ray, 63, *68*, 71, 227, 239, 261
    appendicitis, in, 9
    in adult respiratory distress syndrome, *181*, 182, 211
    blood, 41
    in eclampsia, 82
    fetus and, 21
    fluid status, measuring, *28*
    following injury, 21
    in intestinal obstruction, 12-13
    IUD, 239
    in molar pregnancy, 212
    in pancreatitis, 16
    in peptic ulcer perforation, 15
    in pregnancy, 21
    in pulmonary aspiration, 261
    in pulmonary edema, 207
    in septic shock, *180*

VINCRISTINE	INAPPROPRIATE ADH
	PERIPHERAL NEUROPATHY
ADRIAMYCIN	CARDIOMYOPATHY
CISPLATIN	OTOTOX
CIS, MTX	NEPHROTOXICITY

Other titles of related interest from
MEDICAL ECONOMICS BOOKS

Management of Common Problems in Obstetrics and Gynecology
Edited by Daniel R. Mishell Jr., MD, and Paul F. Brenner, MD
ISBN 0-87489-306-2

Management of High-Risk Pregnancy
Edited by John T. Queenan, MD
ISBN 0-87489-221-X

Protocols for High-Risk Pregnancies
Edited by John T. Queenan, MD, and John C. Hobbins, MD
ISBN 0-87489-275-9

Drugs Used With Neonates and During Pregnancy, Second Edition
Ina Lee Stile, PharmD, Thomas Hegyi, MD, and Mark Hiatt, MD
ISBN 0-87489-342-9

Drug Interactions Index
The late Fred Lerman, MD, and Robert T. Weibert, PharmD
ISBN 0-87489-266-X

For information, write:
Customer Service Manager
MEDICAL ECONOMICS BOOKS
Oradell, New Jersey 07649